Molecular Mechanisms in Cancer

Edited by Metin Budak and Rajamanickam Rajkumar

Published in London, United Kingdom

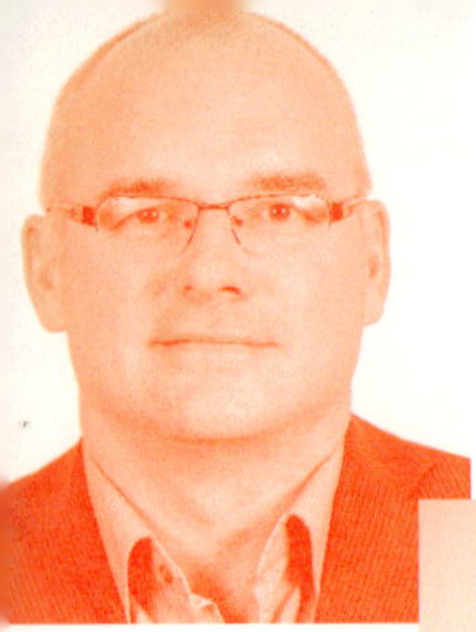
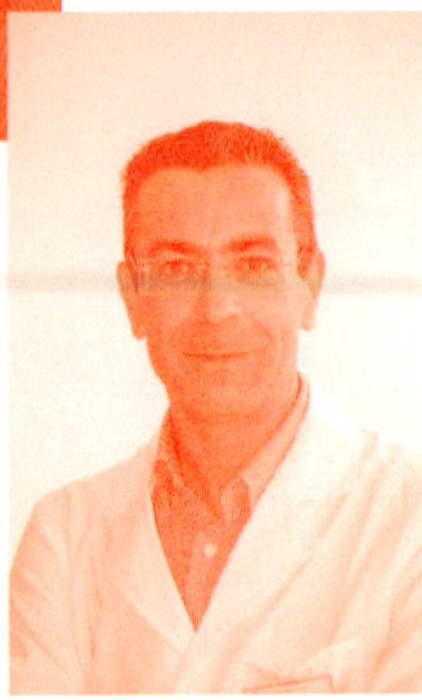
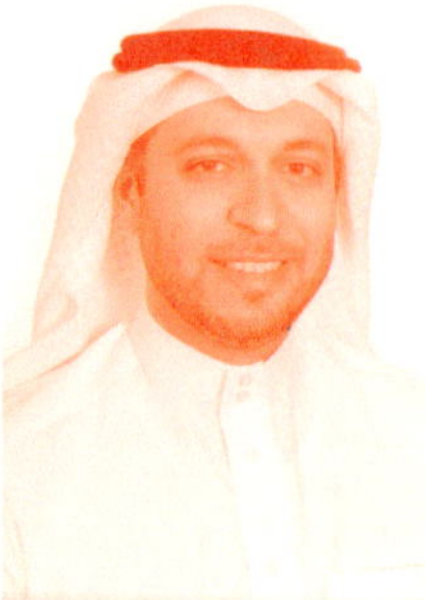
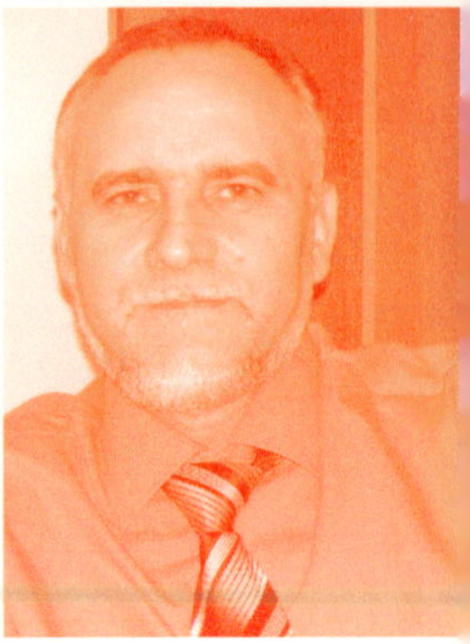
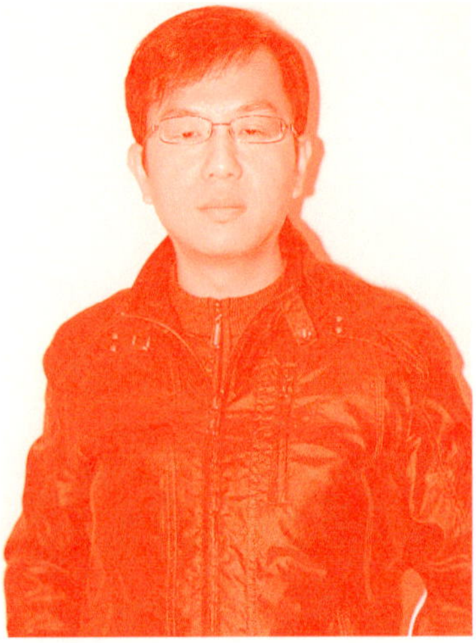
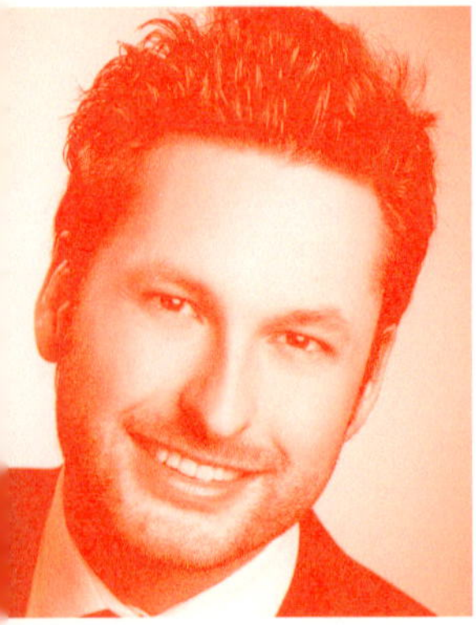
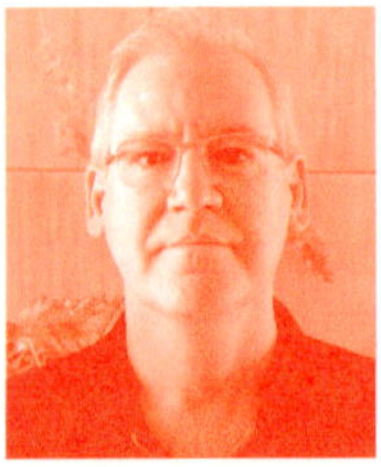

IntechOpen

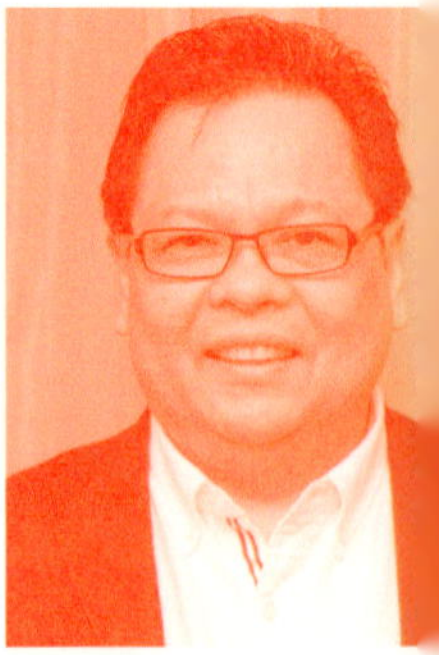
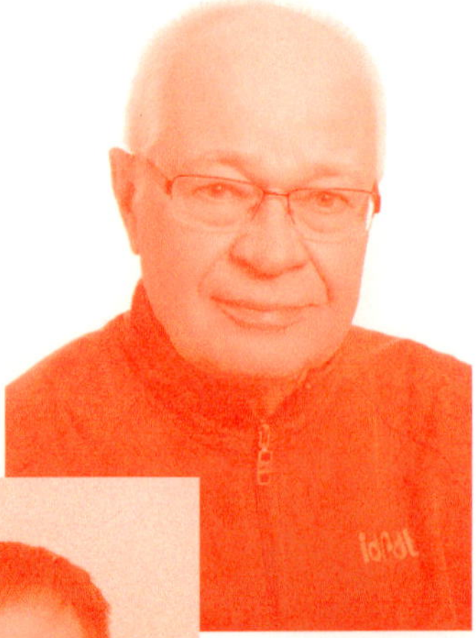
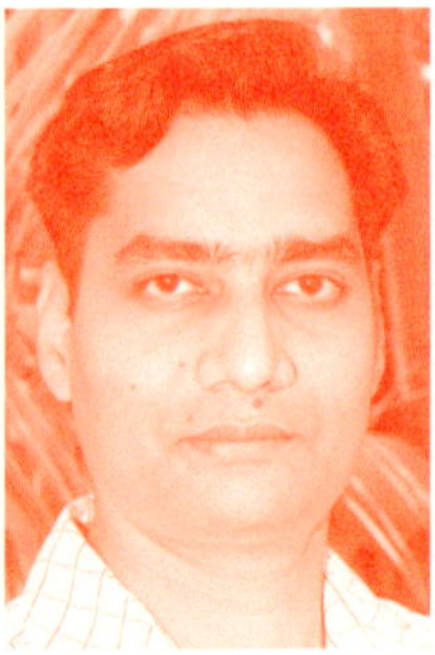
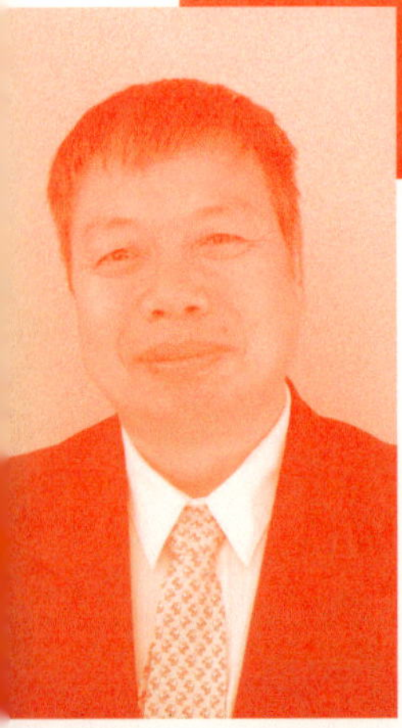
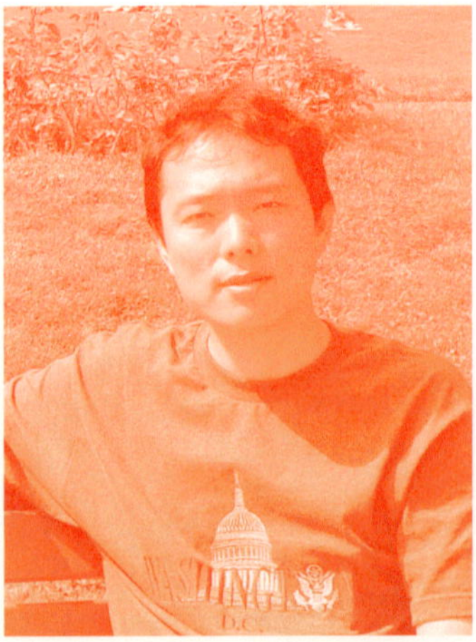
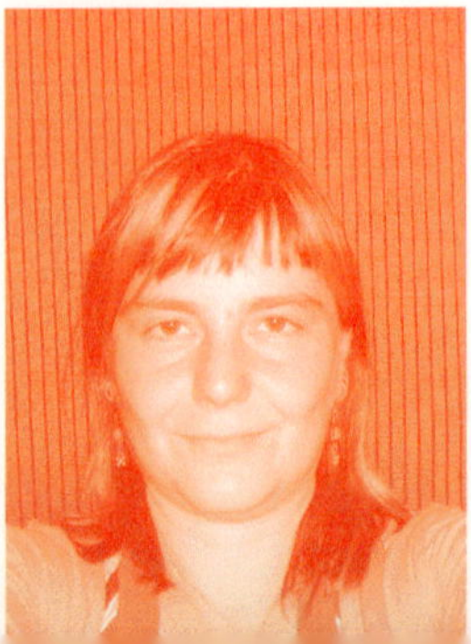

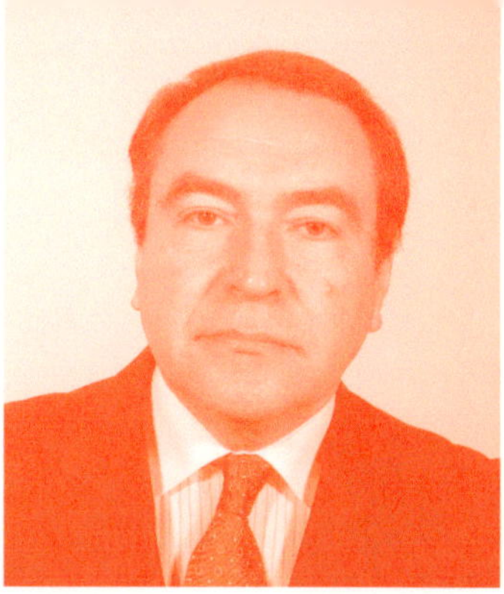
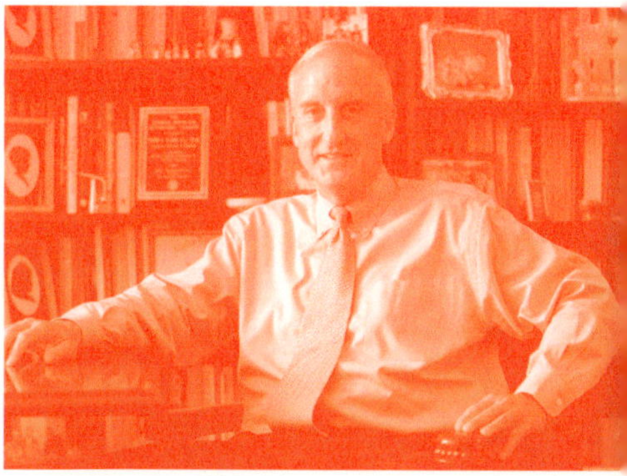
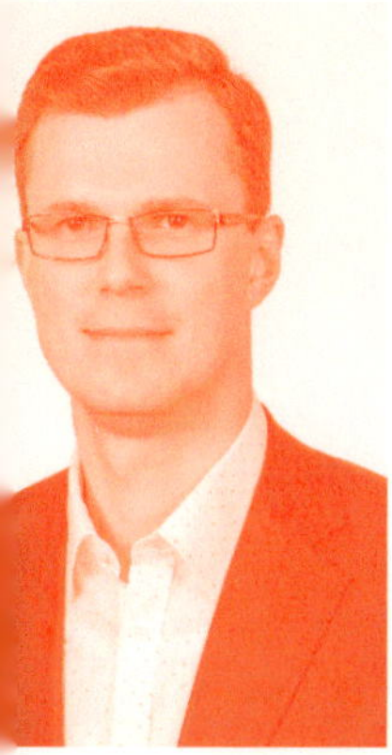
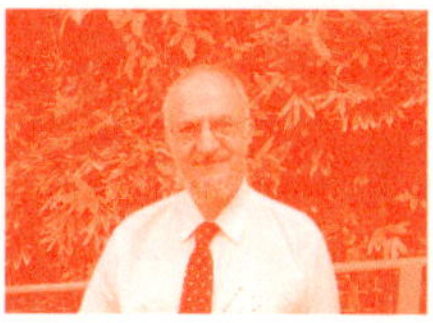
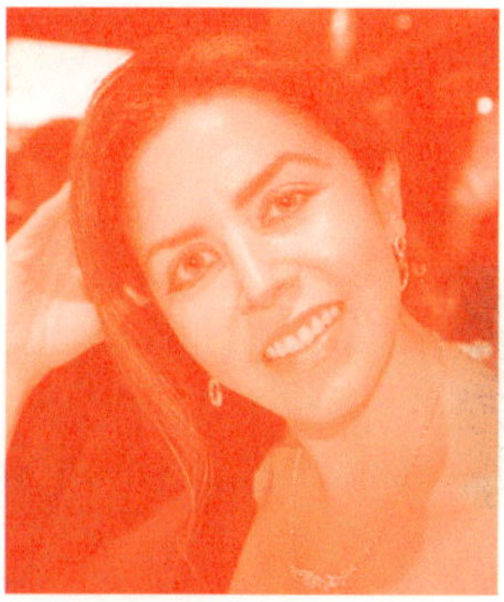

Supporting open minds since 2005

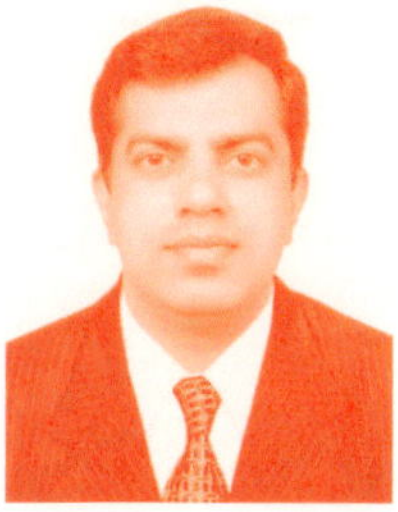
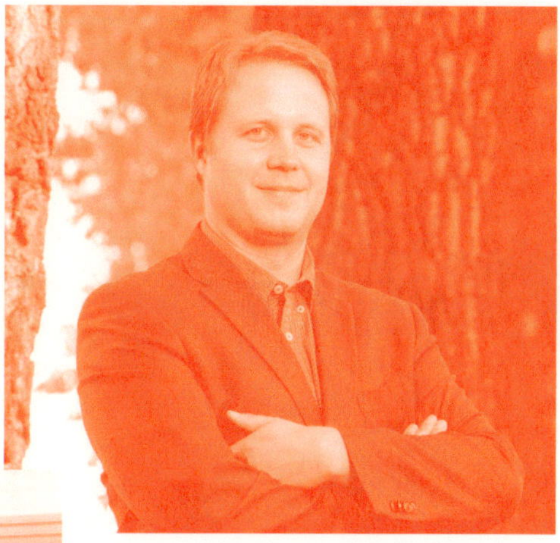
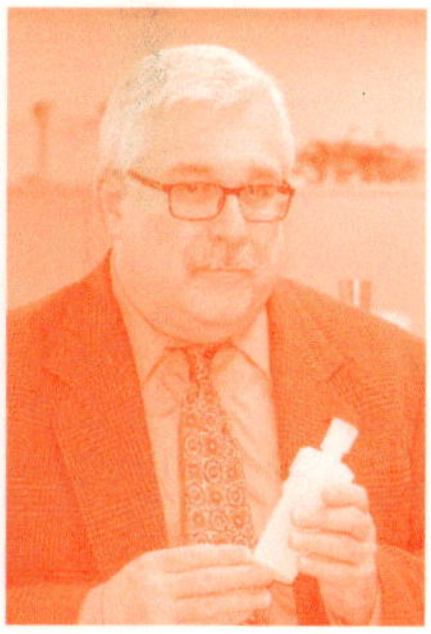
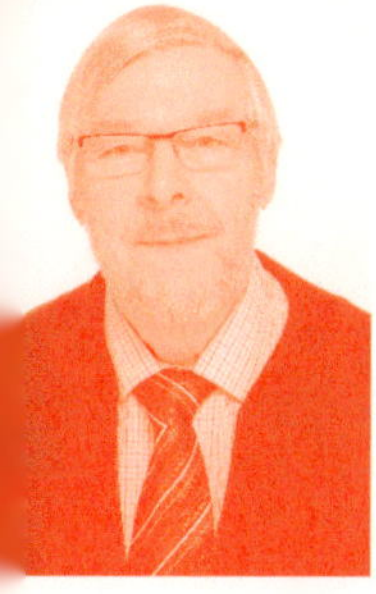
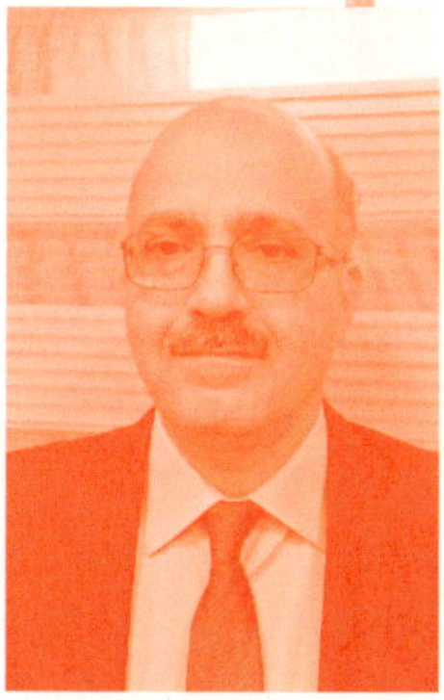
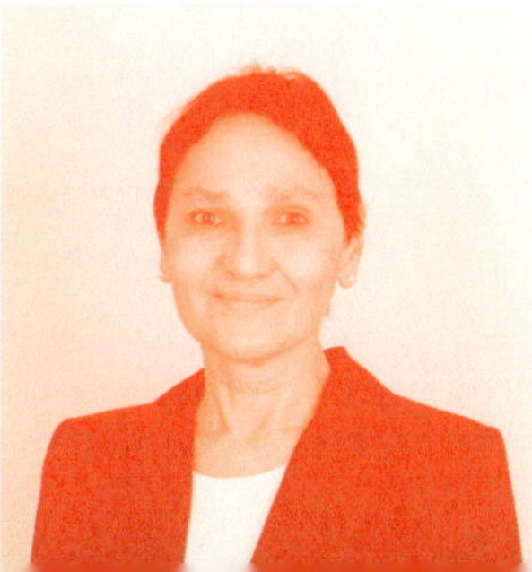
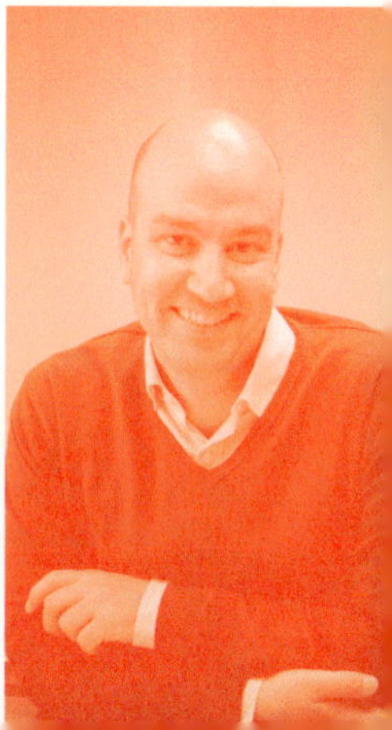

Molecular Mechanisms in Cancer
http://dx.doi.org/10.5772/intechopen.94819
Edited by Metin Budak and Rajamanickam Rajkumar

Contributors
Rafiq A Rather, Sonia Thapa, Madhulika Bhagat, Shashank K. Singh, Mehdi Moghanibashi, Parisa Mohamadynejad, Anand B. Pathak, Satyam Satyarth, Metin Budak, Hatice Segmen, Yıldız Gürsel Ürün, Mustafa Yildiz, Florencia Wendkuuni Djigma, Fidèle Tiendrébéogo, Lassina Traoré, Theodora M. Zohoncon, Augustin T. Bambara, Pegdwendé Abel Sorgho, Aboubacar H. Bambara, Abdou Azaque Zoure, Dorcas Obiri-Yeboah, Bagora Bayala, Teega-Wendé Clarisse Ouedraogo, Prosper Bado, Rogomenoma Alice Ouedraogo, Ina M.A. Traoré, Esther M. A. Traoré, Isabelle T. Kiendrebeogo, Albert T. Yonli, Charlemagne M Ouedraogo, Jacques Simpore, Elsa Díaz López, Mehmet Sarier, Abdoul K. Ouattara, Djeneba Ouermi, Tani Sagna, Christelle. W Nadembega, Olga Lompo, Yvette Marie Chantal Gyebre, Cyrille Bisseye, Maimouna Ilboudo, Regine Ilboudo, Catherine Salambanga, Sindimalgdé Patricia Guigma, Frida S. Tovo, Ali Kandé, Luz Irene Pascual Mathey, Rajamanickam Rajkumar

First published in London, United Kingdom, 2022 by IntechOpen
IntechOpen is the global imprint of INTECHOPEN LIMITED, registered in England and Wales, registration number: 11086078, 5 Princes Gate Court, London, SW7 2QJ, United Kingdom
Printed in Croatia

British Library Cataloguing-in-Publication Data
A catalogue record for this book is available from the British Library

Additional hard and PDF copies can be obtained from orders@intechopen.com

Molecular Mechanisms in Cancer
Edited by Metin Budak and Rajamanickam Rajkumar
p. cm.
Print ISBN 978-1-83969-842-2
Online ISBN 978-1-83969-843-9
eBook (PDF) ISBN 978-1-83969-844-6

For EU product safety concerns:
IN TECH d.o.o., Prolaz Marije Krucifikse Kozulić 3, 51000 Rijeka, Croatia, info@intechopen.com or visit our website at intechopen.com.

Meet the editors

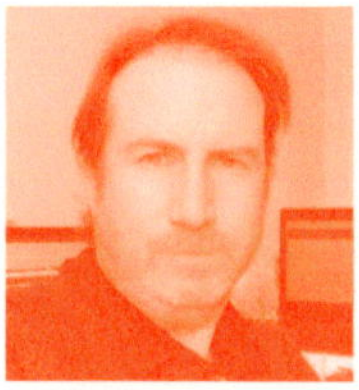

Metin Budak, MSc, Ph.D., is an associate professor and vice director in the Biophysics Department, Faculty of Medicine, Trakya University, Turkey. He has been head of the Molecular Research Lab at the Mirko Tos Ear and Hearing Research Center, Trakya University, since 2018. His specializations are biophysics, molecular biology, epigenetics, genetics, and methylation mechanisms. He has published around twenty-three peer-reviewed papers, two edited books, three book chapters, and thirty-two abstracts. He is a member of the Clinical Research Ethics Committee and Quantification and Consideration Committee of the Medicine Faculty. His research interests include mutations and polymorphisms in cancers, the role of methylation during gene transcription, chromatin DNA packages within the cell, and DNA repair, replication, recombination, and gene transcription.

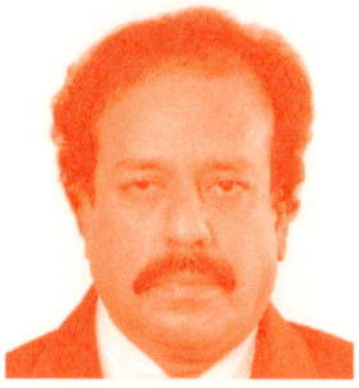

Rajamanickam Rajkumar is an international frontline scientist in cervical cancer and HPV prevention with a Ph.D. in Cancer Epidemiology. He is currently a professor at Meenakshi Medical College, Kanchipuram, India, and a Ph.D. mentor for several medical universities. He was the principal investigator of one of the largest cervical cancer screening programs in India, the International Agency for Research on Cancer (IARC/WHO) funded by The Bill and Melinda Gates Foundation. Dr. Rajkumar conducted the first study in South India on the community prevalence of HPV. He trained in colposcopy and cancer epidemiology in France, Ireland, the United Kingdom, and Singapore. He was a consultant to The Ohio State University Medical Center for cervical cancer screening. He is an honorary member of the Society for Colposcopy & Cervical Pathology of Singapore (SCCPS), Singapore.

Contents

Preface

Molecular Mechanisms in Cancer, created with experts in their fields from different countries, consists of twelve chapters organized into three sections: "Oncogenes," "Tumor Suppressor Genes," and "Viral Oncogenes."

Section 1 includes four chapters that discuss the effects and importance of oncogenes in various cancer types. Chapter 1 examines the roles and importance of alternative mRNA splices in cancer development, changes in intron-exon connections, oncogenic properties, and the roles of eukaryotic polycistronic gene mechanisms in the development of various cancers. Chapter 2 discusses molecular mechanisms in various types of skin cancers as well as the effects of external factors originating from the sun, especially ultraviolet light, and cancers that develop by changing molecular mechanisms. Chapter 3 addresses oncogene and tumor suppressor mechanisms in head and neck squamous cell cancer types and their clinical importance. Chapter 4 describes the potential application of targeted oncogene-dependent gene therapies in cancer treatments.

Section 2 includes three chapters that address the mechanisms of tumor suppressor genes in cancers and their effects on cancer development. Chapter 5 discusses tumor suppressor genes affecting breast cancer, especially the additives of BRCA1 and BRCA2. Chapter 6 examines the roles of the two functions of cellular stress and Nrf2 in cancer development, their contribution to chemoresistance, and their relationship with oxidative stress. Chapter 7 explains molecular changes in benign prostate cancers.

Section 3 includes five chapters that examine the epidemiology of viral oncogenes and their roles in various cancers. Chapter 8 discusses the oncogenic activities and epidemiological behavior of human papilloma viruses (HPVs) in Burkina Faso, West Africa. Chapter 9 provides an overview of the clinical features of viral oncogenic viruses in cervical cancer. Chapters 10 and 11 provide extensive information on the roles of HPV infections in urological cancers. Finally, Chapter 12 discusses the applications of HPV vaccines in different parts of the world and the effects of the ethical or moral behaviors of these societies.

With my respect and thanks to my father, Ali Budak, who provided everything for my education and passed away from cancer.

Metin Budak
Trakya University Faculty of Medicine,
Biophysics Department,
Mirko Tos Ear and Hearing Research Center,
Trakya University,
Edirne, Turkey

Rajamanickam Rajkumar
Meenakshi Medical College Hospital and Research Institute MAHER,
Kanchipuram, Tamil Nadu, India

Section 1

Oncogenes

Chapter 1

Splicing in Cancer

Mehdi Moghanibashi and Parisa Mohamadynejad

Abstract

Defects in splicing, especially alternative splicing have been frequently found in cancers. Mutations in the splicing regulatory elements of important genes involved in cancers or the genes encoding regulatory splicing machinery could play a key role in carcinogenesis. Alterations in regulator factors in splicing have emerged as a new class of oncoproteins and tumor suppressor genes. Understanding the molecular mechanism of how defects in splicing and in particular alternative splicing are involved in carcinogenesis, could lead to new strategies to cancer therapy. Here, we review the molecular mechanism of splicing and regulatory factors involved in alternative splicing, as well as the aberrant splicing that affects cancer hallmarks. Finally, we summarize new approaches in cancer therapy based on splicing.

Keywords: splicing, alternative splicing, spliceosome, oncogene, tumor suppressor gene

1. Introduction

Split genes in eukaryotes were discovered in 1977 for the first time. It was later indicated that the intron sequences should be removed by the spliceosome complex in the splicing process in the nucleus [1].

There are 20,687 protein-coding genes with introns (93%) and 1713 (7%) intron-less protein-coding genes in human genome [2]. It is interesting to note that only ~4% of genes in the schizosaccharomyces cerevisiae contain introns and most of them are single intron genes [3]. The number of introns per gene varies in eukaryotic genomes so that in the human genome is 8.94, and in the fungi (0.05–3.43 introns per gene), plants (0.33–7.30 introns per gene), invertebrates (2.92–7.42 introns per gene) and vertebrates (7.35–10.09 introns per gene) [2].

The length of introns is less than 100 up to 100,000 bp in different genes of various organisms [3]. Unlike lower eukaryotes, there are relatively long introns and short exons in vertebrates [4] but in general, fungal introns are relatively short (93% of the introns in fungi are shorter than 250 nt). However, in invertebrates and plants, the average percentage of short introns (<250 nt) is 48% and 59%, respectively. In contrast, 48% of vertebrate introns are longer than 1000 nt [2].

In the present chapter, we explain the various types of splicing, the molecular mechanism of splicing, regulatory elements and factors in splicing, and finally the alternative splicing and the role of aberrant splicing in cancer are discussed.

2. Mechanism of cis-splicing

The classic and ubiquitous of exons joining from the same pre-mRNA is called cis-splicing. Highly conserved splicing machinery in all eukaryotes shows that splicing is pivotal for all eukaryotic organisms [3]. Five small RNAs (snRNAs), including U1, U2, U4, U5, and U6 (because they are uracil-rich) and approximately 300 related proteins including hnRNPs and SR proteins, make up the spliceosome complexes and are involved in the splicing regulation.

The junction of introns and exons is identified by spliceosome and the "GU-AG" rule is mainly used. Four regions play a key role in splicing, including (a) the GU sequences at the beginning of the introns as 5′ splice-site (5′-SS or donor site), (b) AG dinucleotides at the end of intron referred to 3′ splice-site (3′-SS or acceptor site), (c) the sequences without high conservation in the upstream of the 3′SS called branch point sequence (BPS), and (d) polypyrimidine-rich sequences which is locating between the BPS and the 3′ SS [1].

For conventional splicing, first of all, the complex E (early) is formed by ATP-independent binding of U1 snRNP (small nuclear ribonucleoprotein) to 5′-SS via base-pairing, SF1 (splicing factor 1) to BPS, U2AF2 to polypyrimidine tract, and U2AF1 to 3′-SS. Second, SF1 is replaced by U2 snRNP (with the assistance of U2AF) through the base-pairing to BPS to form complex A. This step is ATP-dependent and reinforced by the SF3a and SF3b protein complexes, as well as U2AF2 and U2AF1. Third, complex B (inactive) is formed by rearranging complex A using recruiting U5/U4/U6 in such a way that U4 and U6 snRNPs bind strongly to each other due to complementary pairing of their RNA components, but U5 snRNP is weakly bound to them (through protein–protein interaction). Following several conformational changes, U1 snRNP leaves mRNA, U6 snRNP binds to 5′-SS, and simultaneously, U4 snRNP leaves mRNA so that U6 and U2 snRNPs pair together through their snRNA, leading to the formation of pre-catalytic (active) spliceosome complex B* (**Figure 1**). Finally, removal of introns and joining of exons are performed using two transesterification reactions by complex C [1] (**Figures 1** and **2**).

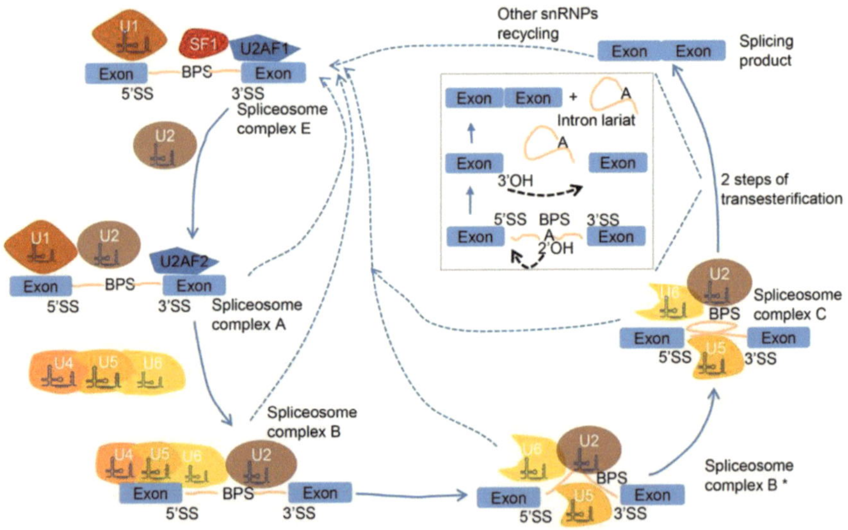

Figure 1.
Various steps of splicing are performed by different snRNAs and snRNPs [5].

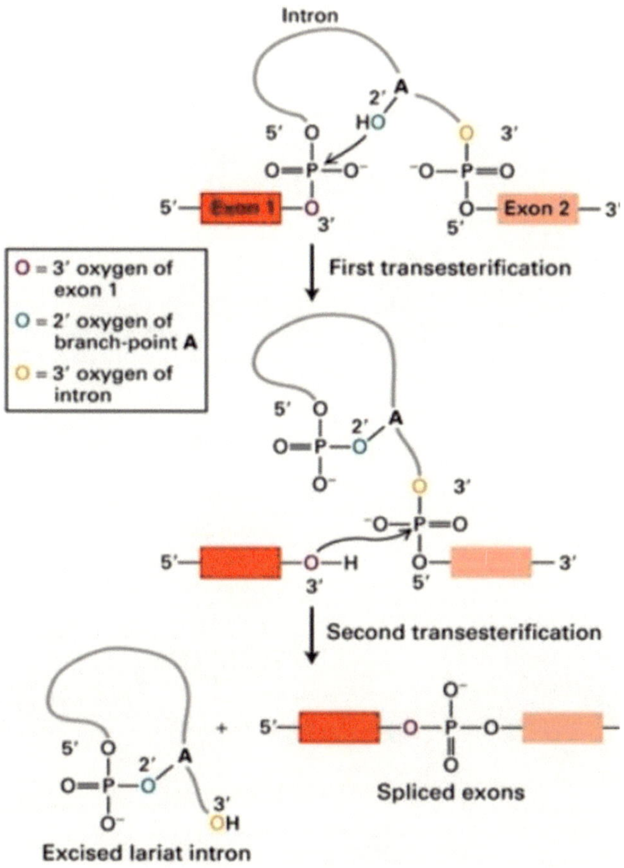

Figure 2.
Molecular mechanism of exon joining [6].

3. Regulation of splicing

Cis-acting elements in RNA constitute a set of rules called "splicing code" that acts as an anchor for trans-acting factors to produce functional transcripts [7]. There is a competition between various splicing factors for the binding to the splicing regulatory elements and in turn the increasing or decreasing the recruitment of spliceosome complexes to premature mRNA.

Generally, the serine/arginine (SR)-rich protein family bind preferentially to exonic splicing enhancer (ESEs) and intronic splicing enhancer (ISEs) sites and play a positive role in the splicing (exon inclusion). However, heterogeneous nuclear ribonucleoproteins (hnRNPs) bind to exonic splicing silencer (ESSs) and intronic splicing silencer (ISSs) elements and generally suppress exon inclusion (**Figure 3**) [1, 5].

In addition to the characteristic domain of RS (arginine/serine dipeptides) in SR proteins, there is an RNA recognition motif (RRM) which is the basis for the classification of SR proteins. In humans, there are 12 types of SR proteins, now called serine/arginine-rich splicing factor (SRSF) 1–12. RS domain of different SR proteins binds to ESE, could directly interact with each other and facilitate the recruitment of spliceosome machinery components including U1 snRNP or U2AF to mRNA, and more importantly, it has been suggested that the SR proteins bound to ESEs play a key role in exon definition in constitutive and alternative splicing.

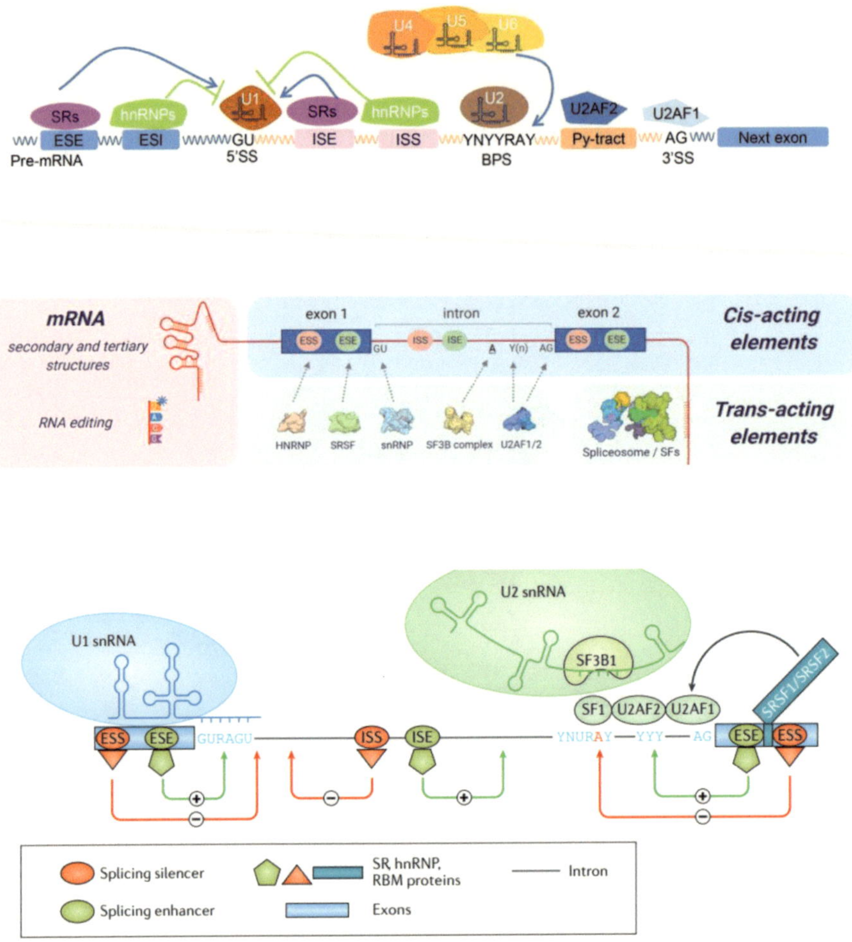

Figure 3.
Control of splicing by cis-acting elements and splicing factors [5, 7, 8].

There are no canonical SR proteins in Saccharomyces cerevisiae and three SR-like proteins including Npl3, regulate splicing efficiency [3].

RRM is also the most common domain in the hnRNPs for the interactions with the premRNA, but hnRNPs also contain another domain called the RGG boxes including Arg-Gly-Gly tripeptides repeats. hnRNP proteins as same as SR proteins, bind directly to a specific site in the target premRNA, but inhibit splicing via blocking the binding of snRNPs to targets or looping out exons [3, 9].

4. Self-splicing

Some introns are spliced without requiring to spliceosome complex (self-splicing), including group I introns (found in bacteria, bacteriophages and eukaryotes including organelle and nuclear genomes) and group II introns (found in bacteria, archaea, and eukaryotic organelles). In both, trans-esterification reactions need to excise the intron and ligate the exons.

The difference between them is that the splicing reaction is initiated by a guanosine cofactor and an internal adenosine in group I and group II introns, respectively. Also, during splicing, group II introns form a lariat like structure, whereas group I introns do not (**Figure 4**) [10].

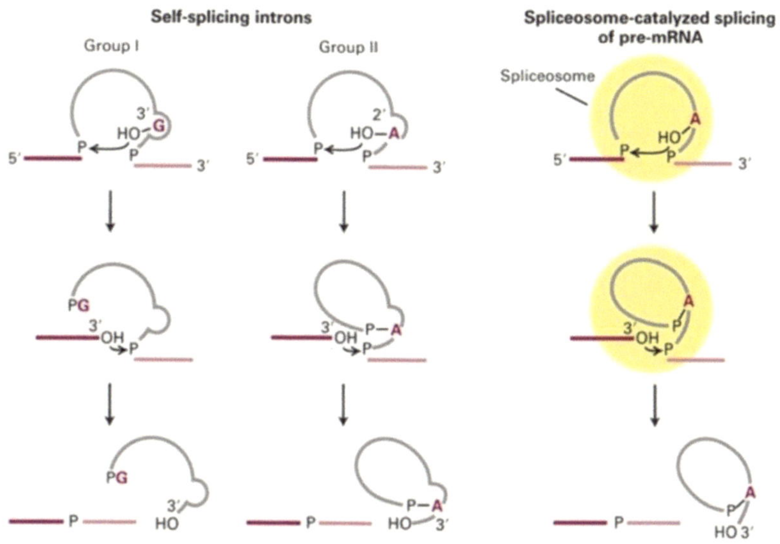

Figure 4.
Comparison of a self-splicing group I, group II introns and spliceosome-catalyzed splicing [10].

5. Trans-splicing

In addition to cis-splicing, there is another type that joins exons on the separate pre-mRNAs and results in the chimeric mRNAs originating from two different genes so-called trans-splicing and commonly occurs in unicellular organisms and caenorhabditis elegans. Interestingly, acyl-CoA-cholesterol acyltransferase 1, RGS12 and CYP3A genes produce mRNA that derived from different genes in human [11].

6. Alternative splicing (AS)

Different combination of exons in a special type of splicing, called alternative splicing, which lead to the formation of multiple protein isoforms from a single pre-mRNA and promotes the transcriptome and proteome complexity. A recent analysis of the Encyclopedia of DNA Elements (ENCODE) project 1 has been revealed that the human genome consists of approximately 21,306 protein-coding genes [12, 13] and it is estimated that 92–94% of human genes harbor alternative splicing [3, 14, 15].

The most common type of alternative splicing mechanism (40% of events) is exon skipping (also called cassette exon) [4] in which one or several exons are not included in the final mRNA (**Figure 5a**) but the rarest mechanism of AS is mutually exclusive exons (**Figure 5d**) [17]. Changing in the selection of either 3′- or 5′-splice sites are other mechanisms of AS (**Figure 5b** and **c**). The fifth type of alternative splicing is intron retention (**Figure 5e**), in which an intron remains in the mature mRNA (the most common after the exon skipping). Applying alternative promoters and unusual polyadenylation are other alternative splicing mechanisms (**Figure 5f** and **g**) [16]. Various trans-acting factors, as well as specific cis-acting elements, play a key role in alternative splicing.

Expression alteration in splicing trans-acting factors and mutations (also, polymorphisms) including single-base substitutions, deletion, insertion, and translocation in cis-elements and trans-regulatory factors that encodes genes involved in splicing, would cause abnormal splicing and lead to diseases and

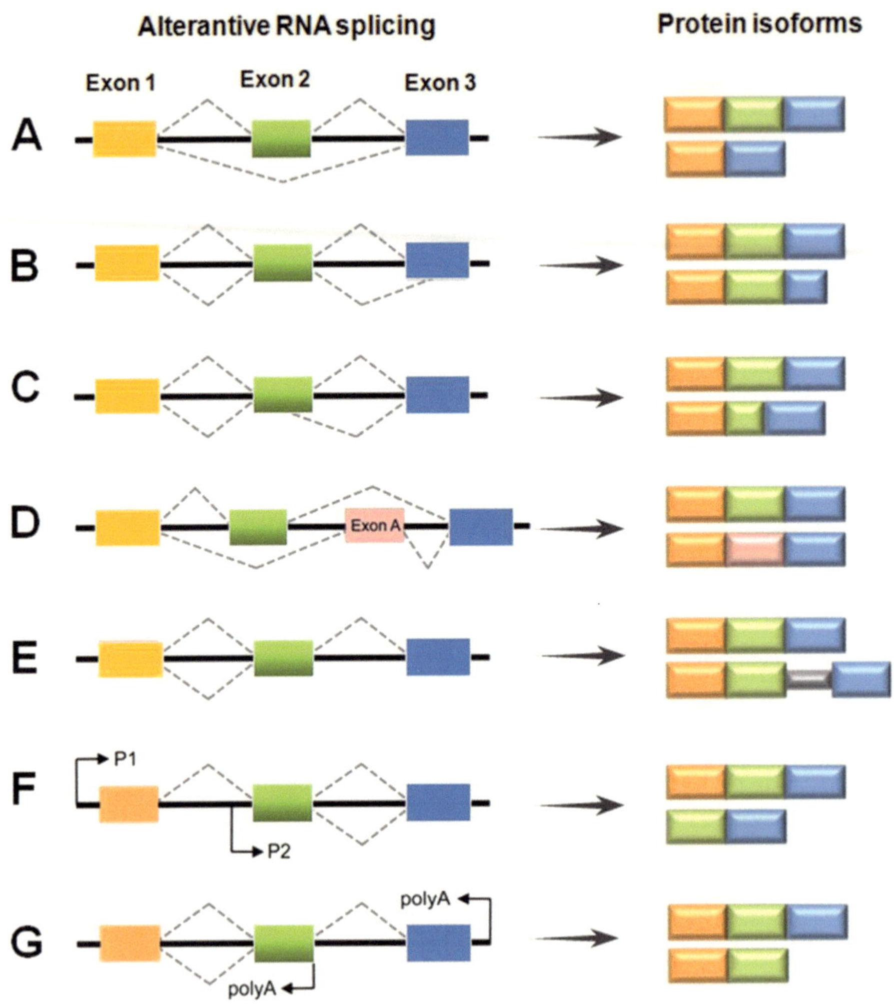

Figure 5.
Schematic representation of different types of alternative splicing [16].

cancer. In addition, the post-modification of trans-regulatory factors and chromatin remodeling could affect splicing by altering the recognition of splicing factors and splicing sites (**Figure 6**) [5].

7. Role of splicing in cancers

Gene duplication and overexpression of SRSF1 were the first evidences that alternative splicing plays an important role in tumor growth [18]. Recently, it has been reported that splicing may be correlated with the various types of cancers, and in particular, alternative splicing can affect various aspects of cancer hallmarks [8, 19] (**Figure 7**) and splicing modulators have emerged as a new class of oncoproteins and tumor suppressor genes. Importantly, RNA sequencing analysis has shown that one of the common mechanisms of tumor suppressor genes inactivation in cancers is intron retention [20].

Recently, RNA-seq studies have been reported that one of the major differences between transcriptome of normal and cancerous tissues are caused by aberrant splicing with AML and hepatocellular carcinoma show the highest and lowest

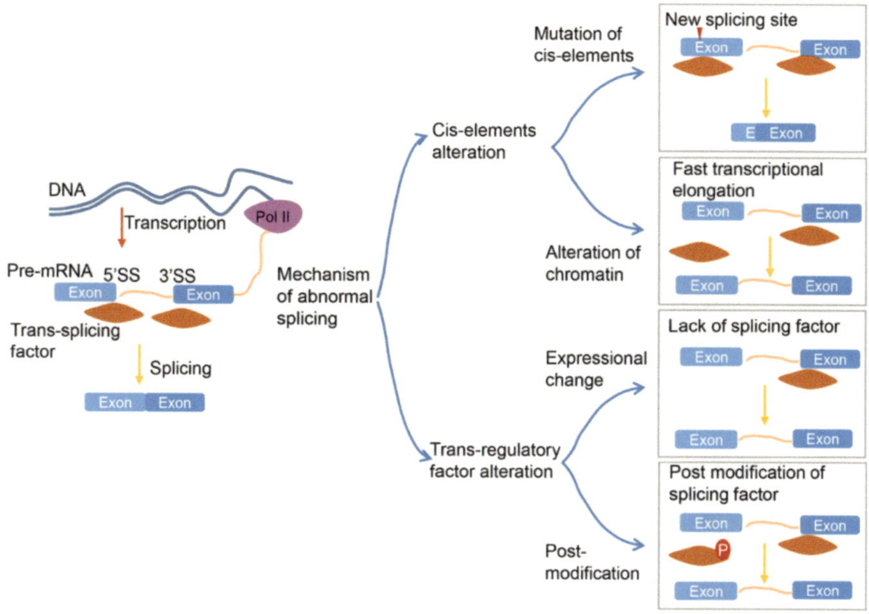

Figure 6.
Various mechanisms for aberrant splicing [5].

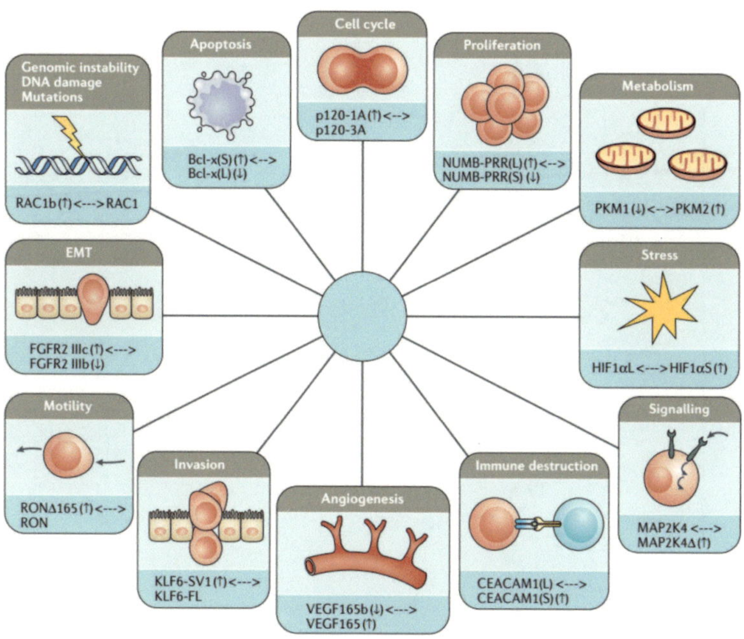

Figure 7.
Effects of aberrant alternative splicing on different hallmarks of cancer. Arrows up: Most contributor, arrows down: Least contributor, EMT (epithelial–mesenchymal transition) [8].

frequency of alternative splicing alteration compared to the corresponding normal tissues, respectively. The most extensive study ever performed on the splicing profile of various types of cancers involving more than 8700 patients from The Cancer Genome Atlas (TCGA) data, shows that alternatively splicing in cancerous tissues is 30% more than normal tissues [7]. Expression dysregulation and frequent somatic mutations in the splicing factors coding genes have been identified in more than 2% of tumors in several cohorts of patients, including TCGA data (**Figure 8**) [21].

7.1 Deregulation of splicing factors expression

A wide range of factors involved in splicing and regulation of alternative splicing has been shown to be dysregulated in gene expression level. For example, serine and arginine-rich splicing factor 1 (SRSF1), a key player of alternative splicing, is involved in tumorigenesis promotion by splicing of RAC1, Tyrosine-protein kinase (SYK), MKI67 and HNRPLL genes. Specifically, in colorectal cancer, SRSF1 and other members of the SR family, including SRSF3, SRSF6, SRSF7 and SRSF10, are overexpressed and referred to as oncogenes [5, 22].

Bcl-x protein, which plays a key role in the regulation of intrinsic pathway of apoptosis, harbor alternative splicing and can obtain two different isoforms Bcl-xl (involved in apoptosis inhibition) and Bcl-xs (participated in apoptosis promotion) [23]. PTB protein 1 preferentially promote Bcl-xs isoform that leads to apoptosis, but down-regulation of PTB protein 1 could produce Bcl-xl, which inhibits apoptosis and result in tumorigenesis [24].

Some aspects of the oncogenic role of C-Myc in tumors, are changing splicing patterns. For example, it can overexpress the ITGA6A variant [the pro-proliferative isoform of integrin subunit α6 gene (ITGA6)] compared to ITGA6B isoform

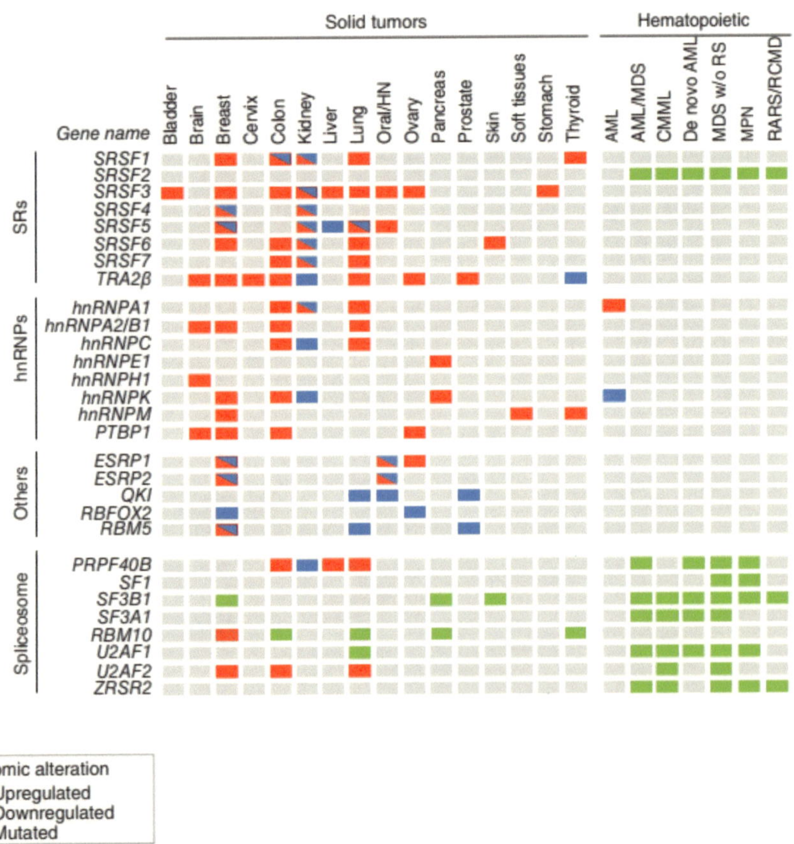

Figure 8.
Frequently alteration of splicing-factors in human cancers. MDS: Myelodysplastic syndrome; CMML: Chronic myelomonocytic leukemia; HN: Head and neck; w/o RS: With or without ringed sideroblasts; RARS/RCMD: Refractory anemia with ringed sideroblasts and refractory cytopenia with multilineage dysplasia and ringed sideroblasts; MPN, myeloproliferative neoplasm [21].

in the colon cancer, which is mediated by epithelial splicing regulatory protein 2 (ESRP2) [22].

Tumor cells preferentially metabolize glucose via the aerobic glycolysis pathway compared to normal cells. Conversion of phosphoenolpyruvate (PEP) to pyruvate is performed by PKM (Pyruvate kinase) enzyme in the last step of glycolysis. PKM is encoded by PKLR (expressed mainly in the liver and hematopoietic cells) and PKM (expressed in most tissues) genes in which both of them harbor alternative splicing [25, 26]. Alternatively, splicing of the PKM gene results in PKM1 isoforms (mainly in normal cells) and PKM2 isoforms (mainly in tumor cells) [27, 28]. The polypyrimidine tract-binding protein (PTB), hnRNPA1 and hnRNPA2 genes are overexpressed by C-Myc and lead to upregulation of PKM2 isoform of pyruvate kinase (PKM) through splicing changing and lead to cell proliferation (**Figure 9**) [29, 30].

Vascular endothelial growth factor A (VEGF-A) is one of the key proteins in the angiogenesis process in tumor progression. The VEGF- A encoding gene produces various isoforms (angiogenic and antiangiogenic) using alternative 3′ and 5′-SSs in exons 6, 7, and 8 that can regulate angiogenesis (**Figure 10**) [31]. Interestingly, angiogenic VEGF isoforms are induced by Serine/arginine-rich protein-specific splicing factor kinase (Srpk1) and SRSF1 protein, which are activated by Wilms' tumor suppressor 1 (Wt1) protein [32].

7.2 Mutation in cis-acting elements and genes encode for trans-acting factors

It has been suggested that various mutations, including silent or synonymous mutations, maybe results in intron retention (often in tumor suppressor genes and lead to premature stop codon) or exon skipping through create and loss of exonic splicing enhancers, silencers, or create novel splice sites [7]. It has been reported that 40% of patients with hereditary non-polyposis colorectal cancer carry the MLH1 mutation, and interestingly, the most common mutation in this gene is located at splicing sites [33] which was in line with bioinformatics analysis results [34]. The most somatic mutations in the splicing factors encoding genes have been observed in bladder cancer and uveal melanoma [7].

Recently, in several cancers, a recurrent mutation in the U1 snRNA encoding gene has been found, which mainly affects the third base of U1 snRNA at the splice

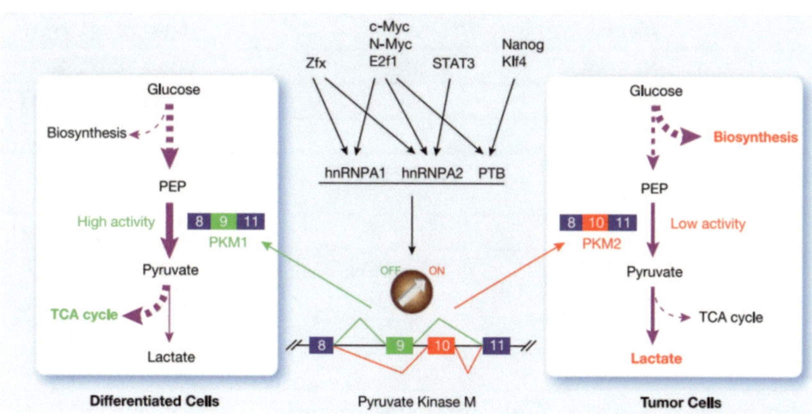

Figure 9.
Regulation of metabolic shift between oxidative phosphorylation and aerobic glycolysis through alternative splicing of PKM gene. In tumors, c-Myc and possibly other factors are involved in the upregulation of the hnRNPA1, A2, and PTB genes which result in exon 9 exclusion and exon 10 inclusion and PKM2 generation. PEP to pyruvate conversion is catalyzed less efficiently by PKM2 compared to PKM1, resulting in enhancement of metabolites for anabolic metabolism [28].

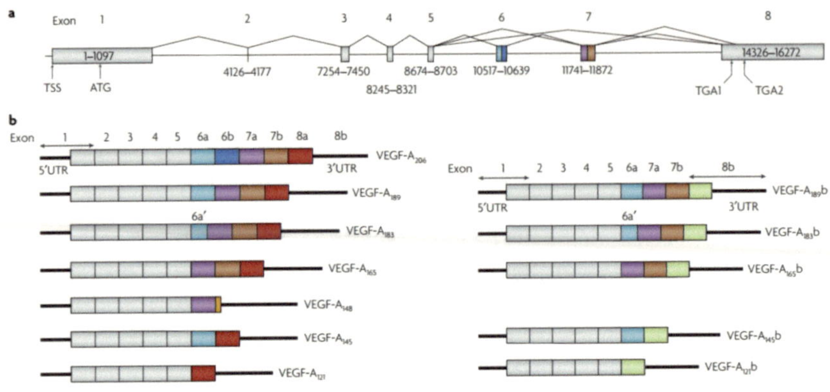

Figure 10.
The structure of the VEGF-A gene includes eight exons (a) and producing of various isoforms by alternative splicing (b). Two mRNA isoform families, pro-angiogenic (VEGF-Axxx, b. left) and anti-angiogenic (VEGF-Axxxb, b. right) are generated by alternative splicing. (xxx shows the amino acid number of the mature protein). The transcriptional start site (TSS), translational start site (ATG) in exon 1, and alternative stop codons within exon 8 (TGA1 and TGA2) are indicated [31].

site recognition sequence that pairs directly with 5′SS. In addition, mutated SF3B1 (**Table 1**) recognizes different BPS and results in cryptic 3′ splice sites selection. Also, the SRSF2 and U2AF1 mutations alter splice site recognition in a sequence-dependent manner and results in alternative 3′ splice site selection and altered exon inclusion, respectively (**Figure 11** and **Table 1**) [7, 8]. It has been suggested that

Mutation type	Gene	Spliceosome component	Top 3 commonly mutated cancer types*
	SF3B1		UVM, UCEC, BLCA
	U2AF1	U2 snRNP	UCS, LAML, UCEC
	PHF5A		KICH, SKCM, LUSC
Hotspot	*SRSF2*	SR protein	LAML, UVM, UCEC
	HNRNPCL1	hnRNP	SKCM, UCEC, STAD
	PCBP1	hnRNP	READ, COAD, BLCA
	HNRNPD		UCEC, DLBC, UCS
	HNRNPDL		UCEC, COAD, STAD
	HNRNPL	hnRNP	COAD, UCEC, SKCM
	PCBP2		UCEC, SKCM, READ
	CCAR1		UCEC, SKCM, BLCA
Loss of function	*RBM10*	A complex	UCEC, LUAD, BLCA
	TCERG1		UCEC, COAD, SKCM
	DDX50	B^{act} complex	UCEC, STAD, LUAD
	FUBP3		UCEC, COAD, SKCM
	FRA10AC1	C complex	UCEC, READ, UCS
	CDC5L	PRP19	UCEC, STAD, SKCM

**BLCA - Bladder Urothelial Carcinoma, COAD - Colon adenocarcinoma, DLBC - Lymphoid Neoplasm Diffuse Large B-cell Lymphoma, KICH - Kidney Chromophobe, LAML - Acute Myeloid Leukemia, LUAD - Lung adenocarcinoma, LUSC - Lung squamous cell carcinoma, READ - Rectum adenocarcinoma, SKCM - Skin Cutaneous Melanoma, STAD - Stomach adenocarcinoma, UCEC - Uterine Corpus Endometrial Carcinoma, UCS - Uterine Carcinosarcoma, UVM - Uveal Melanoma.*

Table 1.
Mutation of splicing factors encoding genes in cancers [7].

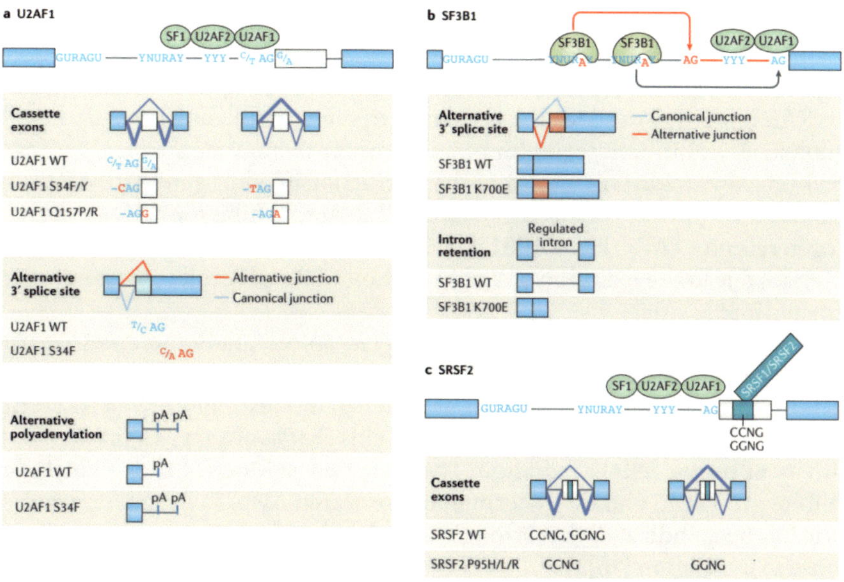

Figure 11.
Effects of cancer-associated mutations in splicing factors on alternative splice site selection. Processing patterns favored by the mutations are shown by thicker lines. WT: Wild type [8].

these mutations may also affect the protein-protein interaction domains and lead to alteration of splicing factors interaction with nucleosomes, which plays an important role in driving splice site definition [7].

8. Splicing and resistance to drugs in cancers

Response of the tumors to therapy may be affected by splicing and resistance to treatment may be reinforced by alternative splicing [35]. Alternative splicing could induce resistance to drugs in cancer through changing factors that are involved in the metabolism of drugs including uptake, transportation and inactivation (**Figure 12**).

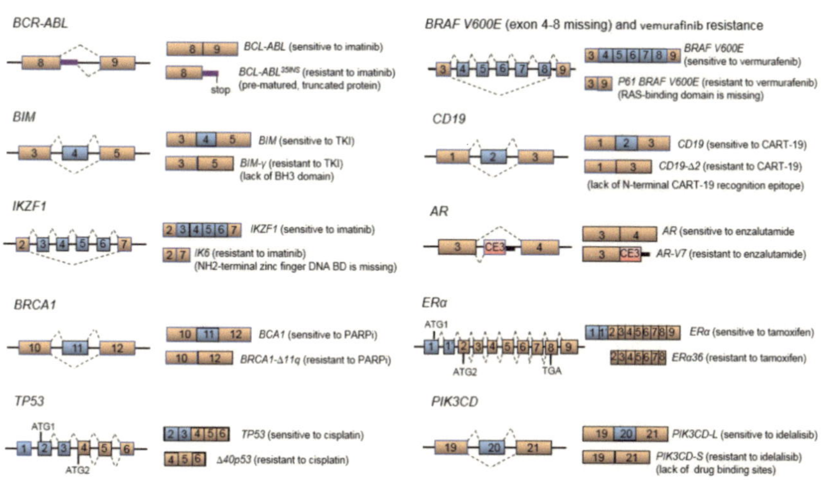

Figure 12.
Aberrant alternative splicing in some oncogenes and resistance to therapy in cancers. ATG1 and ATG2: Start codon for full-length and short mRNA. TGA: Stop codon [36].

One of the most mutated genes in melanoma cancer is BRAF that V600E mutation is the most prevalence mutation in this gene and result in a variant without exons 4–8 (give rise to lack of the RAS-binding domain of BRAF rendered cells insensitive to RAF inhibition) and lead to resistance to vemurafenib in 30% patients of melanoma. One of the strategies for prostate cancer therapy is using antiandrogen specially enzalutamide (antagonist of the interaction of androgens with AR) and abiraterone (blocker of androgen biosynthesis) to inhibit the activity of the androgen receptor (AR). HNRNPA1 could drive a splice variant of AR called ARv7 arises due to the inclusion of a cryptic exon CE3 and result in antiandrogen treatment [7, 36].

In addition to chemo and hormone therapy in cancers, radiotherapies are used for treatment and several factors involved in tumor sensitivity to ionizing radiation that some of them affected by alternative splicing. Interestingly, p73 (a transcription factor) is one of the most important proteins that could act as a marker for the sensitivity of tumor cells to radiation. There are two isoforms of the p73 including the full-length TAp73 and the N-terminally truncated ΔNp73 which truncated isoform has been indicated that strongly associated with poor survival and negative response to irradiation [16].

9. Cancer therapy based on splicing modulation

Recently, new strategies have been used to correct splicing errors and overcome drug resistance. In different levels could be applying various molecules to reverse aberrant splicing. Blocking of splicing factors and kinases which phosphorylated them is one of the strategies for correct splicing (**Figure 13**) [36].

However, using splice switching oligonucleotides (SSOs) is the best-known method for therapy based on splicing [36]. For example, masking the proximal 5′ splice site by an antisense oligonucleotide (ASO) in BCL-X could shift splicing and induce apoptosis in tumor cells. The same strategy is used for reverse aberrant splicing of MDM4 and FAS mRNAs and inhibit p53 degradation and enhanced-cell death, respectively (**Figure 14**) [18]. In addition, ESEs and ESSs which are binding sites for SRSF and HNRNP proteins could be blocked by SSOs and affect splicing events [36].

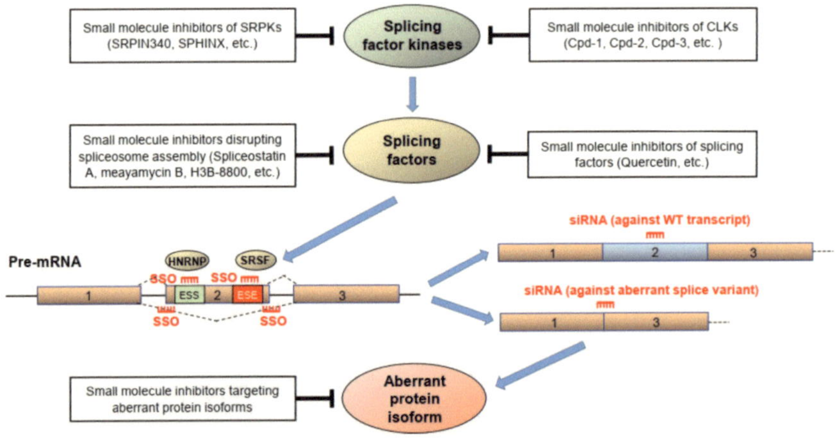

Figure 13.
Various potential strategies for therapeutic approaches to correct splicing errors [36].

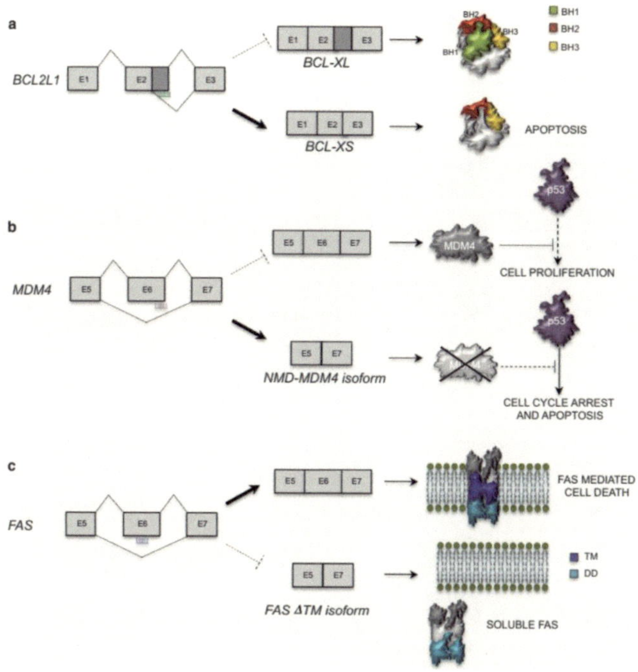

Figure 14.
Cancer therapies based on antisense oligonucleotide-mediated splicing modulation [18].

10. Conclusion

In conclusion, aberrant splicing, especially alternative splicing, can play an important role in carcinogenesis in all hallmarks of cancer (**Figure 15**). Recently, data from TCGA have been reported that many of the key player genes involved

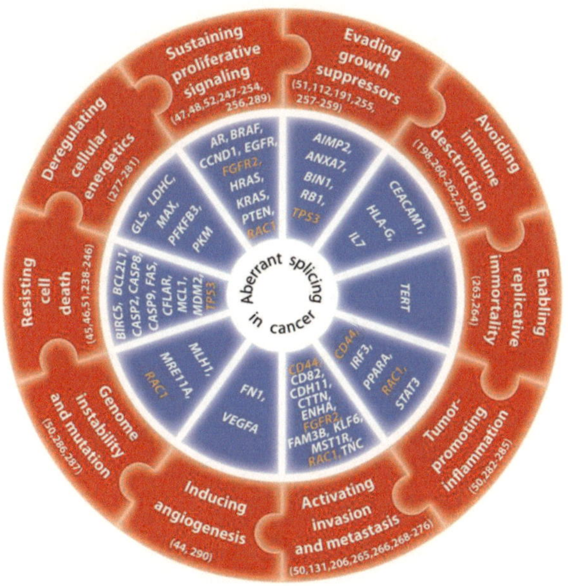

Figure 15.
The implication of alternative splicing of important genes (blue background) in the regulation of hallmarks of cancer (red background) [37].

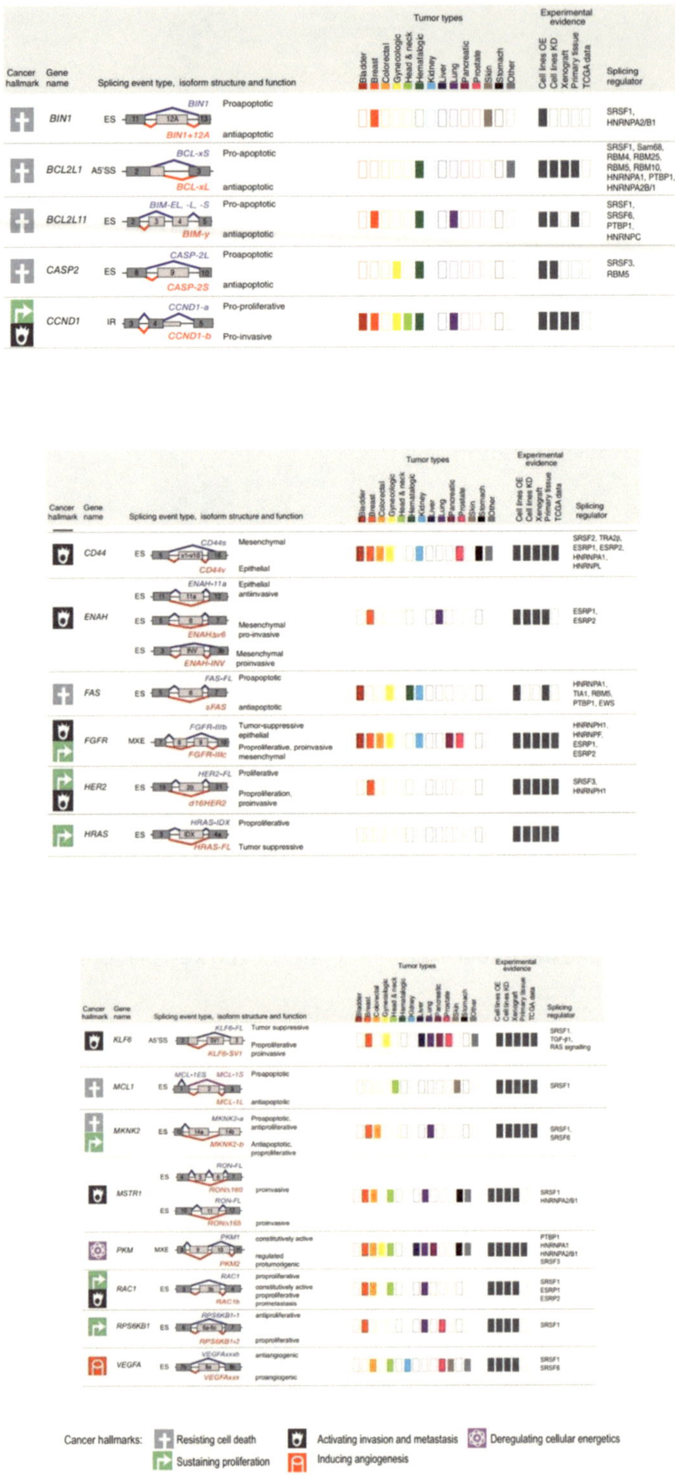

Figure 16.

Tumor-associated isoforms of the important genes in cancers. ES, exon skipping; MXE, mutually exclusive exons; 5'ASS, 5' alternative splice site selection; IR, intron; retention.OE, overexpression; KD, knockdown. Other tumors include: adrenal, gallbladder, ampullary, bone, and brain; gynecological tumors include: ovarian, cervical, and uterine; head and neck tumors include: Oral, head and neck, tongue, esophageal, and thyroid.. ES, exon skipping; MXE, mutually exclusive exons; 5'ASS, 5' alternative splice site selection; IR, intron retention [21].

in cancers are affected by alternative splicing (**Figure 16**). It has recently been suggested that some misspliced RNA transcripts of non-coding RNAs (ncRNAs), including long ncRNAs (lncRNAs) and circular RNAs (circRNAs), may also contribute to tumorigenesis [38, 39]. One of the isoforms of protein phosphatase 1 regulatory subunit 10 (PPP1R10, also called PNUTS) gene generated by alternative splicing is lncRNA-PNUTS, which act as a competitive sponge for miR-205 in breast cancer [40]. In addition, PCGEM1 and BC200 lncRNAs interact with splicing factors such as hnRNPA1, hnRNPA2/B1 and U2AF65 and regulate the alternative splicing of the AR and BCL-x genes, respectively. Moreover, MALAT1 as an LncRNA, regulates alternative splicing by affecting the sub nuclear localization of SR proteins [21]. The role of alternative splicing in carcinogenesis and new strategies for cancer therapy based on reverse abnormal splicing or blocking aberrant splicing are emerging areas of cancer research.

Author details

Mehdi Moghanibashi[1]* and Parisa Mohamadynejad[2]

1 Department of Genetics, School of Medicine, Kazerun Branch, Islamic Azad University, Kazerun, Iran

2 Department of Biology, Faculty of Basic Sciences, Shahrekord Branch, Islamic Azad University, Shahrekord, Iran

*Address all correspondence to: mehdimoghani@yahoo.com

References

[1] Zhang Y, Qian J, Gu C, Yang Y. Alternative splicing and cancer: A systematic review. Signal Transduction and Targeted Therapy. 2021;**6**(1):78. DOI: 10.1038/s41392-021-00486-7

[2] Li Y, Xu Y, Ma Z. Comparative analysis of the exon-intron structure in eukaryotic genomes. Yangtze Medicine. 2017;**1**(1):50-64. DOI: 10.4236/ym.2017.11006

[3] Busch A, Hertel KJ. Evolution of SR protein and hnRNP splicing regulatory factors. Wiley Interdisciplinary Reviews: RNA. 2012;**3**(1):1-12. DOI: 10.1002/wrna.100

[4] Keren H, Lev-Maor G, Ast G. Alternative splicing and evolution: Diversification, exon definition and function. Nature Reviews. Genetics. 2010;**11**(5):345-355. DOI: 10.1038/nrg2776

[5] Chen Y, Huang M, Liu X, Huang Y, Liu C, Zhu J, et al. Alternative splicing of mRNA in colorectal cancer: New strategies for tumor diagnosis and treatment. Cell Death & Disease. 2021;**12**(8):752. DOI: 10.1038/s41419-021-04031-w

[6] Sperling J, Azubel M, Sperling R. Structure and function of the pre-mRNA splicing machine. Structure. 2008;**16**(11):1605-1615. DOI: 10.1016/j.str.2008.08.011

[7] Sciarrillo R, Wojtuszkiewicz A, Assaraf YG, Jansen G, Kaspers GJL, Giovannetti E, et al. The role of alternative splicing in cancer: From oncogenesis to drug resistance. Drug Resistance Updates. 2020;**53**:100728. DOI: 10.1016/j.drup.2020.100728

[8] Bonnal SC, López-Oreja I, Valcárcel J. Roles and mechanisms of alternative splicing in cancer—Implications for care. Nature Reviews. Clinical Oncology. 2020;**17**(8):457-474. DOI: 10.1038/s41571-020-0350-x

[9] Bates DO, Morris JC, Oltean S, Donaldson LF. Pharmacology of modulators of alternative splicing. Pharmacological Reviews. 2017;**69**(1):63-79. DOI: 10.1124/pr.115.011239

[10] Vallès Y, Halanych KM, Boore JL. Group II introns break new boundaries: Presence in a bilaterian's genome. PLoS One. 2008;**3**(1):e1488. DOI: 10.1371/journal.pone.0001488

[11] Horiuchi T, Aigaki T. Alternative trans-splicing: A novel mode of pre-mRNA processing. Biology of the Cell. 2006;**98**(2):135-140. DOI: 10.1042/BC20050002

[12] ENCODE Project Consortium. An integrated encyclopedia of DNA elements in the human genome. Nature. 2012;**489**(7414):57-74. DOI: 10.1038/nature11247

[13] Vaquero-Garcia J, Barrera A, Gazzara MR, González-Vallinas J, Lahens NF, Hogenesch JB, et al. A new view of transcriptome complexity and regulation through the lens of local splicing variations. eLife. 2016;**5**:e11752. DOI: 10.7554/eLife.11752

[14] Wang ET, Sandberg R, Luo S, Khrebtukova I, Zhang L, Mayr C, et al. Alternative isoform regulation in human tissue transcriptomes. Nature. 2008;**456**(7221):470-476. DOI: 10.1038/nature07509

[15] Pan Q, Shai O, Lee LJ, Frey BJ, Blencowe BJ. Deep surveying of alternative splicing complexity in the human transcriptome by high-throughput sequencing. Nature Genetics. 2008;**40**(12):1413-1415. DOI: 10.1038/ng.259

[16] Di C, Syafrizayanti ZQ, Chen Y, Wang Y, Zhang X, Liu Y, et al. Function, clinical application, and strategies of pre-mRNA splicing in cancer. Cell Death and Differentiation. 2019;**26**(7): 1181-1194. DOI: 10.1038/s41418-018-0231-3

[17] Jin Y, Dong H, Shi Y, Bian L. Mutually exclusive alternative splicing of pre-mRNAs. Wiley Interdisciplinary Reviews: RNA. 2018;**9**(3):e1468. DOI: 10.1002/wrna.1468

[18] Paronetto MP, Passacantilli I, Sette C. Alternative splicing and cell survival: From tissue homeostasis to disease. Cell Death and Differentiation. 2016;**23**(12):1919-1929. DOI: 10.1038/cdd.2016.91

[19] Biamonti G, Infantino L, Gaglio D, Amato A. An intricate connection between alternative splicing and phenotypic plasticity in development and cancer. Cell. 2019;**9**(1):34. DOI: 10.3390/cells9010034

[20] Brady LK, Wang H, Radens CM, Bi Y, Radovich M, Maity A, et al. Transcriptome analysis of hypoxic cancer cells uncovers intron retention in EIF2B5 as a mechanism to inhibit translation. PLoS Biology. 2017;**15**(9): e2002623. DOI: 10.1371/journal.pbio.2002623

[21] Urbanski LM, Leclair N, Anczuków O. Alternative-splicing defects in cancer: Splicing regulators and their downstream targets, guiding the way to novel cancer therapeutics. Wiley Interdisciplinary Reviews: RNA. 2018;**9**(4):e1476. DOI: 10.1002/wrna.1476

[22] Groulx JF, Boudjadi S, Beaulieu JF. MYC regulates α6 integrin subunit expression and splicing under its pro-proliferative ITGA6A form in colorectal cancer cells. Cancers (Basel). 2018;**10**(2):42. DOI: 10.3390/cancers10020042

[23] Kuan CY, Roth KA, Flavell RA, Rakic P. Mechanisms of programmed cell death in the developing brain. Trends in Neurosciences. 2000;**23**(7):291-297. DOI: 10.1016/s0166-2236(00)01581-2

[24] Bielli P, Bordi M, Di Biasio V, Sette C. Regulation of BCL-X splicing reveals a role for the polypyrimidine tract binding protein (PTBP1/hnRNP I) in alternative 5′ splice site selection. Nucleic Acids Research. 2014;**42**(19): 12070-12081. DOI: 10.1093/nar/gku922

[25] Jurica MS, Mesecar A, Heath PJ, Shi W, Nowak T, Stoddard BL. The allosteric regulation of pyruvate kinase by fructose-1, 6-bisphosphate. Structure. 1998;**6**(2):195-210. DOI: 10.1016/s0969-2126(98)00021-5

[26] Takenaka M, Noguchi T, Sh S, Hirai H, Yamada K, Matsuda T, et al. Isolation and characterization of the human pyruvate kinase M gene. European Journal of Biochemistry. 1991;**198**:101-106

[27] Christofk HR, Vander Heiden MG, Harris MH, Ramanathan A, Gerszten RE, Wei R, et al. The M2 splice isoform of pyruvate kinase is important for cancer metabolism and tumour growth. Nature. 2008;**452**(7184):230-233. DOI: 10.1038/nature06734

[28] Chen M, Zhang J, Manley JL. Turning on a fuel switch of cancer: hnRNP proteins regulate alternative splicing of pyruvate kinase mRNA. Cancer Research. 2010;**70**(22):8977-8980. DOI: 10.1158/0008-5472.CAN-10-2513

[29] David CJ, Chen M, Assanah M, Canoll P, Manley JL. HnRNP proteins controlled by c-Myc deregulate pyruvate kinase mRNA splicing in cancer. Nature. 2010;**463**(7279):364-368. DOI: 10.1038/nature08697

[30] Mazurek S. Pyruvate kinase type M2: A key regulator of the metabolic

budget system in tumor cells. The International Journal of Biochemistry & Cell Biology. 2011;**43**(7):969-980. DOI: 10.1016/j.biocel.2010.02.005

[31] Harper SJ, Bates DO. VEGF-A splicing: The key to anti-angiogenic therapeutics? Nature Reviews. Cancer. 2008;**8**(11):880-887. DOI: 10.1038/nrc2505

[32] Wagner KD, El Maï M, Ladomery M, Belali T, Leccia N, Michiels JF, et al. Altered VEGF splicing isoform balance in tumor endothelium involves activation of splicing factors Srpk1 and Srsf1 by the Wilms' tumor suppressor Wt1. Cell. 2019;**8**(1):41. DOI: 10.3390/cells8010041

[33] Lagerstedt-Robinson K, Rohlin A, Aravidis C, Melin B, Nordling M, Stenmark-Askmalm M, et al. Mismatch repair gene mutation spectrum in the Swedish Lynch syndrome population. Oncology Reports. 2016;**36**(5):2823-2835. DOI: 10.3892/or.2016.5060

[34] Xiong HY, Alipanahi B, Lee LJ, Bretschneider H, Merico D, Yuen RK, et al. RNA splicing. The human splicing code reveals new insights into the genetic determinants of disease. Science. 2015;**347**(6218):1254806. DOI: 10.1126/science.1254806

[35] Abou Faycal C, Gazzeri S, Eymin B. RNA splicing, cell signaling, and response to therapies. Current Opinion in Oncology. 2016;**28**(1):58-64. DOI: 10.1097/CCO.0000000000000254

[36] Wang BD, Lee NH. Aberrant RNA splicing in cancer and drug resistance. Cancers (Basel). 2018;**10**(11):458. DOI: 10.3390/cancers10110458

[37] Sveen A, Kilpinen S, Ruusulehto A, Lothe RA, Skotheim RI. Aberrant RNA splicing in cancer; expression changes and driver mutations of splicing factor genes. Oncogene. 2016;**35**(19):2413-2427. DOI: 10.1038/onc.2015.318

[38] Romero-Barrios N, Legascue MF, Benhamed M, Ariel F, Crespi M. Splicing regulation by long noncoding RNAs. Nucleic Acids Research. 2018;**46**(5):2169-2184. DOI: 10.1093/nar/gky095

[39] Gawronski AR, Uhl M, Zhang Y, Lin YY, Niknafs YS, Ramnarine VR, et al. MechRNA: Prediction of lncRNA mechanisms from RNA-RNA and RNA-protein interactions. Bioinformatics. 2018;**34**(18):3101-3110. DOI: 10.1093/bioinformatics/bty208

[40] Grelet S, Link LA, Howley B, Obellianne C, Palanisamy V, Gangaraju VK, et al. A regulated PNUTS mRNA to lncRNA splice switch mediates EMT and tumour progression. Nature Cell Biology. 2017;**19**(9):1105-1115. DOI: 10.1038/ncb3595. Epub 2017 Aug 21. Erratum in: Nature Cell Biology. 2017;19(12):1443

Chapter 2

Molecular Genetic Mechanisms in Cancers of Keratinocytic Origin

Yıldız Gürsel Ürün

Abstract

Keratinocytic cancers (KC) comprise a group of diseases that have a broad spectrum clinically and pathologically. At one end of the spectrum are benign proliferations (acanthomas), and at the other end are malignant tumors with aggressive growth and metastatic potential. Traditionally, about 80% of KC cases have basal cell carcinoma (BCC) and 20% have cutaneous squamous cell carcinoma (cSCC). Both tumors have different phenotypic features due to different oncogenic pathways. cSCC is biologically different and requires a different approach due to the higher risk of local recurrence, metastasis and death. Genetic factors play an important role in the development of KC. Family and family history studies, the presence of KC as a feature of rare hereditary syndromes, and genetic association studies give us clues in this regard. More than 20 genetic syndromes associated with KC have been described. Some syndromes are associated with multiple BCC, some with multiple cSCC, and some with both BCC and cSCC. Environmental risk factors include exposure to ultraviolet light radiation and immunosuppression in both tumors. Exposure to ionizing radiation is most common in BCC, while smoking and photosensitive drug use are among the environmental risk factors for cSCC. Molecular, epidemiological, and clinical studies will help better understand the cellular processes involved in tumorigenesis, and develop new strategies for treating and preventing KCs.

Keywords: basal cell carcinoma, squamous cell carcinoma, skin cancer, molecular genetics, environmental carcinogens

1. Introduction

Keratinocytic cancers (KC) comprise a group of diseases that have a broad spectrum clinically and pathologically. Keratinocytic cancers are very common and, despite their low mortality rate, represent a significant public health problem [1]. Traditionally, about 80% of KC cases have basal cell carcinoma (BCC) and 20% have cutaneous squamous cell carcinoma (cSCC) [2]. KC have a complex etiology involving environmental, phenotypical and genetic risk factors [3]. Molecular, epidemiologic, and clinical studies have led to a greater understanding of the cellular events that occur during tumorigenesis, epidemiologic risk factors, and have provided new strategies for treatment and prevention of keratinocyte carcinomas [4]. In the next part of the chapter, BCC- and cSCC-related risk factors and molecular mechanisms associated with tumorigenesis are discussed in detail.

2. Basal cell carcinoma

BCC is a skin tumor thought to arise from the pluripotent cells of the pilosebaceous unit, and there are several clinical types [5]. It is the most common malignancy in fair-skinned populations worldwide [6]. The mortality rate of BCCs is low, but it is an important cause of morbidity, mainly due to local destruction [7]. The incidence and prevalence of BCC increase with age, due to both increasing sun exposure and an aging population [8]. The highest incidence of BCC has been reported in the following countries: Australia, followed by the United States (US) and Europe [9, 10]. In the United States, an increase in an incidence of 4–8% per year has been noted [11]. BCC is more common in men than women, with a male-to-female ratio of approximately 2:1 [12]. The natural course of BCC is a lesion that usually begins as a small, barely visible papule and over the years grows into a nodule or plaque that sometimes ulcerates without showing aggression [13]. When the histologic subtypes of BCC were classified by the World Health Organization according to the risk of recurrence, they were divided into two groups: (1) those with lower risk: nodular, superficial, pigmented, infundibulocystic (a variant of BCC with adnexal differentiation), fibroepithelial; (2) those with higher risk: basosquamous carcinoma, BCC with sclerosing/morpheic, infiltrating, sarcomatoid differentiation, and micronodules [14]. The development of BCC is the result of the interaction of many genes and environmental factors. Most genes involved in BCC pathogenesis have a uniform mutational signature that results in the ultraviolet (UV)-induced Deoxyribonucleic acid (DNA) damage [15].

2.1 Etiopathogenesis

More than 99% of cases of basal cell carcinoma are sporadic. In the absence of an overtly inherited disease-causing mutation, both environmental factors and the sum of an individual's genetic variations culminate in BCC development [16]. Among the most important risk factors for basal cell carcinoma is exposure to UV radiation [13]. Further risk factors include age, male gender, skin type I and II according to Fitzpatrick (individuals with genetically determined low skin pigmentation), history of BCC, pharmacological therapy, long-term exposure to arsenic, exposure to ionizing radiation, long-lasting immunosuppression, and genetic syndromes [15, 17]. Scarring and chronic ulceration are particularly significant for developing BCCs in non-chronic UV-exposed areas [17]. Chronic exposure to immunosuppressive agents due to organ transplantations linearly increases the risk of developing BCC over time [8]. The main carcinogenic factor is UV, which explains why most tumors are found in sun-exposed skin areas [13]. Indeed, BCC harbors the highest mutated human tumors (65 mutations/megabases) [18, 19] and a high percentage of UV-induced mutations (C:T or CC:TT transitions in dipyrimidine regions) [20]. Sunburns that occur after intense, episodic sun exposure increase the risk for BCC [21]. Both UVA and UVB play a role in skin carcinogenesis by causing DNA damage and immunosuppression. UVB is directly absorbed by the DNA molecule and causes UV-induced DNA damage. In one study, 75.7% of UV-induced DNA coding mutations resulted in the formation of cyclobutane dimers as a consequence of chronic UVB damage [22]. UVA induces cellular reactive oxygen species (ROS) that cause oxidative DNA damage [21–25]. Basal cell carcinomas are common in the elderly population given cumulative sun exposure and exogenous factors. Age-related deterioration of biological functions leads to chronic inflammation, decreased immune system function, genomic instability, and decreased DNA repair capacity. Therefore, aging skin is characterized by the accumulation and presence of DNA damage and senescent cells. The chronic inflammatory state leads to changes in the integrity of the dermal matrix. All these processes increase the rate of malignancy development with age [15]. The incidence of BCC is generally higher in men than in women, possibly due to occupational exposure to the sun and increased recreational activity in men. However, this difference is less pronounced today, possibly due to lifestyle changes-smoking or tanning beds [24, 25]. People with a previous history of BCC have a higher risk of developing both keratinocytic cancers (KC) and melanoma [15]. These patients have a 10-fold increased risk compared with the general population [26]. A prospective cohort study of 1426 patients showed that 40.7% of them developed a new KC within 5 years after the first lesion and 82% of them developed a new KC within 5 years after more than one lesion [27].

Medications taken by patients pose a risk for the development of BCC. Many drugs such as tetracyclines, thiazide diuretics, nonsteroidal anti-inflammatory drugs (NSAIDs), and retinoids are potentially photosensitizing. Therefore, these drugs elicit phototoxic, photoallergic skin reactions and, when combined with UV radiation, act as carcinogens that increase the risk of skin cancer [28]. Adults taking tetracycline who were exposed to UV light in their youth have an increased risk of BCC [29]. Angiotensin receptor blockers, an antihypertensive drug, have been shown to increase BCC risk by promoting angiogenesis and cancer progression [30]. A Dutch study found an increased risk of BCC in long-term users of loop diuretics, with no association with thiazides and potassium-sparing agents [31]. However, the available data are insufficient to draw firm conclusions about the association between the use of different types of antihypertensive drugs and skin cancer risk. Organ transplant patients have an increased risk of KC due to the immunosuppressive agents they receive. The incidence of BCC in transplant patients has increased tenfold. HIV seropositivity doubles the risk for BCC [32]. The fact that approximately 20% of lesions occur on skin sites not exposed to sunlight is an indication that extrinsic factors other than UV play a role in the pathogenesis of BCC. Other known extrinsic factors include ionizing radiation, arsenic, tar, psoralen and UVA (PUVA), and nitrogen mustard [33, 34]. Ionizing radiation (radiotherapy, X-rays, occupational exposure, whole-body irradiation treatments, atomic bombing) increases the risk of BCCs and possibly cSCCs in various carcinogenic ways. This occurs through various carcinogenic mechanisms such as DNA damage, genomic instability, and cell apoptosis [35, 36].

2.2 Inherited susceptibility to BCC

Some individuals have an increased susceptibility to developing BCC due to genetic syndromes, germline single-nucleotide polymorphisms (SNPs), and genetic traits [37]. A recent study found an overall heritability of 14.0% for KC and 17.0% for BCC in data based on genome-wide array data and self-reported KC history [38]. In the absence of other predisposing factors, especially when multiple BCCs occur at a young age, a possible association with genodermatoses should be considered [17]. The genodermatoses most commonly associated with BCC include Gorlin-Goltz syndrome (also known as Nevoid Basal Cell Carcinoma Syndrome), Bazex-Dupre-Christol syndrome, Rombo syndrome, Generalized Follicular Basaloid Hamartoma syndrome, and Happle-Tinschert syndrome [5]. Nineteen rare syndromes have been described in BCC due to the inheritance of highly penetrant germline mutations. These syndromes, their associated mutations and molecular pathways are listed in **Table 1** [37]. Genetic alterations associated with basal cell carcinoma were first described in Gorlin-Goltz syndrome, an inherited predisposition. In the pathogenesis of this syndrome, there are abnormalities associated with the long arm of the patched (PTCH1) gene on chromosome 9 (q22.3-q31) without significant heterogeneity [40]. The prevalence is reported to be approximately 1:56,000 [17]. Affected patients have multiple developmental anomalies, multiple BCCs, and odontogenic keratocysts of the jaw at an early age; the risk of developing medulloblastoma increases in early childhood [39, 41]. BCCs occur on average by age 25, typically in sun-exposed areas, with few to thousands of lesions [39]. Although, most cases are inherited in an autosomal dominant manner, approximately 26% (8–41) of cases develop as de novo [42]. In most cases, this syndrome is caused by mutations on chromosome 9q22.3 that inactivate the PTCH1-containing germline; these inactivating mutations lead to premature termination of the PTCH protein. A second somatic mutation, e.g., caused by UV radiation, can lead to malignancy by loss of the second copy (the loss of heterozygous expression) of the

Syndrome	Gene(s)	Gene function(s)
Gorlin-Goltz syndrome (Nevoid Basal Cell Carcinoma syndrome)	PTCH1, SUFU, PTCH2	HH pathway members
Bazex-Dupré-Christol syndrome	UBE2A, ACTRT1	DNA repair and regulation of cell cycle, HH pathway
Rombo syndrome	Unknown	Rombo syndrome gene is not known; it is involved in DNA repair and/or cell cycle regulation and may play a role during hair follicle growth and differentiation
Generalized follicular basaloid hamartoma syndrome	Unknown	Unknown
Happle-Tinschert syndrome	Unknown	Unknown
Muir-Torre syndrome	MSH2, MLH1, MSH6, and PMS2	DNA mismatch repair
Cowden syndrome	PTEN	PI3K-AKT signaling pathway
Brooke-Spiegler syndrome	CYLD	NF-κB and EGFR pathways regulator
Cartilage-hair hypoplasia	RMRP	Immune response
Xeroderma pigmentosum	XPA-XPG, XPV, POLH	Nucleotide excision repair
Bloom syndrome	BLM (RECOL3)	Chromosomal stability
Werner syndrome	WRN (RECOL2), LMNA	Chromosomal stability
Rothmund-Thomson syndrome	RECOL4, C160rf57	Chromosomal stability
Schopf-Schulz-Passarge syndrome	WNT10A	WNT/β-catenin signaling pathway, cell proliferation and migration
Oculocutaneous albinism	TYR, OCA2, TYRP1, SLC45A2 (MATP), SLC24A5, C10orf11, 4q24	Melanin synthesis
Hermansky-Pudlak syndrome	HPS1-HPS8	Melanin synthesis
Epidermodysplasia verruciformis (Lewandowsky-Lutz dysplasia)	TMC6 (EVER1), TMC8 (EVER2	Immune response and signal transduction in the endoplasmic reticulum
Schimmelpenning syndrome	Unknown	Unknown
Phacomatosis pigmentokeratotica	Unknown	Unknown

Adapted from Choquet et al. [37] and Kilgour et al. [39].

Table 1.
Genetic syndromes associated with inherited susceptibility to BCC.

tumor suppressor gene [39]. Other less common mutated genes include PTCH2 and suppressor of fused (SUFU) gene, which play a role in Gorlin syndrome [43]. Bazex-Dupre-Christol syndrome is another genetic syndrome associated with the Hedgehog (HH) pathway. The development of multiple BCCs is associated with congenital hypotrichosis, follicular atrophoderma, and milia [44]. The prevalence is less than 1:1,000,000 [17]. The disease is inherited in an X-linked dominant manner, and mutations commonly occur in the actin-related protein T1 (ACTRT1) gene. The mutation in ACTRT1 ultimately leads to increased GLI transcription factors 1 (GLI1)-induced oncogenic transcription, responsible for the abnormal HH pathway [45]. Rombo syndrome is a very rare autosomal dominant syndrome. In addition to the development of BCCs, this syndrome is accompanied by acrocyanosis, keratosis pilaris, atrophoderma vermiculatum, hypotrichosis as well as hypohidrosis. The prevalence is less than 1: 1,000,000 and it is difficult to distinguish from Bazex-Dupré-Christol syndrome [17].

Susceptibility to BCC may be due to inherited deficiencies in DNA repair. Xeroderma pigmentosum (XP) is an autosomal recessive disorder caused by inherited mutations in any of 8 possible genes required for nucleotide excision repair (NER). Damaged DNA is recognized in actively transcribed genes via the transcription-dependent repair (TCR) pathway and in the rest of the genome via the slower global genome repair (GGR) pathway. Mutations in any of these proteins in the TCR, NER, or GGR pathways result in abnormalities in DNA repair. The classic phenotype of XP manifests in early childhood in the form of freckles before age 2, severe burns after minimal sun exposure, and early-onset skin cancer [46]. XP patients have a > 10,000-fold increased lifetime risk of non-melanocytic skin cancer and a > 2000-fold increased risk of melanoma compared to the general population [47]. Besides xeroderma pigmentosum, the other genetic abnormalities Bloom, Werner, and Rothmund-Thomson syndromes have a predominantly increased risk for BCC and an increased risk for cSCC. The genes involved in these syndromes impair nucleotide excision repair and chromosome stability [37]. In addition to genetic disorders, certain inherited phenotypic traits have also been shown to increase BCC risk [39]. People with fair skin, light eyes and hair, childhood freckles, inability to tan, and Northern European ancestry are known to have an increased risk of developing BCC [21, 48].

2.3 Genetic polymorphism

Genome-wide association studies (GWAS) have played a key role in identifying polygenic effects that mediate susceptibility to BCC [16]. Over the past decade, GWAS has accelerated the discovery of genetic determinants [37]. GWAS studies of SCC and BCC in a European population have identified 33 loci associated with susceptibility to BCC. Taken together, these 33 loci account for 10.98% of the heritability of BCC [37, 39]. In addition to specific mutations of BCC, germline polymorphisms in genes that determine pigmentary characteristics, such as the melanocortin-1 receptor (MC1R), the human homolog of agouti signaling protein (ASIP), and tyrosinase (TYR), have also been associated with increased risk of BCC [49–51]. MC1R encodes a G-protein-coupled transmembrane receptor that activates adenylate cyclase to produce intracellular cyclic adenosine monophosphate (cAMP) in response to stimulation by α-melanocyte-stimulating hormone (α-MSH). Signal transduction by cAMP induces the maturation of phenomelanosomes to eumelanosomes and is responsible for the darker pigmentation and thus the increased UV resistance. The MC1R gene is highly polymorphic in fair-skinned individuals [51]. Several studies have found that pigmentation-independent mechanisms, even after controlling for skin phototype and hair color, significantly increase BCC risk in some of the common variants [50, 51]. GWAS studies have also identified the IRF4, HERC2, LPP, BNC2, EXOC2, RALY, and SLC45A2 genes as important risk loci for BCC, along with other pigmentation genes [39]. While most of these loci are associated with increased risk, ORs of less than one has been reported for SLC45A2, BNC2, and HERC2, suggesting a lower risk [52]. Polymorphism studies on tumor suppressor genes have mainly focused on the tumor suppressor gene p53 (TP53). One polymorphism encoding the TP53 gene, rs78378222, is highly significant for BCC with an overall OR of 2.16. The s78378222 polymorphism affects the AATAAA polyadenylation of the signal of the 30 untranslated regions of the TP53 gene, changing it to AATACA. These results are related to an interrupted polyadenine tail of TP53 mRNA, which is required for stabilization and nuclear export [53]. Genes that determine epidermal differentiation and cytoskeletal organization have also been identified as carrying polymorphisms associated with increased BCC susceptibility [17, 39]. The keratin5 (KRT5) gene, together with its heterodimeric partner keratin14 (K14), produces the K5 protein. These proteins are essential proteins for the cytoskeletal intermediate filament network in the basal keratinocyte. The rs11170164 polymorphism results in a G138E substitution in the KRT5 gene and increases BCC risk [54]. Recently, attention has focused on gene polymorphisms affecting the NOTCH signaling pathway. The NOTCH signaling pathway plays an essential role in regulating keratinocyte proliferation and differentiation; this pathway is associated with skin abnormalities and skin cancer [55]. P53 is thought to induce NOTCH signaling and further promote NOTCH by inhibiting AP-1, a p53 inhibitor. NOTCH signaling regulates keratinocyte proliferation through two mechanisms: first, it inhibits p63, a transcription factor essential for epidermal growth, and second, it increases the expression of cyclin-dependent kinase inhibitor 1A (CDKN1A), a cell cycle inhibitor [39]. NOTCH signaling regulates keratinocyte differentiation through increased expression of transcriptional regulators such as the IRF6 and Hes/Hey genes [55, 56]. Polymorphism of genes (*FOXP1* and *IRF4*) in transcription factor regions that repress NOTCH signaling causes increased susceptibility to BCC [39].

Chromosomal instability is a known risk factor for KC, including BCC [37]. Chromosomal instability is believed to increase tumor adaptation and survival through genetic variation [57]. In addition, several studies have identified polymorphisms in telomere length-related genes that pose a risk for BCC [39]. Studies of gene polymorphisms affecting DNA repair also provide information. Lin et al. examined SNPs in 165 genes of the DNA repair pathway, identified no variants of XPA, MUS81, and NABP2 in three major repair genes, and associated these three variants with a significantly increased risk of BCC risk. The former variant decreased BCC risk (OR 0.93), whereas the latter two increased risk (ORs 1.06 and 1.11, respectively) [58]. Immunity and inflammation of the skin are known to influence the risk of skin cancer, including BCC [39]. Polymorphisms in the human leukocyte antigen (HLA) region have been associated with increased BCC susceptibility, as have IRF4 and UBAC2, which play a role in immune regulation [37]. In 2009, Welsh et al. examined the CT60 GG genotype of the cytotoxic lymphocyte-associated antigen-4 (CTLA-4) gene. They showed that this genotype reduced BCC risk. CTLA-4 is known to play a critical role in UV-induced skin immunosuppression, as it is expressed on t-regulatory cells that are upregulated by UV radiation. The CT60 GG genotype has been shown to result in decreased t-regulatory cell function, UV-induced immunosuppression, and consequently increased antitumor capacity [59]. Moreover, gene polymorphisms are associated with different phenotypes of BCC and modulation of BCC risk. Such a phenotype was observed in young men, in patients with multiple BCC clusters localized to the trunk and not exposed to the sun [60]. This phenotype was associated with germline polymorphisms of genes encoding the liver detoxification enzymes cytochrome p450 2D6 and glutathione S-transferase, as well as with germline polymorphisms of the vitamin D receptor and TNF-α [39].

2.4 Somatic mutations implicated in BCC tumorigenesis

Hedgehog is a signaling pathway in the skin that maintains the stem cell population and controls the development of hair follicles and sebaceous glands [39]. Abnormal activation of this pathway controls many aspects of tumorigenesis, including stages of initiation, progression, and relapse, in part by directing a cancer stem cell phenotype.

2.4.1 Hedgehog signaling pathway

Abnormal activation of the HH signaling pathway is a hallmark of the pathogenesis of BCC. The HH pathway is a highly conserved signaling pathway that plays a critical role in embryogenesis, cell differentiation, and cell proliferation. During embryogenesis, this signaling pathway regulates the morphogenesis of the epidermis and its appendages. Hedgehog is responsible for maintaining and controlling the growth of swollen stem cells. In addition, it is responsible for hair follicle growth and epidermal regeneration in the postnatal period, as well as the protection of bulge stem cells [15]. The HH family includes many intracellular signaling proteins and was first described in Drosophila melanogaster (fruit fly). The HH mutation in the fruit fly causes the embryo to have a spiny appearance reminiscent of a curled hedgehog and is called a hedgehog [61]. The HH signaling pathway consists of several key components: HH ligands, the transmembrane receptor proteins PTCH1 and PTCH2, smoothened proteins (SMO), and GLI1, GLI2, and GLI3 [62]. The PTCH gene encodes a receptor that mediates HH signaling. The intracellular PTCH1/Hh signaling pathway is required for cell growth, regulation, and differentiation. PTCH mutations have been detected not only in Gorlin-Goltz syndrome but also in sporadic BCC cases [5]. Activation of the HH pathway begins with the binding of the HH ligand to a transmembrane receptor complex consisting of the PTCH and SMO proteins. When the HH ligand binds to PTCH, the HH-PTCH complex is cleaved by lysosomes, which suppress SMO and preregulate the pathway's downstream signaling cascade through several proteins, including the SUFU. As a result, GLI family proteins are released, which are normally sequestered from the cytoplasm. GLI acts as a transcription factor. When secreted, it migrates to the nucleus and triggers the transcription of genes involved in cell renewal, cell fate and survival, and angiogenesis [20, 63]. In addition, GLI1 forms a feedback loop that automatically regulates HH signaling via modulation of PTCH1 [64]. PTCH protein has a negative regulatory effect on HH and suppresses PTCH SMO in the resting state. Oncogenic mutations affecting PTCH and SMO proteins lead to activation of the HH signaling pathway, which in turn causes epidermal hyperplasia and basal keratinocyte proliferation [65]. The PTCH-1 mutation plays a role in BCC carcinogenesis; PTCH-2 is effective in BCC pathogenesis only when together with the PTCH-1 mutation [5]. Activation of the noncanonical HH signaling pathway via GLI transcription factors occurs independently of the aforementioned signaling pathway. In this pathway, the binding of HH-PTCH1 and SMO is passed on. GLI activation is positively regulated by KRAS, TGF-β, PI3K-AKT, and PKC-α and negatively regulated by p53, PKA, and PKC-δ [66]. HH pathway activation is regulated at the genetic level by inactivating PTCH1 mutations identified in 90% of sporadic BCCs and by SMO activating mutations in about 10%. In about half of PTCH1 mutations, the "UV signature" includes C-T and tandem transitions CC-TT.

However, the source of UV radiation needs to be adjusted for these mutations, as other factors, such as oxidative stress, are involved in the mutagenesis of this gene. Both point mutations and somatic copy number aberrations (SCNAs) in the PTCH1 gene have been frequently reported in BCC [13] In summary, like PTCH tumor suppressor genes, SMO serves as a proto-oncogene and inactivation of PTCH or activation of SMO plays a role in the pathogenesis of BCC [5].

2.4.2 TP53 gene

The second most common event associated with BCC pathogenesis is the inactivation of the TP53 gene. The TP53 tumor suppressor gene is involved in cell cycle arrest and activation of programmed cell death [67]. In a mouse model study investigating the pathogenesis of BCC, it was shown that in X-ray-induced BCCs, inactivation of the P53 gene in interfollicular keratinocytes upregulates HH pathway activity through increased SMO expression [68]. Somatic mutations in TP53 are common in all human cancers, and non-synonymous mutations in BCC occur sporadically in approximately 61% of cases. Similar to PTCH1, most mutations in TP53 are UV-signed in the majority of BCCs [39].

2.4.3 Hippo-YAP signaling genes

The Hippo signaling pathway is critical for limiting tissue growth. It consists of a cascade of kinases that repress a downstream transcriptional co-activator, Yes-associated protein (YAP), by phosphorylation. The YAP1 protein is the major downregulatory effector of the Hippo pathway [69]. Genetic studies in mouse models suggest that the Hippo pathway plays a role in stabilizing skin growth and differentiation [70]. Moreover, elevated nuclear YAP1 levels lead to the massive proliferation of proliferative basal epidermal cells [71]. Premature stop mutations in the LATS1 gene, one of the kinases required for coding in the Hippo pathway, were reported in 16% of BCCs. Similarly, loss of functional mutations in the TPN14 gene, a tumor suppressor gene that acts as a negative regulator of YAP, was observed in 23% of BCC patients [72].

2.4.4 MYCN/FBXW7 signaling

bHLH transcription factor (MYCN) is a member of the MYC family of transcriptional activators and functions as a potential downstream effector of the HH pathway [73]. Alterations in the levels of MYC family transcription factors affect cell growth, proliferation, differentiation and apoptosis [74]. MYCN missense mutations have been identified in 30% of BCCs. Most mutations are located in the MYC box 1 domain, which is involved in the interaction with the tumor suppressor FBXW7. Functional studies have shown that there are four common N-MYC substitutions (T58A, P59L, P60L and P63L) that impair binding to FBXW7 and result in excess N-MYC protein expression [72].

2.4.5 TERT-promoter

Telomerase is a ribonucleoprotein complex. It maintains telomere length by telomere DNA repeats (TTAGGG) synthesized at the 30 ends of chromosomes to reverse the progressive shortening of DNA with each cell division. Telomerase consists of a reverse transcriptase protein (TERT) encoded by the hTERT gene and an RNA component (hTERC) that serves as a template for DNA telomere synthesis. Activation of the promoter-mediated hTERT gene has been shown to generate de novo binding sites for the family of E26 transformation-specific (ETS) transcription factors, thereby increasing telomerase expression and preventing cancer cell senescence or apoptosis [75]. TERT promoter mutations have been detected in high frequency in many different cancers such as melanoma, non-melanoma skin cancer, bladder cancer, and glioma, as they negatively affect TERT gene expression [76]. UV-related mutations of the TERT gene affecting the promoter region are found in 39–74% of patients with BCC [20].

2.4.6 DPH3-OXNAD1 bidirectional promoter

Similar to TERT, recurrent mutations were also found in the bidirectional promoter of the diphthamide biosynthesis protein 3 (DPH3) and NAD-binding domain containing 1 *(OXNAD1)* genes at non-coding positions close to the transcription start site. The DPH3 gene diphthamide, a modified histidine residue found in eukaryotic elongation factor 2, is required for protein synthesis [39]. Inactivation of DPH3 is characterized by the loss of a tumor cell's ability to metastasize; thus, the gene has a tumor-suppressive effect [77]. UV-signed genetic somatic mutations in the DPH3 and OXNAD1 genes have been detected in 42% of BCC [78].

2.4.7 Other potential BCC-associated genes

In a large cohort study, mutations in two cancer-associated genes, PPP6C and STK19, were observed to be associated with BCC tumorigenesis at high frequency [72]. PPP6C regulates cell cycle progression in human cells by controlling cyclin D1. STK19 is a kinase with an unknown function involved in transcriptional regulation [20, 77]. The PPP6C mutation was observed in 15% of patients with BCC and the STK19 mutation in 10%. Other genes commonly mutated in BCC include ARID1A, CASP8, CSMD1, GRIN2A, KRAS, NOTCH1, NOTCH2, NRAS, PIK3CA, PREX2, and RAC1. However, no statistically significant association was demonstrated between these genes and BCC. Two independent exome sequencing studies reported a high frequency of loss-of-function mutations in NOTCH1 (29% and 50%, respectively) and NOTCH2 (26% and 67%, respectively) genes, suggesting that they play a tumor-suppressive role in BCC [22, 72].

2.5 Epigenetic modifications

MicroRNAs (miRNAs) are small regulatory RNAs that act at multiple transcriptional, posttranscriptional, and epigenetic levels. Expression levels of altered miRNAs are associated with BCC progression and non-coding RNA (ncRNA) regulation and play a role in tumor promotion [15]. Studies have found that the expression levels of miRNAs differ in different BCC subtypes. For example, the expression of miR-183, a miRNA that inhibits metastasis to other organs, is significantly lower in infiltrative BCC than in nodular BCC [79]. In nodular BCC, the upregulated miR-141 is associated with the 200a and 200c, C-MYC-, WNT and beta-catenin signaling pathways [79]. MiR-203 and miR-451a function as tumor suppressors. HH and epidermal growth factor receptor (EGFR) signaling suppress the effect of miR-203 on c- JUN and thus cell proliferation [80]. The expression of miRNA-451a has been shown to decrease significantly in both human and mouse BCC patients. Inhibition of primary miRNA-451a increases cell growth via its target TBX1. Conversely, overexpression of miRNA-451a in tumor cells leads to cell cycle arrest by suppressing cell growth [81]. The OncomiR-1 cluster (miR-17-92) shows a regulatory role in SHH signaling in a mouse model of PTCH1, and the corresponding miRNAs were overexpressed in human BCCs [82]. Some long ncRNAs (lncRNAs) (such as ANRIL) are differentially expressed in BCCs [83].

2.6 Tumor microenvironment

Most BCC tumors develop from a surrounding fibromyxoid stroma. It likely provides a permissive tumor microenvironment (TME) by protecting the tumor from the immune system [84]. Indeed, an enhanced tumor-stromal response and local host immunosuppression have been noted in BCCs with high-risk histopathological subtypes [85]. Previous studies have shown a shift toward a Th2 response, an increase in T-regulatory lymphocytes, and the presence of cancer-associated fibroblasts in BCC TME [86]. However, high-throughput sequencing of T-cell receptors has not identified clonal tumor-specific populations of tumor-infiltrating lymphocytes in BCC [87]. The recent study by Lefrançois et al. [86] supports the above information. This study also found that tumor inflammation induced by macrophage activity is associated with advanced BCCs and lymphocytic infiltration plays an important role in nonadvanced tumors, possibly related to an adaptive antitumor response. In TMJ studies related to HH, the major pathway in the pathogenesis of BCC, the paracrine HH pathway is thought to be a complex mechanism involving cancer-related fibroblasts, leading to angiogenesis, fibrosis, immune evasion, and neuropathic pain [88]. Further studies are needed to clarify this issue. In summary, the cancer-associated genes and the various pathways contributing to BCC carcinogenesis suggest a heterogeneous genetic origin. Understanding the molecular genetics of BCC carcinogenesis is important for developing new targeted therapies, increasing treatment efficacy, and overcoming tumor resistance.

3. Cutaneous squamous cell carcinoma

Cutaneous squamous cell carcinoma is the second most common KC [89]. Data from the Rochester Epidemiology Project, conducted by the Mayo Clinic, show an overall 263% increase in cSCC incidence between 1976 and 1984 and 2000–2010 [90]. In the United Kingdom, the age-standardized incidence of primary cSCC was 77 per 100,000 between 2013 and 2015, with an average annual increase of 5% [91]. This increase has been associated with higher sun exposure levels, tanning bed use, an increase in the aging population and advances in skin cancer detection [92, 93]. The incidence of cSCC is higher in men than in women (3:1 ratio) and increases significantly with age [75, 94]. cSCC results from the uncontrolled proliferation of atypical epidermal keratinocytes due to mutations in genes involved in epidermal homeostasis. It is well known that tumor development is a gradual process that defines different histological and pathological stages, from a premalignant lesion, actinic keratosis (AK), to invasive cSCC [95]. However, similar mutations can also be found in normal keratinocytes, especially in chronically sun-exposed skin [96]. Therefore, other factors-including epigenetic alterations, viral infections, or microenvironmental changes-promote the development and progression of cSCC [97]. cSCC lesions typically occur on chronically sun-exposed sites such as the face, lips, ears, and bald scalp and are characterized by hyperkeratotic, often ulcerated plaques or nodules [75]. The histopathologic classification of cSCC includes keratoacanthomas, acantholytic, spindle cell, verrucous, adenosquamous, and clear cell cSCC [14]. Tumors classified as desmoplastic, acantholytic, and de nova are at higher risk of metastasis to the skin. In addition, less differentiated tumors are associated with a poorer prognosis [98]. In addition to histopathological features, other features determine the high risk of cSCC and the risk of metastasis: 1. subclinical metastasis, 2. depth of invasion (>2 mm), 3. high-risk anatomical localization (face, ear, pre/postauricular, genital, hands and feet), 4. perineural involvement, 5. recurrence, 6. multiple cSCC tumors, 7. immunosuppression [98, 99]. It is well known that the mortality rate for cSCC in the south and the central United States is similar to that for renal and oropharyngeal carcinomas and melanomas [94].

3.1 Etiopathogenesis

The etiology of cSCC is multifactorial. Environmental, immunologic, and genetic factors all play a role [95]. Cumulative exposure to ultraviolet radiation under the influence of the sun and/or tanning devices is the most important causative factor [100, 101]. Epidemiological studies suggest that cumulative sun exposure (mainly UVB radiation) is the most important environmental cause of cSCC. In contrast, intense, intermittent sun exposure (e.g., sunburn, childhood exposure) is the most important risk factor for BCC and melanoma [102, 103]. Although, ionizing radiation is considered a potential risk factor for cSCC, studies have not fully proven this [37]. One study found that therapeutic radiation increased the total number of BCCs but had no effect on SCCs [36]. Another study found an increased risk of both BCC and SCC at sites with prior radiation [104]. Chronic immunosuppression due to organ transplant medications, chronic leukemias and lymphomas, and HIV infection has been shown to be a major risk factor for cSCC and, to a lesser extent, BCC [105–107]. In contrast to the general population, heart and lung transplant recipients, in particular, tend to develop cSCC more frequently than BCC [108]. The tumorigenic effect of immunosuppression is thought to be related to weak immune surveillance of keratinocytes that do not clear precancerous lesions [109]. While class I HLA proteins are expressed in patients with cSCC, these proteins are not expressed in patients with BCC; therefore, potential immunosuppression has been reported to lead to the development of more cSCC [110]. Patients with chronic lymphocytic leukemia who lack competent cell-mediated and humoral immunity also have an 8- to 10-fold increased risk of developing cSCC [111]. Chronic inflammation increases the risk of cSCC development and progression [37]. 1% of all skin cancers and 95% of patients with cSCC develop on chronically inflamed skin such as scars, burns, and ulcers [112]. Chronic inflammation produces ROS and reactive nitrogen intermediates that lead to DNA damage, which leads to genomic instability and tumorigenesis, resulting in the development of cSCC [113].

Human Papillomavirus (HPV) is a double-stranded DNA virus that infects the squamous epithelium. HPVs are classified into 5 genera (alpha, beta, gamma, mu, and nu) [95]. The β-subtype of HPV has been associated with an increased risk of cSCC [114]. A meta-analysis study reported increased rates of cSCC with HPV types 5, 8, 15, 17, 20, 24, 36, and 38 [115]. However, a study comparing HPV viral load and HPV mRNA expression in tumorous and normal tissues found no difference in HPV viral load between tumors from individuals with cSCC and healthy tissues, and HPV mRNA expression was not detected in tumorous tissues [116]. Nevertheless, HPV is not transcriptionally active in cSCC. HPV likely plays an important role in the pathogenesis of cSCC, during the onset of the disease, not during its progression [117]. In HIV-infected individuals, the development of cSCC depends on the number of CD4+ T cells and viral load. A 2017 study found that the risk of developing SCC increased by 222% in patients with a CD4+ T-cell count <200 cells/mL and a viral load $\geq 10{,}000$ copies/mL [107].

Medications also increase the risk of developing cSCC. We can examine drugs in three categories: immunosuppressive drugs, B-Raf proto-oncogene, serine/threonine kinase (BRAF) inhibitors, and photosensitive drugs. Several immunosuppressive agents increase the risk of KC through direct mutagenic effects, regardless of their immunosuppressive role [37]. Because of the increasing effect of azathioprine on UVA photosensitivity, the KC risk is increased by increased oxidative DNA damage [118]. In a large whole-exome sequencing study of 40 primary cSCCs from immunosuppressed and immunocompetent patients, a novel signature mutation (signature 32) associated with chronic exposure to azathioprine was identified in 27 of the tumor samples. The calcineurin inhibitor cyclosporine has a direct tumorigenic effect [119]. Cyclosporine has been observed to increase tumor growth in mice with severe combined immunodeficiency [120]. Another study showed that cyclosporine-mediated inhibition of calcineurin (and thus a nuclear factor of activated T cells) prevents p53-dependent cellular senescence [121]. Patients receiving BRAF inhibitors, targeted therapies for the treatment of melanoma, have been found to have an increased development of cSCC, approximately 15–30%. The mechanism of carcinogenesis for these inhibitors is likely to be those pre-existing mutations in RAS or RTK that lead to the proliferation of cancer cells, secondary to activation of the MAPK pathway [122]. cSCC has been associated with photosensitive drug use. Long-term treatment with voriconazole, an antifungal drug, leads to SCC development in immunocompromised patients, including children [123]. Phototoxic eruptions due to voriconazole have been documented in almost all patients who develop SCC [123, 124]. The use of thiazide, an antihypertensive drug among photosensitive drugs, and cSCC development should be discussed. Although, Gandini et al. [125] found no association between this treatment and SCC in their meta-analysis, Tang et al. [126] defined a possible association in their meta-analysis. In addition, treatments with PUVA are known to increase cSCC risk due to their mutagenic and immunosuppressive effects. The risk of SCC increases moderately in those receiving fewer than 150 PUVA treatment sessions, whereas the risk of SCC increases greatly in those receiving more than 350 treatment sessions [127]. Epidemiologic studies have yielded conflicting results regarding the role of smoking as a risk factor for SCC. A 2012 systematic review and meta-analysis found that smoking was associated with a 50% increased risk of SCC in never smokers [128]. In 2017, an Australian cohort study reported that the rate of SCC was twice as high in smokers compared with never smokers after adjusting for factors such as age, gender, education, skin color, tanning ability, number of freckles, childhood sunburn, and cumulative sun exposure [129]. Further studies are needed to investigate the effects of cigarette smoking on KC risk.

3.2 Inherited susceptibility to cSCC

A large cohort study in Sweden concluded that people whose siblings or parents had invasive cSCC had a two- to three-fold higher risk of receiving the same diagnosis [130]. Similar skin phenotypes, shared environmental exposures, and genetic factors may contribute to familial risk [131]. In a population-based study, after adjusting for phenotypic and environmental risk factors for cSCC, individuals with a family history of KC were found to have a 4-fold higher risk of cSCC [132]. The genetic syndromes associated with cSCC are summarized in **Table 2**. Epidermolysis bullosa syndromes (EBS) are a group of mechanobullous skin diseases characterized by bullae that occur with little or no trauma. EBS-associated SCCs usually develop over chronic wounds or scars, tend to be multiple and aggressive, and increase with age [133]. Oculocutaneous albinism (OCA) is a group of autosomal recessive melanin biosynthesis disorders characterized by generalized pigment reduction of the skin, eyes, and hair. Patients with OCA are at increased risk for early-onset skin cancers, most commonly SCC [134]. Epidermodysplasia verruciformis is a rare disease characterized by hypersensitivity to HPV strains 5 and 8 and SCC [135].

In 2016, three GWAS cSCC risk studies of European origin were published, identifying 16 genetic risk loci [136–138]. In the first GWAS study, 11 loci associated with cSCC risk were reported at the genome-wide significance level ($P < 5 \times 10^{-8}$). These included FOXP1, TPRG1/TP63, SLC45A2, IRF4, HLA-DQA1, BNC2/CNTLN,

Syndrome	Gene(s)	Gene function(s)
Epidermolysis bullosa	KRT5, KRT14, LAMB3, COL17A1, COL7A1, FERMT1 KIND1	Keratinization, collagen formation, cell junction organization, extracellular matrix organization
Fanconi anemia	BRAC1, BRAC2, BRIP1, ERCC4, FAAP20, FAN1, FANCA-FANCM, MAD2L2, PALB2, RAD51, RAD51C, SLX4, UBE2T, and XRCC2	Fanconi anemia pathway
Dyskeratosis congenita (Zinsser-Engman-Cole syndrome)	ACD, CTC1, DKC1, NHP2, NOP10, PARN, RTEL1, TERC, TERT, TINF2, and WRAP53	Telomere maintenance and trafficking
Multiple self-healing squamous epithelioma (Ferguson-Smith disease)	TGFBR1	TGF-β signal transduction
Huriez syndrome	Unknown	Unknown
Xeroderma pigmentosum	XPA-XPG, XPV, POLH	Nucleotide excision repair
Bloom snydrome	BLM (RECQL3)	Chromosomal stability
Werner syndrome	WRN (RECOL2), LMNA	Chromosomal stability
Rothmund-Thomson syndrome	RECOL4, C160rf57	Chromosomal stability and telomere maintenance and trafficking
Schöpf-Schultz-Passarge syndrome	WNT10A	WNT/β-catenin signaling pathway and cell proliferation and migration
Epidermodysplasia verruciformis (Lewandowsky-Lutz dysplasia)	TMC6 (EVER1), TMC8 (EVER2	Immune response and signal transduction in endoplasmic reticulum
Oculocutaneous albinism	TYR, OCA2, TYRP1, SLC45A2 (MATP), SLC24A5, C10orf11, 4q24	Melanin synthesis
Hermansky-Pudlak syndrome	HPS1-HPS8	Melanin synthesis

Table 2.
Genetic syndromes associated with inherited susceptibility to cSCC.

TYR, OCA2, HERC2, DEF8, and ASIP/RALY [136]. The second study focused on the DEF8 locus [138]. The third and most recent GWAS study determined SLC45A2, IRF4, BNC2/CNTLN, TYR, OCA2, HERC2, and ASIP/RALY, as well as the intergenic region on chromosome 2p22, AHR, SEC16A, CADM1, and MC1R [137]. As a result of these studies, cSCC-related nucleotide polymorphisms were identified in MC1R, ASIP/RALY, TYR, SLC45A2, and OCA2 genes, CADM1 in the metastasis suppressor gene, and AHR, a transcription factor regulating cell proliferation, in SEC16A'a gene associated with secretion and cellular proliferation [101]. SLC45A2, IRF4, TYR, HERC2, DEF8, and RALY identified for cSCC are known to be multiple risk loci near the pigmentation gene, supporting the role of lighter pigmentation and exposure to UV radiation in the developmental risk of cSCC [137]. The relationship between genetic variants in the FOXP1 and IRF4 regions is also associated with Notch signaling in cSCC [37].

3.3 Somatic mutations

Recent studies have shown that somatic mutations are much more common in cSCC than in other SCCs and melanomas [139]. cSCC has 5 times more mutations than other malignancies, such as lung mutations, and 4 times more mutations than melanomas [139, 140]. The accumulation of these mutations and other cellular alterations transforms the skin into cSCCs with an increased degree of dysplasia [94]. Most cSCCs carry a UV mutational signature with characteristic C > T or CC > TT dinucleotide mutations, although some may be passenger mutations also found in surrounding photoaged skin [141]. Genes altered in cSCC include mutations in UV-induced TP53, CDKN2A, NOTCH1, and NOTCH2, which are involved in cell cycle control, and in epigenetic regulators KMT2C, KMT2D, TET2, and TGF-β receptors, leading to their inactivation [101]. The most frequently altered tumor suppressor genes in cSCC are TP53, CDKN2A, NOTCH1, and NOTCH2. In addition, a network of dysregulated molecular signaling pathways, including EGFR signaling cascades affecting RAS/RAF/MEK/ERK and PI3K/AKT/mTOR signaling pathways, has been shown to play a critical role in the carcinogenesis of cSCC [75].

3.3.1 TP53, CDKN2A, NOTCH1, NOTCH2 molecular alterations

TP53 mutations occur in 54–95% of cSCC and often show a consistent C > T or CC > TT UV signature. Resistance to apoptosis and clonal growth in keratinocytes in the TP53 gene as a consequence of UV-mediated DNA damage [142, 143]. Variants in the TP53 gene frequently occur in AKs and precancerous lesions such as cSCC in situ and thus represent the first event of carcinogenesis. The CDKN2A gene encodes the alternatively spliced proteins p16INK4a and p14ARF. These proteins regulate cell cycle progression and are involved in retinoblastoma and proliferation by TP53, respectively. Loss of this locus with heterozygous or point mutations has been detected in 21–62% of cSCC patients [119, 139, 144–146]. Hypermethylation of the CDKN2A promoter was reported in 35–78% of patients [147].

NOTCH receptor mutations are an important tumor suppressor mechanism in cSCC and appear to play an important role in HRas proto-oncogene, GTPase (HRAS)-induced skin carcinogenesis [146]. The NOTCH family includes the single-pass transmembrane receptor. This receptor consists of an extracellular ligand-binding domain containing multiple EGF-like repeats (EGF-LR) and an intracellular domain that mediates transcription of the target gene. Loss of NOTCH signaling leads to impaired differentiation, increased stem cell activity, and the development and progression of cSCC [56, 139, 146]. NOTCH1 or NOTCH2 mutations have been identified in approximately 80 percent of cSCC and occur early in cSCC carcinogenesis [146, 148]. Activating HRAS mutations, NOTCH1 mutations, and CDKN2A mutations have been found in high frequency in cSCC from patients treated with BRAF inhibitors [146].

3.3.2 Overexpression of EGFR and MET tyrosine kinases receptors

The EGFR gene encodes the ErbB transmembrane glycoprotein receptor, which belongs to the tyrosine kinase receptor family. Ligand binding to EGFR causes the receptor to downregulate several signaling pathways such as MAPK/ERK and PI3K/AKT/mTOR. These signaling pathways control cell maturation, proliferation, inhibition of angiogenesis, and apoptosis [75]. The overall incidence of EGFR mutations in cSCC varies from 2.5 to 5% [144, 149, 150]. Overexpression of EGFR protein has been associated with poor prognosis and lymph node metastases in cSCC [151]. In recent studies, overexpression of this protein has been associated with a reduction in degradation and dephosphorylation mechanisms [152]. MET is a tyrosine kinase receptor that upregulates the RAS/RAF/MEK/ERK signaling pathway and its overexpression [75]. This signaling pathway has been shown to contribute to proliferation, invasion, migration, drug resistance, and angiogenesis in a variety of human tumors [153]. A recent study pointed out that treatment with capmatinib, a selective MET inhibitor, was able to prevent the upregulation of hepatocyte growth factor- stimulated EGFR protein, demonstrating the cooperation of MET and EGFR in cSCC carcinogenesis [154].

3.3.3 RAS-RAF-MEK-ERK pathway

RAS molecules are a family of GTP-binding proteins and are among the most frequently mutated genes in human cancers. RAS is an up-activator of the RAF/MEK/ERK1/ERK2 kinase pathway, and activating mutations in RAS promote SCC formation [155]. The active GTP-RAS complex promotes the formation of RAF dimers, which in turn activate the MEK-ERK cascade through phosphorylation. ERK interacts with multiple cytosolic targets and many nuclear substrates, including kinases, cytoskeletal proteins, and transcription factors. Signals for cell proliferation, differentiation, survival, migration, angiogenesis, and chromatin remodeling are triggered [75]. Recycling cycles are controlled by the MAPK cascade [156]. The MAPK pathway has been shown to play a role in cSCC development, and the MAPK inhibitor sorafenib has been associated with cSCC development in patients using BRAF inhibitors such as vemurafenib and dabrafenib [157, 158]. As for RAS genes, harbor activating RAS mutations (HRAS) are associated with cSCC. According to recent data, 21% of cSCC-associated somatic mutations were associated with HRAS [159].

Macrophage migration inhibitory factor (MIF) is a proinflammatory cytokine that contributes to cell proliferation by inducing ERK phosphorylation and MAPK pathway activation [160]. MIF also functions as a negative regulator of P53 [161]. MIF has been determined to be overexpressed in cSCC lesions compared to normal tissue [162]. In addition, ERK is involved in regulating the transcriptional activity of E-twenty-six 1 (ETS) 1 [163]. ETS-1 belongs to the family of ETS transcription factors, which are characterized by the presence of a conserved ETS DNA-binding domain. ETS-1 transcribes numerous target genes, including metalloprotease family members critical for extracellular matrix remodeling and angiogenesis, and regulates genes required for cell proliferation and survival [4]. ETS-1 has been detected to be immunohistochemically overexpressed in its poorly differentiated and metastatic form in SCC [164].

3.3.4 PI3K/AKT/mTOR pathway

The PI3K/AKT/mTOR pathway has common inputs and interacts with the MAPK pathway. Once activated, PI3K converts PIP2 to PIP3, which leads to activation of the serine/threonine kinase AKT, also known as protein kinase B, which in turn activates mTOR [75]. mTOR functions as a physiological sensor for nutrients and cell division and regulates growth by promoting RNA translation and protein synthesis [75, 165]. The PI3K/AKT/mTOR signaling cascade is negatively regulated by PTEN [166]. Activation of this signaling pathway results in SCC development and progression [167]. This condition is mainly controlled by loss of function of the PTEN gene or activation or amplification of mutations in the PIK3CA gene, which encodes the catalytic subunit of PI3K [75]. In the PI3K/AKT/mTOR pathway, molecular alterations of PTEN are observed in 7–25% of patients with cSCC due to inactivating mutations and resulting hyperactivation and homozygous loss [119, 145].

3.3.5 Telomerase pathway

Telomerase consists of reverse transcriptase (TERT) protein component encoded by the hTERT gene. The activation of the hTERT gene that occurs through promoter mutations has been shown to create de novo binding sites for the ETS transcription factors family, thus promoting telomerase expression and preventing senescence or apoptosis of cancer cells [75]. TERT promoter mutations were found in 31.6% of cSCC and are frequently associated with recurrent (OR = 6.75) and metastatic (OR = 15.89) lesions [75, 168].

3.4 Genetic polymorphisms

In cSCC, nearby loci, including the human leukocyte antigen locus at 6p21, and loci containing genes involved in germline pigmentation pathways with SNPs, GWAS studies identified an intronic SNP in non-pigment loci such as FOXP1 (3p13), an intergenic SNP at 3q28 near T63, an intergenic SNP at 9p22, and the SNP rs12203592 in IRF4 [136, 137, 169, 170]. In a study using 21 published SNPs based on GWAS, the risk attributable to the multilocus population was calculated to be 62%, suggesting that the risk for cSCC would be reduced by 62% if the effects of all risk alleles were removed from a population [171]. In the new GWAS meta-analysis conducted in 2020, eight new susceptibility loci for cSCC were discovered. These loci included genes involved in cancer progression (SETDB1: rs10399947, CASP8/ALS2CR12: rs10200279, WEE1: rs7939541), immune regulation (BACH2: rs10944479), keratinocyte differentiation (TRPS1:rs7834300, KRT5: rs11170164 and rs657187) and pigmentation: rs1325118) [170]. Another polymorphism that increases cSCC development is methylenetetrahydrofolate reductase polymorphisms related to the folate mechanism [172]. In a cohort of renal transplant recipients, the risk of developing cSCC was statistically significantly increased in those carrying the common MTHFR:C677T polymorphism in the folate pathway [173]. In a cohort of 694 transplant patients, cSCC was reported to develop earlier in these patients due to a polymorphism in the rs12203592 T allele of the gene encoding IRF4, which plays a role in the activation of melanin synthesis via tyrosinase [169]. Polymorphisms in thiopurine S-methyltransferase, which regulates azathioprine inactivation, have not been found to increase cSCC risk in studies [172].

3.5 Epigenetic modifications

Environmental factors can alter the epigenetic state of cells. Epigenetic changes include DNA methylation and histone modification (i.e., methylation, acetylation, phosphorylation, ubiquitination, and chromatin remodeling) [174]. A link between cSCC and gene-specific promoter hypermethylation has been established. Specifically, the CDKN2A gene is involved in positive cell cycle regulation, ASC is associated with apoptosis in G0S2 and the DAPK1 gene, and SFRPs and FRZBs are associated with Wnt signaling in the transcription factor and the adhesion molecules cadherin CDH1 and CDH13 [175–178]. PE-cadherin (CDH1) promoter hypermethylation was found in cSCC (85%), in situ cSCC (50%), AK (44%), and normal skin (22%). Downregulation of E-cadherin has been associated with increased tumor invasion, increased metastatic potential, and advanced stage of cSCC [178, 179]. Several enzyme families catalyze different types of histone modifications. The best known are the modifications, acetylation and methylation of H3 histones; it is H4 that directly alters chromatin condensation and gene transcription. Acetylation is catalyzed by histone acetyltransferases (HATs); histone deacetylases (HDACs) remove the acetyl group, allowing chromatin condensation and thus gene inactivation [95]. HAT up-regulation of p300 plays an important role in the development and progression of cSCC [180].

Methylation of the amino acids lysine and arginine occurs by histone methyltransferases, and the effect of the modification depends on which residue is modified. For example, trimethylation of histone H3 on lysine 4 (H3K4me3) activates transcription, whereas lysine 27 or lysine 9 on histone H3 represses transcription [181]. Polycomb group proteins (PcG) are an important family of histone modifiers that have been extensively studied in skin cancer. The PcG enzyme EZH2 is the primary histone methyltransferase and controls the proliferative potential of self-renewing keratinocytes by suppressing the CDK2A locus. EZH2 is frequently mutated in cancer and its overexpression is associated with cSCC progression [182–184]. Type 2 lysine methyltransferase, together with the enzymes KMT2C and KMT2D, forms a transcriptional core complex and provides histone H3 modification. Mutations in KMT2C and KMT2D have been found in both primary cSCC (36% and 31%, respectively) and metastatic tumors (43% and 62%, respectively) [185].

3.6 Tumor microenvironment

The tumor microenvironment, age-associated secretory phenotype, or SASP (i.e., cytokines, growth factors, and metalloproteinases) is a complex molecular system composed of a heterogeneous population of cells (tumor cells and adjacent stromal cells (fibroblasts, endothelial cells, inflammatory and immune cells) [95]. The TME plays an important role in the carcinogenesis of cSCC. The newly developing neoplastic keratinocytes of cSCC interact with other stromal cell types. It interacts with the local microenvironment and regulates the cell-cell relationship by acting as a tumor promoter and via epigenetic reprogramming, DNA damage, promotion of hypoxia, angiogenesis, activation of cancer-associated fibroblasts (CAFs), recruitment of regulatory immune cells, and inhibition of antitumor immune surveillance [97, 186, 187]. Organotypic culture studies have shown that the epidermal component formed by epidermal hyperplasia of aged epidermal keratinocytes requires the presence of CAF to penetrate the matrix [188].

Human leukocyte antigen variants and the programmed cell death protein 1/ programmed cell death ligand-1 axis (PD-1/PD-L1) also play a role in the tumor microenvironment [189, 190]. Expression of PD-L1 is also involved in primary cSCC. PD-L1 has been detected in approximately 26% of primary cSCC and 50% of metastatic lesions [101]. In cSCC, p63 regulates the transcriptional expression of the proinflammatory cytokines IL -1, IL -6, IL −8, tumor-associated angiogenesis, and lymphangiogenesis by altering the expression of human beta-defensins. All these findings suggest that p63 contributes globally to cSCC development by regulating the tumoral environment [191–193].

4. Conclusion

In conclusion, the development and progression of BCC and cSCC are associated with various alterations such as genetic mutations, epigenetic modifications, viral infections, or microenvironmental changes that affect epidermal hemostasis. Future studies will better explain the etiopathogenesis of BCC and cSCC, and thus contribute to the development of disease prevention and targeted therapies.

Abbreviations

AHR	aryl hydrocarbon receptor
AKT	serine/threonine-protein kinase
ARID1A	AT rich interactive domain 1A
ASC	apoptosis-associated speck-like protein containing a CARD

BNC2	basonuclin 2
CADM1	cell adhesion molecule 1
CASP8	caspase-8
CDKN2A	cyclin dependent kinase inhibitor 2A
C-MYC	transcriptional regulator Myc-like
CNTLN	centlein
CSMD1	CUB and Sushi multiple domains 1
DAPK1	death-associated protein kinase 1
DEF8	differentially expressed in FDCP 8
EXOC2	exocyst complex component 2
EZH2	enhancer of zeste 2 polycomb repressive complex 2 subunit
FBXW7	F-box and WD repeat domain containing 7
FOXP1	forkhead box P1
FRZB	frizzled-related protein
GRIN2A	glutamate ionotropic receptor NMDA type subunit 2A
HERC2	HECT and RLD domain containing E3 ubiquitin protein ligase 2
HES	hairy/enhancer of split
HEY	HES-related genes such as hairy/enhancer of split related with YRPW motif
HLA-DQA1	major histocompatibility complex, class II, DQ alpha 1
IRF4	interferon regulatory factor 4
IRF6	interferon regulatory factor 6
KMT2C	lysine methyltransferase 2C
KMT2D	lysine methyltransferase 2D
KRAS	KRAS proto-oncogene, GTPase
LATS1	large tumor suppressor kinase 1
LPP	LIM domain containing preferred translocation partner in lipoma
MC1R	melanocortin 1 receptor
MET	MET proto-oncogene, receptor tyrosine kinase
MUS81	MUS81 structure-specific endonuclease subunit
NABP2	nucleic acid binding protein 2
NOTCH1	Notch receptor 1
NOTCH2	Notch receptor 2
NRAS	NRAS proto-oncogene, GTPase
PI3K/AKT/Mtor	phosphatidylinositol 3-kinase/serine/threonine-specific protein kinases/mammalian target of rapamycin
PI3K	phosphatidylinositol 3-kinase
PIK3CA	phosphatidylinositol-4,5-bisphosphate 3-kinase catalytic subunit alpha
PIP2	phosphatidylinositol (4,5)-bisphosphate
PIP3	phosphatidylinositol (3,4,5)-trisphosphate
PKA	cAMP dependent protein kinase
PKC-α	protein kinase C-alpha
PKC-δ	protein kinase C-delta
PREX2	phosphatidylinositol-3,4,5-trisphosphate-dependent Rac exchange factor 2
RALY	RALY heterogeneous nuclear ribonucleoprotein
RAS/RAF/MEK/ERK	Ras/Raf/mitogen-activated protein kinase/extracellular-signal-regulated kinase (ERK)
RTK	receptor tyrosine kinase

SEC16A	SEC16 homolog A, endoplasmic reticulum export factor
SFRP	secreted frizzled-related protein
SLC45A2	solute carrier family 45, member 2
TBX1	T-box transcription factor 1
TET2	tet methylcytosine dioxygenase 2
TGF-β	transforming growth factor beta
TNF-α	tumor necrosis factor alpha
TPRG1	tumor protein p63 regulated 1
UBAC2	UBA domain containing 2
WNT/β-catenin	wingless signaling transduction beta catenin
XPA	Xeroderma pigmentosum complementation group A (XPA, DNA damage recognition and repair factor)

Author details

Yildiz Gürsel Ürün
Faculty of Medicine, Department of Dermatology, Trakya University, Edirne, Turkey

*Address all correspondence to: ygurselu@gmail.com

References

[1] LeBoit P, Burg G, Weedon D, Sarasin A. WHO Classification of Tumours. Pathology and Genetics. Skin Tumours. 1st ed. Lyon: IARC Press; 2006

[2] Cameron MC, Lee E, Hibler BP, Barker CA, Mori S, Cordova M, et al. Basal cell carcinoma: Epidemiology; pathophysiology; clinical and histological subtypes; and disease associations. Journal of the American Academy of Dermatology. 2019;**80**(2):303-317

[3] Belbasis L, Stefanaki I, Stratigos AJ, Evangelou E. Non-genetic risk factors for cutaneous melanoma and keratinocyte skin cancers: An umbrella review of meta-analyses. Journal of Dermatological Science. 2016;**84**(3): 330-339

[4] Nagarajan P, Parikh N, Garrett-Sinha LA, Sinha S. Ets1 induces dysplastic changes when expressed in terminally-differentiating squamous epidermal cells. PLoS One. 2009;**4**(1): e4179

[5] Kartal SP, Bayramgürler D. Pathogenesis of basal cell carcinoma. Güncel Dermatoloji Dergisi. 2016;**1**(1): 18-23

[6] Lomas A, Leonardi-Bee J, Bath-Hextall F. A systematic review of worldwide incidence of nonmelanoma skin cancer. The British Journal of Dermatology. 2012;**166**(5): 1069-1080

[7] Kim DP, Kus KJB, Ruiz E. Basal cell carcinoma review. Hematology/Oncology Clinics of North America. 2019;**33**(1):13-24

[8] Lai V, Cranwell W, Sinclair R. Epidemiology of skin cancer in the mature patient. Clinics in Dermatology. 2018;**36**(2):167-176

[9] Staples MP, Elwood M, Burton RC, Williams JL, Marks R, Giles GG. Non-melanoma skin cancer in Australia: The 2002 national survey and trends since 1985. The Medical Journal of Australia. 2006;**184**(1):6-10

[10] Holm AS, Nissen CV, Wulf HC. Basal cell carcinoma is as common as the sum of all other cancers: Implications for treatment capacity. Acta Dermato-Venereologica. 2016;**96**(4):505-509

[11] Mudigonda T, Pearce DJ, Yentzer BA, Williford P, Feldman SR. The economic impact of non-melanoma skin cancer: A review. Journal of the National Comprehensive Cancer Network. 2010;**8**(8):888-896

[12] Asgari MM, Moffet HH, Ray GT, Quesenberry CP. Trends in basal cell carcinoma incidence and identification of high-risk subgroups, 1998-2012. JAMA Dermatology. 2015;**151**(9): 976-981

[13] Peris K, Fargnoli MC, Garbe C, Kaufmann R, Bastholt L, Seguin NB, et al. Diagnosis and treatment of basal cell carcinoma: European consensus-based interdisciplinary guidelines. European Journal of Cancer. 2019;**118**:10-34

[14] Elder D, Massi D, Scolyer R, Willemze R. Keratinocytic/epidermal tumours. World Health Organization (WHO) Classification of Skin Tumours. 2018;**11**:23-64

[15] Fania L, Didona D, Morese R, Campana I, Coco V, Di Pietro FR, et al. Basal cell carcinoma: From pathophysiology to novel therapeutic approaches. Biomedicines. 2020;**8**(11):449

[16] Adolphe C, Xue A, Fard AT, Genovesi LA, Yang J, Wainwright BJ. Genetic and functional interaction network analysis reveals global

enrichment of regulatory T cell genes influencing basal cell carcinoma susceptibility. Genome Medicine. 2021;**13**(1):19

[17] Lang BM, Balermpas P, Bauer A, Blum A, Brölsch GF, Dirschka T, et al. S2k guidelines for cutaneous basal cell carcinoma—Part 1: Epidemiology, genetics and diagnosis. Journal der Deutschen Dermatologischen Gesellschaft. 2019;**17**(1):94-103

[18] Atwood SX, Sarin KY, Whitson RJ, Li JR, Kim G, Rezaee M, et al. Smoothened variants explain the majority of drug resistance in basal cell carcinoma. Cancer Cell. 2015;**27**(3): 342-353

[19] Sharpe HJ, Pau G, Dijkgraaf GJ, Basset-Seguin N, Modrusan Z, Januario T, et al. Genomic analysis of smoothened inhibitor resistance in basal cell carcinoma. Cancer Cell. 2015;**27**(3):327-341

[20] Pellegrini C, Maturo MG, Di Nardo L, Ciciarelli V, Gutiérrez García-Rodrigo C, Fargnoli MC. Understanding the molecular genetics of basal cell carcinoma. International Journal Molecular Sciences. 2017;**18**(11):2485

[21] Zanetti R, Rosso S, Martinez C, Nieto A, Miranda A, Mercier M, et al. Comparison of risk patterns in carcinoma and melanoma of the skin in men: A multi-Centre case-case-control study. British Journal of Cancer. 2006;**94**(5):743-751

[22] Jayaraman SS, Rayhan DJ, Hazany S, Kolodney MS. Mutational landscape of basal cell carcinomas by whole-exome sequencing. The Journal of Investigative Dermatology. 2014;**134**(1):213-220

[23] Nehal KS, Bichakjian CK. Update on keratinocyte carcinomas. The New England Journal of Medicine. 2018;**379**(4):363-374

[24] Boyd AS, Shyr Y, King LE Jr. Basal cell carcinoma in young women: An evaluation of the association of tanning bed use and smoking. Journal of the American Academy of Dermatology. 2002;**46**(5):706-709

[25] Bassukas ID, Tatsioni A. Male sex is an inherent risk factor for basal cell carcinoma. Journal of Skin Cancer. 2019;**2019**:8304271

[26] Marcil I, Stern RS. Risk of developing a subsequent nonmelanoma skin cancer in patients with a history of nonmelanoma skin cancer: A critical review of the literature and meta-analysis. Archives of Dermatology. 2000;**136**(12):1524-1530

[27] Wehner MR, Linos E, Parvataneni R, Stuart SE, Boscardin WJ, Chren MM. Timing of subsequent new tumors in patients who present with basal cell carcinoma or cutaneous squamous cell carcinoma. JAMA Dermatology. 2015;**151**(4):382-388

[28] Schmidt SA, Schmidt M, Mehnert F, Lemeshow S, Sørensen HT. Use of antihypertensive drugs and risk of skin cancer. Journal of the European Academy of Dermatology and Venereology. 2015;**29**(8):1545-1554

[29] Gallagher RP, Hill GB, Bajdik CD, Fincham S, Coldman AJ, McLean DI, et al. Sunlight exposure, pigmentary factors, and risk of nonmelanocytic skin cancer. I. Basal cell carcinoma. Archives of Dermatology. 1995;**131**(2):157-163

[30] Cassano N, Di Stefani A, Vena GA, Peris K. Antihypertensive drugs and risk of skin cancer. Giornale Italiano di Dermatologia e Venereologia. 2018;**153**(5):672-684

[31] Ruiter R, Visser LE, Eijgelsheim M, Rodenburg EM, Hofman A, Coebergh JW, et al. High-ceiling diuretics are associated with an increased risk of basal cell carcinoma in a population-based follow-up study.

European Journal of Cancer. 2010;**46**(13):2467-2472

[32] Marzuka AG, Book SE. Basal cell carcinoma: Pathogenesis, epidemiology, clinical features, diagnosis, histopathology, and management. The Yale Journal of Biology and Medicine. 2015;**88**(2):167-179

[33] Gunes A, Akarsu S. Bazoselüler karsinom. Turkiye Klinikleri J Dermatol-Special Topics. 2013;**6**:1-10

[34] Bauer A, Diepgen TL, Schmitt J. Is occupational solar ultraviolet irradiation a relevant risk factor for basal cell carcinoma? A systematic review and meta-analysis of the epidemiological literature. The British Journal of Dermatology. 2011;**165**(3):612-625

[35] Li C, Athar M. Ionizing radiation exposure and basal cell carcinoma pathogenesis. Radiation Research. 2016;**185**(3):217-228

[36] Karagas MR, McDonald JA, Greenberg ER, Stukel TA, Weiss JE, Baron JA, et al. Risk of basal cell and squamous cell skin cancers after ionizing radiation therapy. For the skin Cancer prevention study group. Journal of the National Cancer Institute. 1996;**88**(24):1848-1853

[37] Choquet H, Ashrafzadeh S, Kim Y, Asgari MM, Jorgenson E. Genetic and environmental factors underlying keratinocyte carcinoma risk. JCI Insight. 2020;**5**(10):e134783

[38] Ge T, Chen C-Y, Neale BM, Sabuncu MR, Smoller JW. Phenome-wide heritability analysis of the UK biobank. PLoS genetics. 2017;**13**(4): e1006711

[39] Kiran NK, Tilak Raj TN, Mukunda KS, Rajashekar RV. Nevoid basal cell carcinoma syndrome (Gorlin-Goltz syndrome). Contemporary Clinical Dentistry. 2012;**3**(4):514-518

[40] Smith MJ, Beetz C, Williams SG, Bhaskar SS, O'Sullivan J, Anderson B, et al. Germline mutations in SUFU cause Gorlin syndrome-associated childhood medulloblastoma and redefine the risk associated with PTCH1 mutations. Journal of Clinical Oncology. 2014;**32**(36):4155-4161

[41] Kilgour JM, Jia JL, Sarin KY. Review of the molecular genetics of rasal cell carcinoma; Inherited susceptibility, somatic mutations, and targeted therapeutics. Cancers (Basel). 2021;**13**(15):3870

[42] Akbari M, Chen H, Guo G, Legan Z, Ghali G. Basal cell nevus syndrome (Gorlin syndrome): Genetic insights, diagnostic challenges, and unmet milestones. Pathophysiology. 2018;**25**(2):77-82

[43] Evans DG, Oudit D, Smith MJ, Rutkowski D, Allan E, Newman WG, et al. First evidence of genotype-phenotype correlations in Gorlin syndrome. Journal of Medical Genetics. 2017;**54**(8):530-536

[44] Torrelo A, Sprecher E, Mediero IG, Bergman R, Zambrano A. What syndrome is this? Bazex-Dupre-Christol syndrome. Pediatr Dermatol. 2006;**23**(3):286-290

[45] Bal E, Park H-S, Belaid-Choucair Z, Kayserili H, Naville M, Madrange M, et al. Mutations in ACTRT1 and its enhancer RNA elements lead to aberrant activation of hedgehog signaling in inherited and sporadic basal cell carcinomas. Nature medicine. 2017;**23**(10):1226-1233

[46] Black JO. Xeroderma Pigmentosum. Head and Neck Pathology. 2016;**10**(2):139-144

[47] Bradford PT, Goldstein AM, Tamura D, Khan SG, Ueda T, Boyle J, et al. Cancer and neurologic degeneration

in xeroderma pigmentosum: Long term follow-up characterises the role of DNA repair. Journal of Medical Genetics. 2011;**48**(3):168-176

[48] van Dam RM, Huang Z, Rimm EB, Weinstock MA, Spiegelman D, Colditz GA, et al. Risk factors for basal cell carcinoma of the skin in men: Results from the health professionals follow-up study. American Journal of Epidemiology. 1999;**150**(5):459-468

[49] Gudbjartsson DF, Sulem P, Stacey SN, Goldstein AM, Rafnar T, Sigurgeirsson B, et al. ASIP and TYR pigmentation variants associate with cutaneous melanoma and basal cell carcinoma. Nature Genetics. 2008;**40**(7):886-891

[50] Box NF, Duffy DL, Irving RE, Russell A, Chen W, Griffyths LR, et al. Melanocortin-1 receptor genotype is a risk factor for basal and squamous cell carcinoma. The Journal of Investigative Dermatology. 2001;**116**(2):224-229

[51] Han J, Kraft P, Colditz GA, Wong J, Hunter DJ. Melanocortin 1 receptor variants and skin cancer risk. International Journal of Cancer. 2006;**119**(8):1976-1984

[52] Chahal HS, Wu W, Ransohoff KJ, Yang L, Hedlin H, Desai M, et al. Genome-wide association study identifies 14 novel risk alleles associated with basal cell carcinoma. Nature Communications. 2016;7:12510

[53] Stacey SN, Sulem P, Jonasdottir A, Masson G, Gudmundsson J, Gudbjartsson DF, et al. A germline variant in the TP53 polyadenylation signal confers cancer susceptibility. Nature Genetics. 2011;**43**(11):1098-1103

[54] Stacey SN, Sulem P, Masson G, Gudjonsson SA, Thorleifsson G, Jakobsdottir M, et al. New common variants affecting susceptibility to basal cell carcinoma. Nature Genetics. 2009;**41**(8):909-914

[55] Nowell C, Radtke F. Cutaneous Notch signaling in health and disease. Cold Spring Harbor Perspectives in Medicine. 2013;**3**(12):a017772

[56] Nowell CS, Radtke F. Notch as a tumour suppressor. Nature Reviews. Cancer. 2017;**17**(3):145-159

[57] Vargas-Rondón N, Villegas VE, Rondón-Lagos M. The role of chromosomal instability in cancer and therapeutic responses. Cancers (Basel). 2017;**10**(1):4

[58] Lin Y, Chahal HS, Wu W, Cho HG, Ransohoff KJ, Song F, et al. Association study of genetic variation in DNA repair pathway genes and risk of basal cell carcinoma. International Journal of Cancer. 2017;**141**(5):952-957

[59] Welsh MM, Applebaum KM, Spencer SK, Perry AE, Karagas MR, Nelson HH. CTLA4 variants, UV-induced tolerance, and risk of non-melanoma skin cancer. Cancer Research. 2009;**69**(15):6158-6163

[60] Ramachandran S, Fryer AA, Smith A, Lear J, Bowers B, Jones PW, et al. Cutaneous basal cell carcinomas: Distinct host factors are associated with the development of tumors on the trunk and on the head and neck. Cancer. 2001;**92**(2):354-358

[61] Caro I, Low JA. The role of the hedgehog signaling pathway in the development of basal cell carcinoma and opportunities for treatment. Clinical Cancer Research. 2010;**16**(13):3335-3339

[62] Briscoe J, Thérond PP. The mechanisms of Hedgehog signalling and its roles in development and disease. Nature Reviews. Molecular Cell Biology. 2013;**14**(7):416-429

[63] Ruiz i Altaba A, Sánchez P, Dahmane N. Gli and hedgehog in cancer: Tumours, embryos and stem cells. Nature Reviews. Cancer. 2002;**2**(5):361-372

[64] Katoh Y, Katoh M. Hedgehog target genes: Mechanisms of carcinogenesis induced by aberrant hedgehog signaling activation. Current Molecular Medicine. 2009;**9**(7):873-886

[65] Athar M, Tang X, Lee JL, Kopelovich L, Kim AL. Hedgehog signalling in skin development and cancer. Experimental Dermatology. 2006;**15**(9):667-677

[66] Pietrobono S, Gagliardi S, Stecca B. Non-canonical hedgehog signaling pathway in cancer: Activation of GLI transcription factors beyond smoothened. Frontiers in Genetics. 2019;**10**:556

[67] Aubrey BJ, Strasser A, Kelly GL. Tumor-suppressor functions of the TP53 pathway. Cold Spring Harbor Perspectives in Medicine. 2016;**6**(5):a026062

[68] Wang GY, Wang J, Mancianti ML, Epstein EH Jr. Basal cell carcinomas arise from hair follicle stem cells in Ptch1(+/−) mice. Cancer Cell. 2011;**19**(1):114-124

[69] Zhao B, Li L, Lei Q, Guan KL. The hippo-YAP pathway in organ size control and tumorigenesis: An updated version. Genes & Development. 2010;**24**(9): 862-874

[70] Zhang H, Pasolli HA, Fuchs E. Yes-associated protein (YAP) transcriptional coactivator functions in balancing growth and differentiation in skin. Proceedings of the National Academy of Sciences of the United States of America. 2011;**108**(6):2270-2275

[71] Schlegelmilch K, Mohseni M, Kirak O, Pruszak J, Rodriguez JR, Zhou D, et al. Yap1 acts downstream of α-catenin to control epidermal proliferation. Cell. 2011;**144**(5):782-795

[72] Bonilla X, Parmentier L, King B, Bezrukov F, Kaya G, Zoete V, et al. Genomic analysis identifies new drivers and progression pathways in skin basal cell carcinoma. Nature Genetics. 2016;**48**(4):398-406

[73] Hatton BA, Knoepfler PS, Kenney AM, Rowitch DH, de Alborán IM, Olson JM, et al. N-myc is an essential downstream effector of Shh signaling during both normal and neoplastic cerebellar growth. Cancer Research. 2006;**66**(17):8655-8661

[74] Welcker M, Orian A, Jin J, Grim JE, Harper JW, Eisenman RN, et al. The Fbw7 tumor suppressor regulates glycogen synthase kinase 3 phosphorylation-dependent c-Myc protein degradation. Proceedings of the National Academy of Sciences of the United States of America. 2004;**101**(24):9085-9090

[75] Di Nardo L, Pellegrini C, Di Stefani A, Del Regno L, Sollena P, Piccerillo A, et al. Molecular genetics of cutaneous squamous cell carcinoma: Perspective for treatment strategies. Journal of the European Academy of Dermatology and Venereology. 2020;**34**(5):932-941

[76] Rachakonda PS, Hosen I, de Verdier PJ, Fallah M, Heidenreich B, Ryk C, et al. TERT promoter mutations in bladder cancer affect patient survival and disease recurrence through modification by a common polymorphism. Proceedings of the National Academy of Sciences of the United States of America. 2013;**110**(43): 17426-17431

[77] Wang L, Shi Y, Ju P, Liu R, Yeo SP, Xia Y, et al. Silencing of diphthamide synthesis 3 (Dph3) reduces metastasis of murine melanoma. PLoS One. 2012;**7**(11):e49988

[78] Denisova E, Heidenreich B, Nagore E, Rachakonda PS, Hosen I, Akrap I, et al. Frequent DPH3 promoter mutations in skin cancers. Oncotarget. 2015;**6**(34):35922-35930

[79] Heffelfinger C, Ouyang Z, Engberg A, Leffell DJ, Hanlon AM, Gordon PB, et al. Correlation of global microRNA expression with basal cell carcinoma subtype. G3 (Bethesda). 2012;**2**(2):279-286

[80] Sonkoly E, Lovén J, Xu N, Meisgen F, Wei T, Brodin P, et al. MicroRNA-203 functions as a tumor suppressor in basal cell carcinoma. Oncogene. 2012;**1**(3):e3

[81] Sun H, Jiang P. MicroRNA-451a acts as tumor suppressor in cutaneous basal cell carcinoma. Molecular Genetics & Genomic Medicine. 2018;**6**(6):1001-1009

[82] Sand M, Skrygan M, Sand D, Georgas D, Hahn SA, Gambichler T, et al. Expression of microRNAs in basal cell carcinoma. The British Journal of Dermatology. 2012;**167**(4):847-855

[83] Sand M, Bechara FG, Sand D, Gambichler T, Hahn SA, Bromba M, et al. Long-noncoding RNAs in basal cell carcinoma. Tumour Biology. 2016;**37**(8):10595-10608

[84] Bertheim U, Hofer PA, Engström-Laurent A, Hellström S. The stromal reaction in basal cell carcinomas. A prerequisite for tumour progression and treatment strategy. British Journal of Plastic Surgery. 2004;**57**(5):429-439

[85] Kaur P, Mulvaney M, Carlson JA. Basal cell carcinoma progression correlates with host immune response and stromal alterations: A histologic analysis. The American Journal of Dermatopathology. 2006;**28**(4):293-307

[86] Lefrançois P, Xie P, Gunn S, Gantchev J, Villarreal AM, Sasseville D, et al. In silico analyses of the tumor microenvironment highlight tumoral inflammation, a Th2 cytokine shift and a mesenchymal stem cell-like phenotype in advanced in basal cell carcinomas. Journal of Cell Communication and Signaling. 2020;**14**(2):245-254

[87] Omland SH, Hamrouni A, Gniadecki R. High diversity of the T-cell receptor repertoire of tumor-infiltrating lymphocytes in basal cell carcinoma. Experimental Dermatology. 2017;**26**(5): 454-456

[88] Katoh M. Genomic testing, tumor microenvironment and targeted therapy of Hedgehog-related human cancers. Clinical Science (London, England). 2019;**133**(8):953-970

[89] Lubov J, Labbé M, Sioufi K, Morand GB, Hier MP, Khanna M, et al. Prognostic factors of head and neck cutaneous squamous cell carcinoma: A systematic review. Journal of Otolaryngology - Head & Neck Surgery. 2021;**50**(1):54

[90] Muzic JG, Schmitt AR, Wright AC, Alniemi DT, Zubair AS, Olazagasti Lourido JM, et al. Incidence and trends of basal cell carcinoma and cutaneous squamous cell carcinoma: A population-based study in Olmsted County, Minnesota, 2000 to 2010. Mayo Clinic Proceedings. 2017;**92**(6):890-898

[91] Venables ZC, Nijsten T, Wong KF, Autier P, Broggio J, Deas A, et al. Epidemiology of basal and cutaneous squamous cell carcinoma in the U.K. 2013-15: A cohort study. The British Journal of Dermatology. 2019;**181**(3): 474-482

[92] Marks R. The epidemiology of non-melanoma skin cancer: Who, why and what can we do about it. The Journal of Dermatology. 1995;**22**(11): 853-857

[93] Hacker SM, Flowers FP. Squamous cell carcinoma of the skin. Will heightened awareness of risk factors slow its increase? Postgraduate Medicine. 1993;**93**(8):115-121, 25-6

[94] Que SKT, Zwald FO, Schmults CD. Cutaneous squamous cell carcinoma: Incidence, risk factors, diagnosis, and

staging. Journal of the American Academy of Dermatology. 2018;**78**(2): 237-247

[95] Fania L, Didona D, Di Pietro FR, Verkhovskaia S, Morese R, Paolino G, et al. Cutaneous squamous cell carcinoma: from pathophysiology to novel therapeutic approaches. Biomedicines. 2021;**9**(2):171

[96] Martincorena I, Roshan A, Gerstung M, Ellis P, Van Loo P, McLaren S, et al. Tumor evolution. High burden and pervasive positive selection of somatic mutations in normal human skin. Science. 2015;**348**(6237):880-886

[97] Nissinen L, Farshchian M, Riihilä P, Kähäri VM. New perspectives on role of tumor microenvironment in progression of cutaneous squamous cell carcinoma. Cell and Tissue Research. 2016;**365**(3):691-702

[98] Burton KA, Ashack KA, Khachemoune A. Cutaneous squamous cell carcinoma: A review of high-risk and metastatic disease. American Journal of Clinical Dermatology. 2016;**17**(5):491-508

[99] Paolino G, Donati M, Didona D, Mercuri SR, Cantisani C. Histology of non-melanoma skin cancers: An update. Biomedicines. 2017;**5**(4):71

[100] Kim JYS, Kozlow JH, Mittal B, Moyer J, Olenecki T, Rodgers P. Guidelines of care for the management of cutaneous squamous cell carcinoma. Journal of the American Academy of Dermatology. 2018;**78**(3):560-578

[101] Stratigos AJ, Garbe C, Dessinioti C, Lebbe C, Bataille V, Bastholt L, et al. European interdisciplinary guideline on invasive squamous cell carcinoma of the skin: Part 1. Epidemiology, diagnostics and prevention. European Journal of Cancer. 2020;**128**:60-82

[102] Vitasa BC, Taylor HR, Strickland PT, Rosenthal FS, West S, Abbey H, et al. Association of nonmelanoma skin cancer and actinic keratosis with cumulative solar ultraviolet exposure in Maryland watermen. Cancer. 1990;**65**(12): 2811-2817

[103] Armstrong BK, Kricker A. The epidemiology of UV induced skin cancer. Journal of Photochemistry and Photobiology. B. 2001;**63**(1-3):8-18

[104] Lichter MD, Karagas MR, Mott LA, Spencer SK, Stukel TA, Greenberg ER. Therapeutic ionizing radiation and the incidence of basal cell carcinoma and squamous cell carcinoma. The New Hampshire Skin Cancer Study Group. Archives of Dermatology. 2000;**136**(8): 1007-1011

[105] Onajin O, Brewer JD. Skin cancer in patients with chronic lymphocytic leukemia and non-Hodgkin lymphoma. Clinical Advances in Hematology & Oncology. 2012;**10**(9):571-576

[106] Mehrany K, Weenig RH, Lee KK, Pittelkow MR, Otley CC. Increased metastasis and mortality from cutaneous squamous cell carcinoma in patients with chronic lymphocytic leukemia. Journal of the American Academy of Dermatology. 2005;**53**(6): 1067-1071

[107] Asgari MM, Ray GT, Quesenberry CP Jr, Katz KA, Silverberg MJ. Association of multiple primary skin cancers with human immunodeficiency virus infection, CD4 count, and viral load. JAMA Dermatology. 2017;**153**(9): 892-896

[108] Krynitz B, Edgren G, Lindelöf B, Baecklund E, Brattström C, Wilczek H, et al. Risk of skin cancer and other malignancies in kidney, liver, heart and lung transplant recipients 1970 to 2008—A Swedish population-based study. International Journal of Cancer. 2013;**132**(6):1429-1438

[109] Harwood CA, Toland AE, Proby CM, Euvrard S, Hofbauer GFL, Tommasino M, et al. The pathogenesis of cutaneous squamous cell carcinoma in organ transplant recipients. The British Journal of Dermatology. 2017;**177**(5):1217-1224

[110] Walter A, Barysch MJ, Behnke S, Dziunycz P, Schmid B, Ritter E, et al. Cancer-testis antigens and immunosurveillance in human cutaneous squamous cell and basal cell carcinomas. Clinical Cancer Research. 2010;**16**(14):3562-3570

[111] Velez NF, Karia PS, Vartanov AR, Davids MS, Brown JR, Schmults CD. Association of advanced leukemic stage and skin cancer tumor stage with poor skin cancer outcomes in patients with chronic lymphocytic leukemia. JAMA Dermatology. 2014;**150**(3):280-287

[112] Jellouli-Elloumi A, Kochbati L, Dhraief S, Ben Romdhane K, Maalej M. Cancers arising from burn scars: 62 cases. Annales de Dermatologie et de Vénéréologie. 2003;**130**(4):413-416

[113] Tang L, Wang K. Chronic inflammation in skin malignancies. Journal of Molecular Signaling. 2016;**11**:2

[114] Asgari MM, Kiviat NB, Critchlow CW, Stern JE, Argenyi ZB, Raugi GJ, et al. Detection of human papillomavirus DNA in cutaneous squamous cell carcinoma among immunocompetent individuals. The Journal of Investigative Dermatology. 2008;**128**(6):1409-1417

[115] Chahoud J, Semaan A, Chen Y, Cao M, Rieber AG, Rady P, et al. Association between β-genus human papillomavirus and cutaneous squamous cell carcinoma in immunocompetent individuals—A meta-analysis. JAMA Dermatology. 2016;**152**(12):1354-1364

[116] Arron ST, Ruby JG, Dybbro E, Ganem D, Derisi JL. Transcriptome sequencing demonstrates that human papillomavirus is not active in cutaneous squamous cell carcinoma. The Journal of Investigative Dermatology. 2011;**131**(8):1745-1753

[117] Aldabagh B, Angeles JG, Cardones AR, Arron ST. Cutaneous squamous cell carcinoma and human papillomavirus: Is there an association? Dermatologic Surgery. 2013;**39**(1 Pt 1): 1-23

[118] O'Donovan P, Perrett CM, Zhang X, Montaner B, Xu YZ, Harwood CA, et al. Azathioprine and UVA light generate mutagenic oxidative DNA damage. Science. 2005;**309**(5742): 1871-1874

[119] Inman GJ, Wang J, Nagano A, Alexandrov LB, Purdie KJ, Taylor RG, et al. The genomic landscape of cutaneous SCC reveals drivers and a novel azathioprine associated mutational signature. Nature Communications. 2018;**9**(1):3667

[120] Hojo M, Morimoto T, Maluccio M, Asano T, Morimoto K, Lagman M, et al. Cyclosporine induces cancer progression by a cell-autonomous mechanism. Nature. 1999;**397**(6719):530-534

[121] Wu X, Nguyen BC, Dziunycz P, Chang S, Brooks Y, Lefort K, et al. Opposing roles for calcineurin and ATF3 in squamous skin cancer. Nature. 2010;**465**(7296):368-372

[122] Su F, Viros A, Milagre C, Trunzer K, Bollag G, Spleiss O, et al. RAS mutations in cutaneous squamous-cell carcinomas in patients treated with BRAF inhibitors. The New England Journal of Medicine. 2012;**366**(3): 207-215

[123] Cowen EW, Nguyen JC, Miller DD, McShane D, Arron ST, Prose NS, et al. Chronic phototoxicity and aggressive

squamous cell carcinoma of the skin in children and adults during treatment with voriconazole. Journal of the American Academy of Dermatology. 2010;**62**(1):31-37

[124] McCarthy KL, Playford EG, Looke DF, Whitby M. Severe photosensitivity causing multifocal squamous cell carcinomas secondary to prolonged voriconazole therapy. Clinical Infectious Diseases. 2007;**44**(5):e55-e56

[125] Gandini S, Palli D, Spadola G, Bendinelli B, Cocorocchio E, Stanganelli I, et al. Anti-hypertensive drugs and skin cancer risk: A review of the literature and meta-analysis. Critical Reviews in Oncology/Hematology. 2018;**122**:1-9

[126] Tang H, Fu S, Zhai S, Song Y, Asgari MM, Han J. Use of antihypertensive drugs and risk of keratinocyte carcinoma: A meta-analysis of observational studies. Pharmacoepidemiology and Drug Safety. 2018;**27**(3):279-288

[127] Stern RS. The risk of squamous cell and basal cell cancer associated with psoralen and ultraviolet a therapy: A 30-year prospective study. Journal of the American Academy of Dermatology. 2012;**66**(4):553-562

[128] Leonardi-Bee J, Ellison T, Bath-Hextall F. Smoking and the risk of nonmelanoma skin cancer: Systematic review and meta-analysis. Archives of Dermatology. 2012;**148**(8):939-946

[129] Dusingize JC, Olsen CM, Pandeya NP, Subramaniam P, Thompson BS, Neale RE, et al. Cigarette smoking and the risks of basal cell carcinoma and squamous cell carcinoma. The Journal of Investigative Dermatology. 2017;**137**(8):1700-1708

[130] Hussain SK, Sundquist J, Hemminki K. The effect of having an affected parent or sibling on invasive and in situ skin cancer risk in Sweden. The Journal of Investigative Dermatology. 2009;**129**(9):2142-2147

[131] Kharazmi E, Fallah M, Sundquist K, Hemminki K. Familial risk of early and late onset cancer: Nationwide prospective cohort study. BMJ. 2012;**345**:e8076

[132] Asgari MM, Warton EM, Whittemore AS. Family history of skin cancer is associated with increased risk of cutaneous squamous cell carcinoma. Dermatologic Surgery. 2015;**41**(4):481-486

[133] Fine JD, Johnson LB, Weiner M, Li KP, Suchindran C. Epidermolysis bullosa and the risk of life-threatening cancers: The national EB registry experience, 1986-2006. Journal of the American Academy of Dermatology. 2009;**60**(2):203-211

[134] Nikolaou V, Stratigos AJ, Tsao H. Hereditary nonmelanoma skin cancer. Seminars in Cutaneous Medicine and Surgery. 2012;**31**(4):204-210

[135] Majewski S, Jablonska S. Skin autografts in epidermodysplasia verruciformis: Human papillomavirus-associated cutaneous changes need over 20 years for malignant conversion. Cancer Research. 1997;**57**(19):4214-4216

[136] Asgari MM, Wang W, Ioannidis NM, Itnyre J, Hoffmann T, Jorgenson E, et al. Identification of susceptibility loci for cutaneous squamous cell carcinoma. The Journal of Investigative Dermatology. 2016;**136**(5):930-937

[137] Chahal HS, Lin Y, Ransohoff KJ, Hinds DA, Wu W, Dai HJ, et al. Genome-wide association study identifies novel susceptibility loci for cutaneous squamous cell carcinoma. Nature Communications. 2016;7:12048

[138] Siiskonen SJ, Zhang M, Li WQ, Liang L, Kraft P, Nijsten T, et al.

A genome-wide association study of cutaneous squamous cell carcinoma among European descendants. Cancer Epidemiology, Biomarkers & Prevention. 2016;**25**(4):714-720

[139] Pickering CR, Zhou JH, Lee JJ, Drummond JA, Peng SA, Saade RE, et al. Mutational landscape of aggressive cutaneous squamous cell carcinoma. Clinical Cancer Research. 2014;**20**(24):6582-6592

[140] Comprehensive genomic characterization of squamous cell lung cancers. Nature. 2012;**489**(7417):519-525

[141] Alexandrov LB, Nik-Zainal S, Wedge DC, Aparicio SA, Behjati S, Biankin AV, et al. Signatures of mutational processes in human cancer. Nature. 2013;**500**(7463):415-421

[142] Ziegler A, Jonason AS, Leffell DJ, Simon JA, Sharma HW, Kimmelman J, et al. Sunburn and p53 in the onset of skin cancer. Nature. 1994;**372**(6508): 773-776

[143] Ortonne JP. From actinic keratosis to squamous cell carcinoma. The British Journal of Dermatology. 2002;**146** (Suppl 61):20-23

[144] Al-Rohil RN, Tarasen AJ, Carlson JA, Wang K, Johnson A, Yelensky R, et al. Evaluation of 122 advanced-stage cutaneous squamous cell carcinomas by comprehensive genomic profiling opens the door for new routes to targeted therapies. Cancer. 2016;**122**(2):249-257

[145] Li YY, Hanna GJ, Laga AC, Haddad RI, Lorch JH, Hammerman PS. Genomic analysis of metastatic cutaneous squamous cell carcinoma. Clinical Cancer Research. 2015;**21**(6):1447-1456

[146] South AP, Purdie KJ, Watt SA, Haldenby S, den Breems N, Dimon M, et al. NOTCH1 mutations occur early during cutaneous squamous cell carcinogenesis. The Journal of Investigative Dermatology. 2014; **134**(10):2630-2638

[147] Brown VL, Harwood CA, Crook T, Cronin JG, Kelsell DP, Proby CM. p16INK4a and p14ARF tumor suppressor genes are commonly inactivated in cutaneous squamous cell carcinoma. The Journal of Investigative Dermatology. 2004;**122**(5):1284-1292

[148] Wang NJ, Sanborn Z, Arnett KL, Bayston LJ, Liao W, Proby CM, et al. Loss-of-function mutations in Notch receptors in cutaneous and lung squamous cell carcinoma. Proceedings of the National Academy of Sciences of the United States of America. 2011;**108**(43):17761-17766

[149] Mauerer A, Herschberger E, Dietmaier W, Landthaler M, Hafner C. Low incidence of EGFR and HRAS mutations in cutaneous squamous cell carcinomas of a German cohort. Experimental Dermatology. 2011;**20**(10):848-850

[150] Ridd K, Bastian BC. Somatic mutation of epidermal growth factor receptor in a small subset of cutaneous squamous cell carcinoma. The Journal of Investigative Dermatology. 2010;**130**(3):901-903

[151] Cañueto J, Cardeñoso E, García JL, Santos-Briz Á, Castellanos-Martín A, Fernández-López E, et al. Epidermal growth factor receptor expression is associated with poor outcome in cutaneous squamous cell carcinoma. The British Journal of Dermatology. 2017;**176**(5):1279-1287

[152] Nicholson RI, Gee JM, Harper ME. EGFR and cancer prognosis. European Journal of Cancer. 2001;**37**(Suppl. 4): S9-S15

[153] Matsumoto K, Umitsu M, De Silva DM, Roy A, Bottaro DP.

Hepatocyte growth factor/MET in cancer progression and biomarker discovery. Cancer Science. 2017;**108**(3): 296-307

[154] Bonan NF, Kowalski D, Kudlac K, Flaherty K, Gwilliam JC, Falkenberg LG, et al. Inhibition of HGF/MET signaling decreases overall tumor burden and blocks malignant conversion in Tpl2-related skin cancer. Oncogene. 2019;**8**(1):1

[155] Khavari PA. Modelling cancer in human skin tissue. Nature Reviews. Cancer. 2006;**6**(4):270-280

[156] Liu F, Yang X, Geng M, Huang M. Targeting ERK, an Achilles' heel of the MAPK pathway, in cancer therapy. Acta Pharmaceutica Sinica B. 2018;**8**(4): 552-562

[157] Anforth R, Fernandez-Peñas P, Long GV. Cutaneous toxicities of RAF inhibitors. The Lancet Oncology. 2013;**14**(1):e11-e18

[158] Flaherty KT, Infante JR, Daud A, Gonzalez R, Kefford RF, Sosman J, et al. Combined BRAF and MEK inhibition in melanoma with BRAF V600 mutations. The New England Journal of Medicine. 2012;**367**(18):1694-1703

[159] Bamford S, Dawson E, Forbes S, Clements J, Pettett R, Dogan A, et al. The COSMIC (catalogue of somatic mutations in Cancer) database and website. British Journal of Cancer. 2004;**91**(2):355-358

[160] Leng L, Metz CN, Fang Y, Xu J, Donnelly S, Baugh J, et al. MIF signal transduction initiated by binding to CD74. The Journal of Experimental Medicine. 2003;**197**(11):1467-1476

[161] Conroy H, Mawhinney L, Donnelly SC. Inflammation and cancer: Macrophage migration inhibitory factor (MIF)—The potential missing link. QJM. 2010;**103**(11):831-836

[162] Heise R, Vetter-Kauczok CS, Skazik C, Czaja K, Marquardt Y, Lue H, et al. Expression and function of macrophage migration inhibitory factor in the pathogenesis of UV-induced cutaneous nonmelanoma skin cancer. Photochemistry and Photobiology. 2012;**88**(5):1157-1164

[163] Foulds CE, Nelson ML, Blaszczak AG, Graves BJ. Ras/mitogen-activated protein kinase signaling activates Ets-1 and Ets-2 by CBP/p300 recruitment. Molecular and Cellular Biology. 2004;**24**(24):10954-10964

[164] Keehn CA, Smoller BR, Morgan MB. Ets-1 immunohistochemical expression in non-melanoma skin carcinoma. Journal of Cutaneous Pathology. 2004;**31**(1):8-13

[165] Zoncu R, Efeyan A, Sabatini DM. mTOR: From growth signal integration to cancer, diabetes and ageing. Nature Reviews. Molecular Cell Biology. 2011;**12**(1):21-35

[166] Courtney KD, Corcoran RB, Engelman JA. The PI3K pathway as drug target in human cancer. Journal of Clinical Oncology. 2010;**28**(6):1075-1083

[167] Einspahr JG, Calvert V, Alberts DS, Curiel-Lewandrowski C, Warneke J, Krouse R, et al. Functional protein pathway activation mapping of the progression of normal skin to squamous cell carcinoma. Cancer Prevention Research (Philadelphia, Pa.). 2012;**5**(3):403-413

[168] Campos MA, Macedo S, Fernandes M, Pestana A, Pardal J, Batista R, et al. TERT promoter mutations are associated with poor prognosis in cutaneous squamous cell carcinoma. Journal of the American Academy of Dermatology. 2019;**80**(3):660-9.e6

[169] Asgari MM, Toland AE, Arron ST. IRF4 polymorphism is associated with

cutaneous squamous cell carcinoma in organ transplant recipients: A pigment-independent phenomenon. The Journal of Investigative Dermatology. 2017;**137**(1):251-253

[170] Sarin KY, Lin Y, Daneshjou R, Ziyatdinov A, Thorleifsson G, Rubin A, et al. Genome-wide meta-analysis identifies eight new susceptibility loci for cutaneous squamous cell carcinoma. Nature Communications. 2020;**11**(1): 820

[171] Sordillo JE, Kraft P, Wu AC, Asgari MM. Quantifying the polygenic contribution to cutaneous squamous cell carcinoma risk. The Journal of Investigative Dermatology. 2018;**138**(7): 1507-1510

[172] Skulsky SL, O'Sullivan B, McArdle O, Leader M, Roche M, Conlon PJ, et al. Review of high-risk features of cutaneous squamous cell carcinoma and discrepancies between the American Joint Committee on Cancer and NCCN Clinical Practice Guidelines in Oncology. Head & Neck. 2017;**39**(3):578-594

[173] Laing ME, Dicker P, Moloney FJ, Ho WL, Murphy GM, Conlon P, et al. Association of methylenetetrahydrofolate reductase polymorphism and the risk of squamous cell carcinoma in renal transplant patients. Transplantation. 2007;**84**(1):113-116

[174] Rodríguez-Paredes M, Esteller M. Cancer epigenetics reaches mainstream oncology. Nature Medicine. 2011;**17**(3): 330-339

[175] Murao K, Kubo Y, Ohtani N, Hara E, Arase S. Epigenetic abnormalities in cutaneous squamous cell carcinomas: Frequent inactivation of the RB1/p16 and p53 pathways. The British Journal of Dermatology. 2006;**155**(5):999-1005

[176] Sandoval J, Esteller M. Cancer epigenomics: Beyond genomics. Current Opinion in Genetics & Development. 2012;**22**(1):50-55

[177] Darr OA, Colacino JA, Tang AL, McHugh JB, Bellile EL, Bradford CR, et al. Epigenetic alterations in metastatic cutaneous carcinoma. Head & Neck. 2015;**37**(7):994-1001

[178] Chiles MC, Ai L, Zuo C, Fan CY, Smoller BR. E-cadherin promoter hypermethylation in preneoplastic and neoplastic skin lesions. Modern Pathology. 2003;**16**(10):1014-1018

[179] Tanaka N, Odajima T, Ogi K, Ikeda T, Satoh M. Expression of E-cadherin, alpha-catenin, and beta-catenin in the process of lymph node metastasis in oral squamous cell carcinoma. British Journal of Cancer. 2003;**89**(3):557-563

[180] D'Arcangelo D, Tinaburri L, Dellambra E. The role of p16(INK4a) pathway in human epidermal stem cell self-renewal, aging and cancer. International Journal of Molecular Sciences. 2017;**18**(7):1591

[181] Kouzarides T. Chromatin modifications and their function. Cell. 2007;**128**(4):693-705

[182] Eckert RL, Adhikary G, Rorke EA, Chew YC, Balasubramanian S. Polycomb group proteins are key regulators of keratinocyte function. The Journal of Investigative Dermatology. 2011;**131**(2):295-301

[183] Ezhkova E, Pasolli HA, Parker JS, Stokes N, Su IH, Hannon G, et al. Ezh2 orchestrates gene expression for the stepwise differentiation of tissue-specific stem cells. Cell. 2009;**136**(6): 1122-1135

[184] Hernández-Ruiz E, Toll A, García-Diez I, Andrades E, Ferrandiz-Pulido C, Masferrer E, et al. The Polycomb proteins RING1B and EZH2 repress the tumoral pro-inflammatory function in metastasizing primary cutaneous

squamous cell carcinoma. Carcinogenesis. 2018;**39**(3):503-513

[185] Yilmaz AS, Ozer HG, Gillespie JL, Allain DC, Bernhardt MN, Furlan KC, et al. Differential mutation frequencies in metastatic cutaneous squamous cell carcinomas versus primary tumors. Cancer. 2017;**123**(7):1184-1193

[186] Sasaki K, Sugai T, Ishida K, Osakabe M, Amano H, Kimura H, et al. Analysis of cancer-associated fibroblasts and the epithelial-mesenchymal transition in cutaneous basal cell carcinoma, squamous cell carcinoma, and malignant melanoma. Human Pathology. 2018;**79**:1-8

[187] Dotto GP. Multifocal epithelial tumors and field cancerization: Stroma as a primary determinant. The Journal of Clinical Investigation. 2014;**124**(4):1446-1453

[188] Tinaburri L, Valente C, Teson M, Minafò YA, Cordisco S, Guerra L, et al. The secretome of aged fibroblasts promotes EMT-like phenotype in primary keratinocytes from elderly donors through BDNF-TrkB axis. Journal of Investigative Dermatology. 2021;**141**(4s):1052-62.e12

[189] Yesantharao P, Wang W, Ioannidis NM, Demehri S, Whittemore AS, Asgari MM. Cutaneous squamous cell cancer (cSCC) risk and the human leukocyte antigen (HLA) system. Human Immunology. 2017;**78**(4):327-335

[190] Varki V, Ioffe OB, Bentzen SM, Heath J, Cellini A, Feliciano J, et al. PD-L1, B7-H3, and PD-1 expression in immunocompetent vs. immunosuppressed patients with cutaneous squamous cell carcinoma. Cancer Immunology, Immunotherapy. 2018;**67**(5):805-814

[191] Gatti V, Fierro C, Annicchiarico-Petruzzelli M, Melino G, Peschiaroli A. ΔNp63 in squamous cell carcinoma: Defining the oncogenic routes affecting epigenetic landscape and tumour microenvironment. Molecular Oncology. 2019;**13**(5):981-1001

[192] Allen CT, Ricker JL, Chen Z, Van Waes C. Role of activated nuclear factor-kappaB in the pathogenesis and therapy of squamous cell carcinoma of the head and neck. Head & Neck. 2007;**29**(10):959-971

[193] Suarez-Carmona M, Hubert P, Gonzalez A, Duray A, Roncarati P, Erpicum C, et al. ΔNp63 isoform-mediated β-defensin family up-regulation is associated with (lymph)angiogenesis and poor prognosis in patients with squamous cell carcinoma. Oncotarget. 2014;**5**(7):1856-1868

Chapter 3

Head Neck Squamous Cell Cancer Genomics: Oncogenes, Tumor Suppressor Genes and Clinical Implications

Anand B. Pathak and Satyam Satyarthi

Abstract

Head Neck Squamous Cell Cancer is genomically heterogenous. Common somatic mutations involve TP53, CDKN2A, FAT1, NOTCH1, PIK3CA, KMT2D and NSD1, less frequently others. Epigenetic changes also contribute to HNSCC biology. Alterations in tumor suppressor genes is a major oncogenic event in HNSCC. Genomic heterogeneity exists between different subsites within head neck region and also between the primary and metastatic disease. Intratumor heterogeneity has also been recognized. Based on key genomic alterations, four major molecular subtypes have been identified. Multi-omics analysis has provided further insights into HNSCC biology and shed light on EGFR pathway and immunogenomics. Corelative genomics of tumor cells, stromal cells and immune cells have led to emergence of distinct immune molecular subtypes of HNSCC. Major tumor suppressor genes and oncogenes have a correlation with prognosis, survival and treatment resistance. EGFR pathway is in focus for renewed understanding of resistance to EGFR targeted treatments and novel ways to target EGFR pathways. Increasingly genomic data is being leveraged towards clinical use including HNSCC prevention, prediction of metastases, survival and prognostication, fine tuning use of surgery, chemotherapy and radiation therapy, identifying patients for using immunotherapy, predicting drug resistance and gaining new information from radiological studies. Several novel targeted therapies are being pursued in clinical trials. Molecular co targeting strategies are being developed. Understanding the way tumor suppressor genes and oncogenes shape HNSCC biology and clinical behavior is bringing the much-needed therapeutic breakthrough in this tough to treat disease.

Keywords: Head Neck, Squamous, genomics, clinical, profiling, applications

1. Introduction

Head neck squamous cell carcinomas (HNSCC) include cancers arising in the mucosa of oral cavity, pharynx, larynx, hypopharynx. According to GLOBOCAN 2020 report, worldwide head neck cancer statistics indicate that there are 1,518,133 cases of head neck cancers per year, resulting in approximately 510,771 deaths per year. In Asia there are 944,946 cases of head neck cancers per year, resulting in approximately 347,870 deaths per year. High incidence rates have been reported from developing countries including India, Pakistan, Bangladesh, Taiwan, and Sri Lanka [1].

Treatment of HNSCC is guided uniformly by anatomic location, tumor size, presence or absence of nodal and distant metastases. Oral cavity cancers are primary treated with surgery followed by adjuvant radiation or chemo-radiation based on pathological features. Cancers in the oropharynx, larynx and hypopharynx are primary treated with chemo-radiation with function preservation as the main goal of therapy. Neo-adjuvant chemotherapy is used in locally advanced tumors to improve resectability. EGFR targeting drugs afatinib, Cetuximab and immune check point inhibitors pembrolizumab, nivolumab are the only FDA approved biological treatments today.

Clinicians managing HNSCC face number of challenges today. Some of these include.

- High mortality in spite of optimal use of currently existing therapeutics.
- Lack of clinically meaningful biological classifier of HNSCC other than HPV status.
- Continued emergence of treatment resistance.
- Great variability in clinical outcome despite uniformity in approach.
- Continued reliance on anatomical factors (TNM) to guide treatment.
- High morbidity and poor quality of life after conventional treatments
- Lack of robust biomarkers to select EGFR targeted therapy which seems to be the only existing targeted therapy for HNSCC.
- Lack of effective systemic adjuvant systemic therapies in high-risk patients.
- Lack of genomically directed therapies similar to other oncogene addicted cancers.
- Lack of effective later lines of therapies
- Low response rates to currently approved immune check point inhibitors
- Lack of robust biomarkers to predict nodal, distant metastases and recurrence
- And even lack of predictive biomarkers for selection of conventional treatments, not to mention lack of robust biomarkers for prognosis.

Considerable work has been done on deciphering HNSCC at genomic level. Major alterations in tumor suppressor genes and oncogenes in HNSCC have been identified. Multi-omics studies have shed considerable light on how genomic alterations shape HNSCC biology and clinical behavior. Number of studies are addressing how knowledge about HNSCC genomics/multi-omics can leveraged to address some of the challenges faced by clinicians managing HNSCC. The need to break the ground in HNSCC prevention and therapy has never been so urgent.

This chapter attempts to review key alterations in tumor suppressor genes and oncogenes in HPV negative HNSCC and the potential clinical implications of these alterations. Key insights gained from multi-omics studies will also be highlighted. This review also quotes some of the novel targeting therapies and novel strategies. Specifically, insights gained in EGFR targeting and immune therapies will also be discussed in the context of genomics. Since the amount of literature being published is so large, it is beyond the scope of this review to provide exhaustive coverage on each aspect of head neck cancer genomics. Hence few indicative studies are quoted to elaborate each point to give the reader a basic orientation. This review will focus on HPV- HNSCC.

2. Head neck squamous cell cancer (HNSCC): oncogenes and tumor suppressor genes

The Cancer Genome Atlas (TCGA) provided landscape of somatic genomic alterations by profiling 279 head neck squamous cell carcinomas. Tobacco related head neck squamous cell cancers showed loss of function mutations of TP53, CDKN2A inactivation, Copy number alterations of 3q26/28, 11q13/22. Few subgroups showed alterations in NSD1, WNT pathway genes AJUBA and FAT1, NFE2L2 [2]. HPV positive cases showed mutations of PIK3CA, loss of TRAF3 and amplification of cell cycle gene E2F1.Whole exome sequencing and microarray data showed unstable HNSCC genome showing high copy number alterations including copy number loss and copy number gains. Co amplifications of CCND1, FADD and CTTN and BIRC2 and YAP1 were found. Focal deletions were found in NSD1 and tumor suppressor genes including FAT1, NOTCH1, SMAD4, CDKN2A. Focal amplifications were found in receptor tyrosine kinases (RTKs) like EGFR, ERBB2, FGFR1. There was a small subset of oral cavity cancer characterized by activating mutations in HRAS, inactivating mutations in CASP8 and wild type TP53. This subset has been labeled as 'M' class which is driven by mutations rather than copy number alterations with tumorigenesis involving RAS, cell death pathway and NFkB. Fusion oncogenes like ALK, ROS or RET were not observed. MET exon 14 skipping mutation was uncommon. Loss of tumor suppressor function was more common than protein coding fusion events.

TCGA identified genes which can be grouped into (1) genes responsible for cell survival and proliferation (TP53, HRAS, EGFR, PIK3CA), (2) cell cycle control genes (CDKN2A AND CCND1), (3) cellular differentiation (NOTCH1) and (4) adhesion and invasion signaling (FAT1). Out of the most commonly mutated genes, TP53, CDKN2A, CASP8 AND NSD1 are differentially mutated across anatomic sites in the head neck region.

Frequency wise the common mutations in HNSCC are listed in **Table 1**.

More than 70% of HNSCC harbor mutations in the tumor suppressor p53 (TP53). TP53 mutations have been characterized in several ways. These mutations could be somatic or missense mutations, functional, partially functional or non-functional, and based on the alteration of DNA binding, as disruptive and non-disruptive.

TP53 mutations influence cell cycle, genomic integrity causing aberrant proliferation, disrupted apoptosis and defective DNA repair. TP53 mutation is probably the main actor in HNSCC pathogenesis and occur early in carcinoma. These mutations are also very high in metastatic HNSCC. Mutation rates of TP53 vary across different subsites in head neck. Larynx and hypopharynx have the highest TP53 mutation rate (83.5%), oral cavity and tongue 75.6%. oropharynx including tonsils and base of tongue have the lowest mutation rate 28.6% [3].

CDKN2A is the second most commonly altered gene in HNSCC CDKN2A encodes a CDK4/CDK6 kinase inhibitor which constrains cells from progressing

Mutations	Percentage
TP53	72
CDKN2A	22
FAT1	23
NOTCH1	19
PIK3CA	21
KMT2D	18
NSD1	10
CASP8	9
NFE2L2	6
FBXW7	5
TGFBR2	4
HRAS	4
CUL3	4
RB1	3
HLA-A	3
PTEN	2
TRAF3	1

Table 1.
Somatic mutations (TCGA findings).

through G1 restriction point. CDKN2A mutations are rare in HPV+ HNSCC [3]. Mutations involving NOTCH gene are third most common in HNSCC [3, 4]. NOTCH family members are transmembrane proteins (NOTCH 1-4) and two family of ligands the Jagged and the Delta-like proteins, involved in cell to cell communication and regulations of squamous differentiation.

CCND1 encodes cyclin D1 and regulates G1-to-S phase transition by formation of complexes with cyclin dependent kinases like CDK4 and CDK6. CCND1 is amplified in 30-40% of HNSCC with cyclin D1 overexpression [3]. AJUBA regulates cell division, vertebrate ciliogenesis and left–right axis determination. NSD1 is a tumor suppressor gene. Mutations in KMT2D and HLA-A contribute to a defective immunosurveillance. EGFR is commonly overexpressed in HNSCC and has been explored as a therapeutic target. PIK3CA alterations are common in HNSCC especially in HPV+ cancers. PIK3CA are seen in patients with advanced HNSCC harboring multiple PI3K pathway mutations [3]. MET is a Hepatocyte Growth Factor (HGF) receptor which regulates cancer cell plasticity through reversible programming of epithelia-mesenchymal transition (EMT) [3]. MET overexpression leads to MET/HGF pathway activation and corelates with worse outcome.

2.1 Epigenetics in HNSCC

Epigenetic changes such as DNA methylation, histone acetylation and expression of small non coding RNAs affect gene expression. There is some evidence of importance of epigenetic changes in HNSCC. Global hypomethylation has been linked to poor prognosis. Epigenetic changes is one major method for tumor resistance. Many tumor suppressor genes like CDKN2A, CDH1, MGME, RASSF1A show promoter hypermethylation [5].

2.2 Key oncogenic events in HNSCC

In terms of key driver oncogenic events in HNSCC can be summarized as follows; (**Table 2**).

In the TCGA dataset, most of the tumors that were sequenced were from early-stage surgical samples. The genomic profile of recurrent/metastatic HNSCC could be different. The American Association for Cancer Research has undertaken a project Genomic Evidence Neoplasia Information Exchange (GENIE) which is an international data sharing project allowing multiple international institutions to share their data of cancer sequencing. This combined dataset includes 700 patients with HNSCC, 40% representing patients with metastases. The frequency of common mutations in HNSCC in the three datasets TCGA, AACR GENIE and COSMIC are found comparable and has paved the way for developing targeted therapies [6].

2.3 Genomic heterogeneity of HNSCC at different subsites and between primary and recurrent metastatic tumor

In addition to HPV status as one important biological differential, different subsites of HNSCC seem to harbor differences at genomic level. TP53 mutations are most frequent in Laryngeal/hypopharyngeal sites followed by oral cavity followed by oropharynx [3]. David Vossena et al. did DNA sequencing on 111 HPV negative HNSCC, 55 oral and 56 laryngeal/pharyngeal cancers and identified somatic point

Function	Gene	Event
Tumor Suppressor	TP53	Loss of function mutation
Tumor suppressor	CDKN2A	Mutation, homozygous deletion, protein down regulation
Tumor suppressor	NF1	Mutation, amplification
PI(3)K	PIK3CA	Amplification, mutation
PI(3)K	PTEN	Mutation, protein downregulation
PI(3)K	PIK3R1	mutation
Oncogenes	CCND1	amplification
Oncogenes	MYC	Amplification
Oncogenes	HRAS	Mutation
Receptor Tyrosine Kinases (RTKs)	EGFR	Amplification, mutation, protein up regulation
RTKs	FGFR1	Mostly amplification, rarely mutation
RTKs	ERBB2	Amplification, protein up regulation, mutation
RTKs	IGF1R	Amplification, mutation
RTKs	EPHA2	Mutation
RTKs	DDR2	Amplification, mutation
RTKs	FGFR2	Amplification, mutation
RTKs	FGFR3	Amplification, mutation
RTKs	MET	Amplification, exon 14 skipping mutation

Table 2.
Oncogenic events in HNSCC.

mutations and copy number alterations. They also included sample data from TCGA to expand analysis. Mutational profiles of oral and laryngeal pharyngeal squamous cell carcinoma showed many similarities. However, oral squamous cell carcinoma was significantly enriched for CASP8 and HRAS mutations. Laryngeal/pharyngeal squamous cell cancers were enriched in LAMA and NSD1. Overall, oral squamous cell carcinoma had fewer somatic point mutations and copy number alterations. Laryngeal/pharyngeal squamous cancer scored higher on mutational and genomic scar signatures associated with homologous recombination DNA repair defects explaining differential response to chemoradiation [7].

Recurrent and metastatic HNSCC do share driver mutations with their primaries in addition to accumulating new mutations. High rates of TERT promoter mutations are found in recurrent or metastatic HPV- HNSCC. HPV+ HNSCC may also start exhibiting mutational landscape of HPV- negative tumors after recurrence and metastases. Recurrent HPV+ positive tumors may get enriched in TP53 mutations and lack PIK3CA mutations as compared to primary HPV+ primary tumors [8].

As noted earlier, head neck mucosal squamous cell carcinoma occurs at several subsites. Clinical behavior heterogeneity in terms of response to therapy, metastatic rate is commonly observed. Clinical heterogeneity is observed even within a single subsite. Tumor cells are known to accumulate genetic alterations over time. Some of these are driver mutations and some are passenger mutations. Heterogenic cell clones undergo selection leading to development of aggressive clones with growth advantage. This is one main reason for development of resistance to chemotherapy and radiation therapy. High degree of intratumor heterogeneity leads to tumor progression, inferior treatment outcome and reduced survival. Whole genome analysis of 74 cases of HNSCC used to calculate Mutant Allele Tumor Heterogeneity (MATH) can be a genetic biomarker of high-risk disease. High MATH has been found to have shorter overall survival [9, 10]. Targeted monotherapies are unlikely to be major breakthrough in HNSCC. Rational combination of two or several therapies or effective co-targeting seems to be the way forward.

2.4 Molecular subtypes of HNSCC cancers based on gene expression profiles

Chung et al. and Walter et al. described four distinct molecular classes in HNSCC based on gene expression patterns: basal, mesenchymal, atypical, and classical (**Table 3**) [11, 12]. The basal subtype is characterized by over-expression of genes functioning in cell adhesion including COL17A1, and growth factor and receptor TGFA and EGFR, high expression of transcription factor TP63. The mesenchymal subtype shows over expression of genes involved in immune response and genes associated with epithelial to mesenchymal transition including vimentin, desmin, TWIST1, and HGF. The classical subtype is shows over-expression of genes related to oxidative stress response and xenobiotic metabolism. The atypical subtype shows elevated expression of CDKN2A, LIG1, and RPA2, low expression of EGFR.

2.5 Multi-omics analysis of HNSCC and novel insights

Huang et al. did proteogenomic study on 108 HPV negative HNSCCs in order to gain biological insights and novel treatment strategies [13]. They found correlation between 263 proteins, 173 phosphoproteins and overall survival. Poor prognosis associated proteins/phosphoproteins were enriched in pathways for somatic copy number alteration drivers, DNA replication, cell cycle and RNA processing. They

Molecular subtype	Key features
Classical	TP53 mutation CDKN2A loss 3q amplification Alterations in oxidative stress genes like KEAP1, NFE2L2, CUL3, Smoking history Laryngeal subsite
Basal	NOTCH1 inactivation Decreased SOX2 expression HRAS-CASP8 co-mutation Co-amplified 11q13/q22
Atypical	Lack of chromosome 7 amplification Activating exon 9 mutations (PIK3CA domain)
Mesenchymal	Alterations in innate immunity genes, High expression of CD56 Low frequency of HLA class I mutations

Table 3.
Molecular subtypes of HNSCC and key features.

also found poor prognosis associated with FAT1 truncation or 11q13.3 amplification. Analysis of Rb pathway showed interesting observations. CDKN2A and CCND1 alterations do not always result in increased CCND1 protein and CDK4/6 activity. Rb status was found more effective indicator of CDK4/6 dependent cell cycle activity than genomic or transcriptomic markers.

Similarly, novel insight was obtained in EGFR pathway. EGFR amplification activates EGFR in a ligand independent manner. The EGFR monoclonal antibody works by binding to the extracellular domain of EGFR to prevent ligand induced activity. Therefore, EGFR ligand abundance is more important to activity of anti EGFR moAbs than EGFR amplification or overexpression.

Immune-proteogenomic analysis revealed immunosuppressive somatic copy number alterations. Higher immune cell infiltration was linked to low clinical stage, less smoking and better prognosis. Immune hot tumors showed both cytotoxic immune enzymes and immunosuppressive proteins. This explains why the response to immune check point inhibitors in PD L1 positive HNSCC patients is modest. In immune cold tumors, the low immune infiltration was not driven by lack of tumor antigen sources but deficient Antigen Presentation Machinery (APM) pathway.

Further Huang et al. divided HNSCC tumors into three clusters using multi-omics data. Cluster I was associated with laryngeal site, strong smoking and high chromosome instability (CIN). Proteomic data suggested linkage between aberrant epigenetic activity, smoking and high CIN. This cluster had the worst prognosis. Cluster II showed elevation of several basal factors and high translational activity. Cluster III showed tumors with weak smoking history, higher immune scores and higher stromal scores. So, cluster I, II and III were CIN, Basal and Immune subtypes respectively. In terms of treatment selection, CIN subtype was associated with frequent aberrations of CCND1, CDKN2A and Rb hyper-phosphorylation indicating potential for CDK 4/6 inhibitors. Basal subtype was associated with high EGFR ligand activity suggesting a potential role for anti-EGFR mAbs. The immune subtype could be appropriate for immune checkpoint blockade. Frequency of high level of biomarkers were 32% in CIN tumors, 62% in Basal tumors and 83% in Immune tumors emphasizing the tremendous potential to select appropriate therapy.

New targets for therapy were also identified including KIT, ECER1G, PLAU, SERPINE1, TOP2A, MMPs, several cell cycle and DNA damage related kinases. Multiple C/T and neoantigens were also found in their analysis which could be potential immunotherapy targets.

2.6 Immunogenomics

Thorsson et al. and Tamborero et al. did extensive immunogenomic analysis of many tumors and came out with six molecular immune subtypes: wound healing (C1), IFN gamma dominant (C2), inflammatory (C3), lymphocyte depleted (C4), immunologically quiet (C5) and TGF-beta dominant (C6) [14, 15]. In the TCGA HNSCC cohort, most tumors were C1 with elevated expression of angiogenic genes, high proliferation rate and a Th2 cell bias to the adaptive immune infiltrate or C2 with the highest M1/M2 macrophage polarization, a strong CD8 signal and prominent TCR diversity.

Genomic and neoantigen evolution from primary to first metastases was studied by Charles Schutt et al. between 23 paired primary and recurrent HNSCC tumors [16]. They found 6 genes which predicted neoantigens in 4 or more patients. Neoantigens in shared genes had increased CD3+ and CD8+ T cell infiltration and duration of survival with disease.

Yao Yao et al. in a study involving 5 HNSCC tumors and normal tissue found four immune related genes, PVR, TNFRSF12A, IL21R, SOCS1 to be significantly associated with overall survival [17]. They tried to integrate these four genes with pathological N stage to better predict overall survival. High expression of PVR AND TNFRSF12A indicated poor overall survival whereas high expression of IL21R and SOCS1 indicated better overall survival.

Chen et al. characterized the immune landscape of HNSC by their tumor and stromal compartments to identify novel immune molecular subgroups [18]. In their study, a training cohort of 522 HNSC samples from the Cancer Genome Atlas profiled by RNA sequencing was analyzed. Gene patterns from tumor, stromal, and immune cell genes were separated. Correlations were studied between the expression patterns with a set of immune-related gene signatures, potential immune biomarkers, and clinicopathological features. Validation was done with six independent datasets containing 838 HNSC samples.

Approximately 40% of HNSCs were labeled as immune class based on enriched inflammatory response, enhanced cytolytic activity, and active interferon-c signaling. Within this, some samples had markers of exhausted immune response and some had markers of active immune response. The Exhausted Immune Class was characterized by enrichment of activated stroma and anti-inflammatory M2 macrophage signatures, WNT/transforming growth factor-b signaling pathway activation and poor survival. Active immune class showed enriched proinflammatory M1 macrophage signature, enhanced cytolytic activity, abundant tumor-infiltrating lymphocytes, high human papillomavirus (HPV) infection, and favorable prognosis. Such a subgrouping might help in tailoring immune therapies to appropriate subsets of patients.

Several genomic features may influence response to immune check point inhibitors [19]. High tumor mutational burden is associated with neoepitope presentation and immune hot phenotype leading to enhanced benefit with immune check point inhibitors. NSD1 inactivating mutations, global DNA hypomethylation, aneuploidy, may lead to impaired chemokine signaling and immune effector response leading to an immune cold phenotype and low benefit from immune checkpoint inhibitors. Groups led by Many HNSCC specific studies tried to subtype patients as immune molecular subtypes. Considerable work is also being done to understand immune events occurring in the areas of field cancerization around an oral premalignant lesion raising the hope for using immunotherapy as immunoprevention. Integrated omics studies are also being pursued to understand occurrence of immune related adverse events and development of immune resistance.

3. Head neck cancer genomics: clinical implications

3.1 Clinical and therapeutic implications of major tumor suppressor genes and oncogenes in HNSCC

TP53 mutation which is common in HNSCC has predictive value for disease free and overall survival. There is a correlation between TP53 mutations and resistance to chemotherapy drugs like cisplatin, doxorubicin, paclitaxel also leading to lower rates of pathological complete responses to neoadjuvant chemotherapy. Absence of TP53 mutated DNA in the surgical margins has been found to improve local recurrence free survival. Patients with no TP53 mutated DNA in the surgical margins may be spared post-operative radiation therapy. Disruptive TP53 mutations predict locoregional recurrence.

Mutant TP53 could be targeted in several ways; (1) introduction of wild type TP53 inside the cancer cells, (2) reactivation of some function of wild type TP53 in mutant cancer cells, (3) degradation of mutant TP53, or (4) targeting coexisting genetic alterations such as CDKN2A deletions or PIK3CA activation to induce synthetic lethality.

CDKN2A It is associated with worse survival in recurrent metastatic HNSCC. Frequent alterations of PI3K-AKT- m TOR pathway has raised the hope for therapeutic targets. However, the results with PI3K/AKT/m TOR pathway targeting have been inconsistent.

There could be a scope for combination of PI3K inhibition with chemotherapy and/or radiation. Currently there are trials underway combining buparlisib, copanlisib and alpelisib in combination with radiation, cisplatin and/or cetuximab. mTOR inhibitors sirolimus, everolimus and temsirolimus have limited efficacy in HNSCC. Further work is needed in this area to develop effective strategies. Activated PI3K/Akt also confers resistance to MET inhibition. Therefore, combining MET/PI3K inhibition might be a good strategy. CCND1 amplification has been associated with recurrence and metastases. It may also confer resistance to cisplatin and EGFR inhibitors. CDK4/6 inhibitors abemaciclib and palbocilib are being tested in combination with cetuximab and IMRT in locally advanced HNSCC. Oral squamous cell carcinoma patients with NOTCH pathway mutations are three times more likely to die with recurrent disease. NOTCH1 mutation may sever as biomarker for identification of HNSCC with higher sensitivity to radiotherapy and chemotherapy. Activated NOTCH1 also contributes to resistance of PI3K inhibitors. NOTCH1 inhibition may enhance efficacy of conventional chemotherapeutic agents by targeting head neck cancer stem cells. Exposure to chemotherapeutic agents may lead to selection of recurrent tumors enriched in cancer stem cells. NOTCH1 inhibition may attenuate such an effect [4].

EGFR is commonly overexpressed in HNSCC [20]. It is associated with resistance to radiation therapy and chemotherapy and worse locoregional and disease-free survival. Two agents Cetuximab a monoclonal antibody binding to the extracellular domain of EGFR and Afatinib a small anti molecule tyrosine kinase inhibitor have been approved by FDA [21, 22]. However, currently there is no biomarker to select patients for these drugs. Considerable work has been done to understand resistance mechanisms to anti-EGFR monoclonal antibodies and -EGFR tyrosine kinase inhibitors. These include (1) Metabolic pathways, (2) cross talk with other signaling pathways, (3) dysregulation of EGFR pathway, (4) epithelial mesenchymal transition and nuclear translocation of EGFR. This understanding will help in overcoming EGFR resistance.

There could be several ways to augment EGFR targeting such as (1) combination of EGFR Mab and EGFR TKi, (2) Horizontal targeting multiple HER receptors, (3) Vertical targeting with inhibition of EGFR and other RTKs involved in nuclear translocation of EGFR.

MET alterations are low but important in terms of serving as a target for therapy. Several drugs are available such as tivantinib, cabozantinib, crizotinib to target MET. MET mutations are also associated with EGFR inhibitor resistance and reduced sensitivity to VEGFR TKIs. Dual VEGFR/c-MET inhibition or dual blockade of MET/EGFR could enhance efficacy.

3.2 Genomic data to improve head neck cancer prevention

We know that progression from normal epithelium to fully developed squamous cell cancer occurs through a multistep process often involving a stage of pre-malignant lesions. It has been found that these stages of normal epithelium, pre-malignant lesions and malignant lesions are not only different histologically, but are different in terms of genomics. Some earlier studies using Affymetrix Gene Chips found that progression from normal epithelium to pre-malignant lesions are associated with more transcriptional alterations than progression from pre-malignant lesions to malignant lesions. Moreover, the normal, pre-malignant and malignant lesions cluster differently. Based on this, there could be potential to classify pre-malignant lesions into low risk and high risk with appropriate treatment approach of aggressive treatment of high- risk lesions to prevent occurrence of HNSCC [23].

3.3 Prediction of metastases based on genomic profiling

Currently, presence or absence of neck nodal metastases is the only robust predictor of recurrence and metastases. Therefore, in most cases clinical N0 necks are addressed with surgical neck dissection. This often means treating a great majority of patients with unnecessary surgery. Currently, there is no single gene mutation or genomic profile which can predict recurrence and metastases as effectively as neck nodal status. This could be due to the fact that occurrence of metastases involves multiple genetic, molecular and metabolic pathways in addition to influence of host immune system. Genomic changes necessary for metastases may exist in majority of primary tumor at diagnosis paving the way to develop a robust metastatic gene signature.

Cromer et al. studied patients with hypopharyngeal squamous cell cancers using gene expression and found metastatic prediction accuracy of 92% using 168 gene targets [24].

Roepman et al. studied expression profiles of 82 primary oral cavity and oropharynx squamous cell cancers using 102 genes as predictors and observed predictive accuracy of 86% in comparison to clinical staging accuracy of 68% [25].

In view of the different lymphatic drainage patterns of different anatomical subsites, probably each anatomic subsite will need different genetic signature to predict nodal metastases.

Karpothiou et al. studied 18 HNSCC and corresponding node metastases and non-neoplastic tissue for RT-qPCR for EGFR, VEGF, Claudin7, Maspin, Survivin and SCCA [26]. They found differential gene expression levels in node metastases compared to the primary tumor and some correlation with prognosis.

Zevallos et al. did a retrospective study applying four molecular subtypes of HNSCC namely Basal (BA), Mesenchymal (MS), Atypical (AT) and Classical (CL) to oral cavity and laryngeal squamous cell cancers [27]. They found that early-stage oral cavity cancer with MS subtype was associated with high risk of nodal metastases. In laryngeal cancer, CL subtype was associated with worse overall survival. Oral cavity squamous cell cancers were predominantly BA and MS whereas laryngeal cancers were predominantly CL and AT subtype.

Ribeiro et al. used array comparative genomic hybridization data from HNSCC patients to develop a model to predict HNSCC recurrence/metastasis [28]. In their study of 104 HNSCC patients, this predictive model showed a good accuracy (>80%). Validation was done in an independent population from TCGA data portal. The genomic model included chromosomal regions from 5p, 6p, 8p, 9p, 11q, 12q, 15q and 17p, containing many upstream and downstream signaling pathways associated with cell proliferation and invasion. This model will need further large-scale study and has the potential to individualize clinical management and also identify potential therapeutic targets.

3.4 Survival and prognostication

There is considerable heterogeneity in the outcome of HNSCC patients with similar TNM stage. Number of studies are addressing this question. Investigators from China came out with a six gene signature (PEX11A, NLRP2, SERPINE1, UPK, CTTN, D2HGDH) using bioinformatics analysis of TCGA dataset, as a new prognostic marker for predicting survival of HNSCC patients [29]. They also did Gene Set Enrichment Analysis and found some pathways significantly enriched between high risk and low risk groups. Clinical trials testing such signature will be helpful.

Reddy et al. in a meta-analysis approach identified respective differentials (tongue: 3508, laryngopharynx: 4893, oropharynx: 2386) [30]; validation in TCGA revealed markers with high incidence (altered in >10% of patients) in tongue (n = 331), laryngopharynx (n = 701) and oropharynx (n = 404). Assessment of these genes in clinical sub-cohorts of TCGA indicated that early stage tongue (MTFR1, C8ORF33, OTUD6B) and laryngeal cancers (TWISTNB, KLHL13 and UBE2Q1) were defined by distinct prognosticators. Similarly, correlation with perineural/angio-lymphatic invasion, identified discrete marker panels with survival impact (tongue: NUDCD1, PRKC1; laryngopharynx: SLC4A1AP, PIK3CA, AP2M1). Alterations in ANO1, NUDCD1, PIK3CA defined survival in tongue cancer patients with nodal metastasis (node+ ECS-), while EPS8 is a significant differential in node+ ECS- laryngopharyngeal cancers.

3.5 Genomics and surgery in HNSCC

Goal of head neck cancer surgery includes wide resection of the primary tumor, neck dissection in clinically selected patients with the goal of obtaining adequate negative margins and acceptable functional outcome. Adjuvant therapy depends upon presence or absence of certain histopathological findings like positive margins, angiolymphatic space invasion, perineural invasion, nodal metastases, nodal metastatic burden, extracapsular extension in the involved nodes. How can HNSCC genomics help in precision surgery [31]?

1. Refining indications for surgery: There is often a dilemma in early - stage oral cavity cancers that are clinically N0, whether to do elective neck node dissection. Here genomic characterization of the primary tumor might help in prediction of nodal metastases and help in selection of patients for neck

dissection [32]. Similarly, negative predictive value of transcriptomic signature in early - stage oral cavity cancer might help in avoiding unnecessary neck dissection [33].

2. Surgery for pre-malignant lesions.

Some premalignant lesions progress to malignant lesions. Molecular genomic studies might help to identify such lesions so that they can be resected immediately [34].

3. Some patients with oligometastatic cancer with indolent behavior might be surgical candidates. Genomic studies on tumor dormancy might help identify such patients who could benefit by metastasectomy [35].

4. Genomic prediction of radiosensitivity (discussed below) might help avoid surgery in such patients.

5. Markers of aggressiveness: Genomics might predict for occurrence of extracapsular spread in involved and hence help allocate patients for adjuvant chemoradiation [36].

6. Perineural invasion is a known pathological marker of aggressiveness. Genomic expression profile of perineural invasion indicating aggressiveness might help triage patients for appropriate adjuvant therapies after surgery [37].

7. Genomic analysis of surgical margins.

In-spite of clear surgical margins about 15% patients do recur after surgery. Molecular analysis of the surgical margins might identify such patients and improve surgical resectability [38–41].

8. Many oral cavity cancers involve mandible. Mandibular resections add considerable morbidity and impair quality of life. Genomic studies might help in deciding extent of mandibular resections based on tumor tropism to involve bone [42].

9. Neoadjuvant immunotherapy is being increasing pursued in clinical trials with it's potential to real down stage the tumor and prevent metastases. This might redefine approach to surgery in near future [43–46].

10. Follow up of patients after cancer surgery: Functional genomics might help in optimizing follow of patients after curative surgical resection by identifying markers of aggressiveness. Genomic profile identification of perineural invasion might help in enhanced surveillance of such patients [47]. Patients with intratumor heterogeneity might be at risk of recurrence. Such patients can be identified prospectively [48]. Genomics may also help in prediction of loco-regional relapse. Group led by Davide Gissi analyzed DNA methylation for the following genes: ZAP70, ITGA4, KIF1A, PARP15, EPHX3, NTM, LRRTM1, FLI1, MIR193, LINC00599, MIR296, TERT, and GP1BB in the brushings from the tumor area at diagnosis and from the regenerating area 6 months after surgery in 49 consecutive patients [49]. As per a predefined cut-off value, sample was labeled as positive or negative. At diagnosis 47 out of 49 specimens were found positive. 16 out of 49 patients had positive scores

at six months after resection. 7 patients relapsed and out of these 6 patients had a positive score in the regenerative area after surgery. The presence of a positive score after oral cancer treatment was the most powerful variable related to the appearance of locoregional relapse. The authors concluded that 13-gene DNA methylation analysis by oral brushing may have a clinical application as a prognostic non-invasive tool in the follow-up of patients surgically treated for oral cavity squamous cancers.

3.6 Genomics to help using radiation therapy in HNSCC

Radiation therapy is mainstay of therapy in majority of HNSCC either as an adjuvant after surgery in oral cavity cancers, as principal treatment with or without chemotherapy in non-oral cavity cancers, as palliative or salvage therapy. Currently, radiation therapy strategies are same across anatomic sites based purely on TNM stage. There are no robust biomarkers of prediction of response, resistance and outcome in HPV- HNSCC.

Genomics have the potential to guide radiation response/resistance and predict toxicities. SF2, survival fraction at 2Gy in cell lines was published by Torres-Roca et al [50].

Pramana et al. also found potential to use gene expression profiling to predict outcome after chemo-radiation in head neck cancer [51].

Radiosensitivity index has been shown to predict clinical outcome in HNSCC patients treated with chemo-radiation in clinical trials, with 2 year survival of 86% in radiation sensitive signature versus 61% in resistant signature [52].

Concept of GARD (Genomic adjusted radiation dose) was developed by Jacob Scott et al., using a gene expression-based radiation-sensitivity index and linear quadratic model to derive GARD. GARD based clinical module potentially can allow individualization of radiation therapy and guide new design for genomically guided clinical trials [53].

Tumor hypoxia is known to lead to radiation resistance. Work has been to develop genomic signature to predict tumor hypoxia so that appropriate intervention strategies targeting tumor hypoxia can be developed [54].

Along the same lines immunogenomics might be used to predict outcome of radiation and immune therapies given in different combinations. Biology based radiation adaptation trials are already going in HPV positive HNSCC.

Gene alterations can also predict radiation induced toxicity and identify patients who are super sensitive to radiation therapy. Whitney Sumner et al. analyzed 37 HNSCC patients and found that genetic alterations in BRCA2, ERBB3, NOTCH1, and CCND1 were associated with higher mean grad radiation toxicity [55]. Alterations in TNFAIP3, HNF1A, SPTA1 and CASP8 were found in radiation supersensitive patients. Such an approach will help in improving therapeutic index of radiation therapy in HNSCC.

Overexpression of FOXC2, MDR1, MRP2, ERCC1. PDGF-C, NRG1, survivin are linked to treatment resistance. Amongst the miRNAs, overexpression of miR-371a-p, miR- 34c-50, miR-1323 and downregulation of miR-324-3p, miR-93-3p, miR-4501 has been linked to radio-resistance in nasopharyngeal carcinoma [56].

3.7 Genomics and chemotherapy in HNSCC

Cisplatin remains the most common chemotherapy drug used in HNSCC. However, resistance to cisplatin is common. Number of genomic correlates of cisplatin response/resistance have been identified. Sanne et al. employed an array of 21,121 pools of siRNAs targeting unique human genes in the NCBI RefSeq database and performed in vitro genome-wide functional genetic screen to identify genes that influence the response to cisplatin in HNSCC cells [57]. By siRNA-mediated knockdown, Fanconi anemia/BRCA pathway emerged as the predominant pathway for cisplatin response in HNSCC cells. Goretti Duran et al. investigated thirty-six selected single nucleotide polymorphisms (SNPs) in 29 genes in 110 patients treated with cisplatin-based chemoradiotherapy and found that genetic polymorphisms with activity in intracellular detoxification (GSTP1), DNA repair (ERCC1, ERCC4, ERCC5, RAD51), and multidrug resistance-associated protein (ABCB1, ABCC1, ABCC2) affect drug toxicity in patients with head and neck who received platinum-based CRT [58]. Gene variants and haplotypes of ERCC1 were associated with the risk of developing hematologic toxicity.

Hiroyuki Shimomura et al. examined Non-SMC Condensin I Complex Subunit H (NCAPH) expression in OSCC and performed a functional analysis of human Oral Squamous Carcinoma Cells (OSCC) and found that resistance to cisplatin, carboplatin, and nedaplatin was enhanced by NCAPH in OSCC cells. NCAPH silencing combined with platinum decreased multidrug resistance [59]. There was no association between NCAPH and resistance to paclitaxel, docetaxel, and 5-fluorouracil.

Lot of studies are looking at potential of using circulating tumor cells and circulating tumor DNA to monitor for recurrence and evolution of treatment resistance.

3.8 Genomics and immunotherapies in HNSCC

Immunotherapy is a promising approach and seems to have added a new paradigm to several cancers including HNSCC. However, with currently available immune checkpoint inhibitors, the response rate is low, very few patients derive benefit, many patients fail to respond, some patients develop hyper-progressive disease and patients may develop immune related adverse events in an unpredicted fashion.

In 2016, FDA approved anti PD1 antibodies pembrolizumab and nivolumab [60, 61]. With establishment of nivolumab and pembrolizumab in the treatment of recurrent metastatic HNSCC, there are several studies looking at different ways to combine them with established treatments like surgery, radiation therapy and chemotherapy including cetuximab. These molecules are being tested in the neoadjuvant, concurrent and adjuvant therapeutic spaces in HNSCC. Ipilimumab an anti-CTLA-4 antibody which works well has been shown to reverse resistance to treatment in HNSCC. Ipilimumab given after cetuximab has been shown to reverse resistance to cetuximab. It has been observed that there is increased infiltration with Treg cells following exposure to cetuximab. Ipilimumab eliminates these Treg cells. Several trials are underway looking at combinations of ipilimumab, radiation and nivolumab.

Several genomic features may influence response to immune check point inhibitors [19]. High tumor mutational burden is associated with neoepitope presentation and immune hot phenotype leading to enhanced benefit with immune check point inhibitors. NSD1 inactivating mutations, global DNA hypomethylation, aneuploidy, may lead to impaired chemokine signaling and immune effector response leading to an immune cold phenotype and low benefit from immune checkpoint inhibitors.

3.9 Genomics and drug resistance

3.9.1 Co-relation between genomic alterations and drug resistance

Several studies have found association of drug resistance and genomic alterations listed below. This knowledge might help in selecting appropriate patients for chemotherapy/drugs including targeted drugs and avoiding un-necessary treatment in those who may not benefit from it [3].

Genomic marker	Therapy resistance
TP53	Cisplatin resistance
EGFR	Radiation resistance
CCND1	Gefitinib resistance
NOTCH1	PI3K inhibitor
MET	Resistance to Cetuximab, Erlotinib
PIK3CA	Bio-radiation with cetuximab, PI3K inhibitors MET inhibitors

3.10 Genomics and radiomics

Imaging including contrast enhanced CT scan, MRI scans and recently PET scans are commonly used to accurately stage the patient at diagnosis and also to monitor response and recurrence. Radiomics based on image texture analysis has the potential to provide valuable real time information about tumor biology and response/resistance to treatment. Studies are looking at correlation between radiomics and genomics. Group led by Kerstin Zwirner at Eberhard Karls university in Germany looked at genetic tumor profiles and radiomic features in 20 HNSCC patients treated with primary radio-chemotherapy [62]. They did NGS of the tumor and corresponding normal tissue and analyzed 327 genes. TP53, FAT1 and KMT2D were the most frequently mutated driver genes in their cohort. They found good correlation between reduced radiomic intra-tumor heterogeneity and somatic mutations in FAT1 with small tumor volumes. Radiomic features of heterogeneity did not corelate with somatic mutations in TP53 or KMT2D. Radiomics and genomics remain work under progress.

4. Head neck cancer genomics and newer targets, drugs and strategies in HNSCC

4.1 New targets, ways and drugs in HNSCC

In addition to focusing on common mutations, there are rare mutations with druggable targets worth exploring [6].

1. Rearrangement of Neutrotrophic Tropomyosin Receptor Kinase (NTRK) gene. NTRK 1,2 and 3 fusions are found in 3%, 1.6% and 3% of HNSCC in the AACR GENIE data set. Pan TRK inhibitor Larotrectinib is being tested in these patients.

2. HRAS

HRAS is a farnesyl transferase substrate depending exclusively on farnesylation. HRAS mutations have been found in 4% of HNSCC patients in the GENIE data set. Tipifarnib which is highly selective inhibitor of farnesyl transferase is being tested in HRAS mutated HNSCC.

3. Antibody Drug Conjugate (ADC) are monoclonal antibodies conjugated to cytotoxic agents. Antibody targets a particular cell surface protein and the drug payload is delivered inside the cell. Several ADCs are being tested in HNSCC including ABBV-221, AVID100 which target EGFR, BAY1129980

targeting C4.4a, IMMU-132 which targets TROP-2 antigen and tisotumab vedotin targeting human tissue factor.

4. DNA damage repair. DNA damage response (DDR) pathway is a druggable target. The most glaring example is PARP inhibitors in BRCA1/2 mutated cancers. About 8% of HNSCC cases have alterations in the DDR related genes. There are several DDR pathway inhibitors targeting DNA damage signaling proteins like ATM, ATR, DNA-PK, WEE1, CHK1 and 2.

5. Tumor Mutational Burden (TMB). High tumor mutational burden is associated with increased expression of tumor specific antigens on the cancer cell surface making the cancer more immunogenic. About 25% HNSCC patients have high TMB having >20 mutations per mega-base of DNA making them susceptible to immunotherapy.

6. Dynamic Monitoring of tumor using ctDNA. As the cancer clinically evolves, it's genomic and molecular landscape changes. ctDNA are short fragments of double stranded DNA shed in the blood by the tumor undergoing necrosis and apoptosis. ctDNA may have mutational profile not seen in the normal cells and could represent the changing genomic landscape of tumor in vivo. Serial monitoring of ctDNA could help in detecting early relapse and help appropriately matched therapies to be delivered in real time.

7. FGFR2 and FGFR3 fusion occurs in 1-3% of HNSCC. These patients might benefit by FGFR inhibitors.

Several targeted drugs are being tested in clinical trials. Exhaustive review of these are beyond the scope of this chapter.

4.2 Molecular co-targeting strategies

HNSCC are genetically highly heterogenous. Monotherapies with targeted therapies yield modest benefit with eventual development of resistance. So, combining two or more molecularly targeted agents might emerge as effective therapy.

There could be several ways to do this; (1) targeting molecules within convergent signaling pathways, (2) targeting molecules with non-overlapping mechanisms of action, (3) targeting anti-tumorigenic molecules working synergistically with conventional chemotherapy or radiation therapy. Several clinical trials evaluating this strategy are listed below (**Table 4**) [5].

4.3 Molecular tumor boards in HNSCC

Most HNSCC will have complex genomes making it difficult to select therapy. This might not be corelating with traditional risk factors. There could be multiple driver mutations in a case or part of a tumor. E. g. a patient might be NOTCH1/PIK3CA double mutant. The question could be should this patient receive a WNT pathway inhibitor or PIK3CA inhibitor or both? The treating Head neck cancer clinician will have to document the genomic data, use of targeted drugs and record longitudinal follow up of each case to further develop use of NGS data in the clinic.

Multidisciplinary involvement of head neck surgeons, geneticists, medical oncologists, radiation oncologists, translational biologists will be integral to formulate personalized treatment approaches in head neck cancers.

Clinical trial	Intervention
NCT02124850	Cetuximab + motolimod + Nivolumab
NCT01218048	cetuximab + surgical resection + adjuvant cisplatin, carboplatin, radiation
NCT02277197	ficlatuzumab + Cetuximab
NCT 0957853	Cetuximab + anti IgG1 antibody + surgical resection
NCT 3153982	Ruxolitinib + Surgical resection
NCT02035527	Raf inhibitor + Doectaxel + cisplatin
NCT01051791	Everolimus
NCT01588431	Bevacizumab + Cetuximab + Docetaxel + Cisplatin followed by radiation/surgical resection
NCT02769520	Pembrolizumab
NCT01316757	Erlotinib + Cetuximab + paclitaxel + carboplatin
NCT01016769	Temsirolimus + Paclitaxel + Carboplatin
NCT02741570	nivolumab + ipilimumab + cetuximab + cisplatin + carboplatin +5fluracil
NCT02952586	Avelumab + cisplatin + radiation
NCT02499120	Cetuximab + Palbociclib

Table 4.
Clinical trials evaluating molecular co-targeting strategies.

European Society for Medical Oncology (ESMO) has a designed a scale (ESCAT) to guide the clinician to select a novel targeted drug with highest potential of efficacy in an HNSCC patient. The most Accordingly, compelling actionable molecular alterations in HNSCC included HRAS activating mutations (tipifarnib, farnesyl transferase inhibitor), MSI, high TMB (for immune check point inhibitors), NTRK fusions (TRK tyrosine kinase inhibitors), CDKN2A inactivating alterations (CDK 4/6 inhibitors) and EGFR amplification (afatinib) [63].

4.4 Big data in HNSCC

Big data approach is being explored in head neck oncology integrating data generated from genomic studies, radiomic data generated from CT, MRI and PET scans, data generated from clinical evaluation and optical imaging, data generated from radiation therapy response and toxicity and integration of all other non-genetic data such as epidemiology, diet, habits, stress, socioeconomic factors etc. There is a multicentric study BD2Decide (Big Data Models for personalized head neck cancer decision support) going on to explore Big Data approach. Three main goals for Big Data in HNSCC will be 1) support and augment clinical decisions, 2) generate new knowledge, 3) develop guidelines for HNSCC prevention and management [64].

5. Conclusions

HNSCC is genomically unstable. TCGA has identified key alterations in tumor suppressor genes and oncogenes in HNSCC. TP53 alteration is a key player in HNSCC tumorigenesis and biology. Principally loss of tumor suppressor drives tumorigenesis than oncogene addiction in HNSCC, however, a small subset of oral cavity cancer may be driven by mutations rather than loss of tumor suppressor gene function. Tumor heterogeneity is prominent in HNSCC and is a major challenge in developing effective therapies. Biologic classifier of HNSCC remains to be implemented in the clinic. Clustering of HNSCC according to multi-omics studies may be more clinically meaningful. Immune therapy is a major treatment paradigm in oncology in general including HNSCC. Corelative genomics and immune contexture will help realize the full potential of this approach. Sufficient indication exists linking major genomic alterations in HNSCC and clinical behavior including performance of conventional treatments. Opportunity exists to leverage this knowledge to fine tune currently existing surgical, radiation and chemotherapeutic approaches. EGFR targeting remains important in HNSCC in spite of lack of predictive biomarker and eventual treatment resistance. Mutli-omics studies have shed light on resistance to EGFR targeting and novel ways to target EGFR axis. Several studies are addressing genomically targeted monotherapies, molecular co targeting strategies and ways to escalate and deescalate treatment intensity based on biology. Time has come to implement molecular tumor boards in HNSCC regularly. BIG data approach will certainly help design multi-pronged approach to control HNSCC globally. Tissue repositories, participation in clinical trials and multi-institutional collaboration remains critical to further progress.

Conflict of interest

None.

Author details

Anand B. Pathak* and Satyam Satyarthi
Department of Medical Oncology, National Cancer Institute, Nagpur, India

*Address all correspondence to: cancercarengp@gmail.com

References

[1] Hyuna Sung' Jacques Ferlay' Rebecca L Siegel: Global Cancer Statistics 2020: GLOBOCAN Estimates of Incidence and Mortality Worldwide for 36 Cancers in 185 Countries. CA Cancer J Clin. 2021 May;71(3):209-249. doi: 10.3322/caac.21660

[2] Nature vol 517, 29 Jan 2015, 576-581

[3] Xiaohua Jiang, Jing Ye, Zhihuai Dong : Novel genetic alterations and their impact on target therapy response in head and neck squamous cell carcinoma. Cancer Management and Research 2019:11 1321-1336. Doi:10.2147/CMAR.5187780

[4] Zhi-Li Zhao, Lu Zhang, Cong-Fa Huang: NOTCH1 inhibition enhances the efficacy of conventional chemotherapeutic agents by targeting head neck cancer stem cell Scientific Reports volume 6, Article number: 24704 (2016

[5] (J D Kemmer, D E Johnson, J R Grandis. Leveraging Genomics for head and neck cancer treatment. Journal of Dental Research 2018, vol 97(6) 603-613). Doi:10.1177/0022034518756352

[6] Eoghan Malone and Lillian L Siu : Precision Medicine in Head and Neck Cancer: Myth or Reality? Clinical Medicine Insights: Oncology Volume 12: 1-7. DOI: 10.1177/117955491877958

[7] David M. Vossena, Caroline V.M. Verhagena, Marcel Verheij : Comparative Genomic Analysis of oral versus laryngeal and pharyngeal cancer. Oral Oncology 81(2018) 35-44

[8] Luc G T Morris' Raghu Chandramohan, Lyndsay West : The Molecular Landscape of recurrent and metastatic head neck cancers: Insights from a precision oncology sequencing platform. JAMA Oncol 3(2): 244-255

[9] Serge J. Smeets, Ruud H. Brakenhoff, Bauke Ylstra : Genetic classification of oral and oropharyngeal carcinomas identifies subgroups with a different prognosis Cell Oncol 2009;31(4): 291-300

[10] Swanton C.: Intratumor heterogeneity through space and time. Cancer Res 2012;73(19):4875-4882

[11] Chung CH, Parker JS, Karaca G : Molecular classification of head and neck squamous cell carcinomas using patterns of gene expression. Cancer Cell. 2004; 5(5):489-500

[12] Walter V, Yin X, Wilkerson MD : Molecular subtypes in head and neck cancer exhibit distinct patterns of chromosomal gain and loss of canonical cancer genes. PLoS One. 2013; 8(2): e56823

[13] Chen Huang, Lijun Chen, Sara R Savage : Proteogenomic Insights into the biology and treatment of HPV negative head and neck squamous cell carcinoma. 2021. Cancer Cell 361-379. Doi:10.1016/j.ccell 2020.12.007

[14] Thorsson, V.; Gibbs, D.L.; Brown, S.D : The Immune Landscape of Cancer. Immunity 2018, 48, 812-830 e814

[15] Tamborero, D.; Rubio-Perez, C.; Muinos, F. : A Pan-cancer Landscape of Interactions between Solid Tumors and Infiltrating Immune Cell Populations. Clin. Cancer Res. 2018, 24, 3717-3728

[16] Charles Schutt, Hua Sun, Jaya Sarin Pradhan : Genomic and neoantigen evolution from primary tumor to first metastases in head and neck squamous cell carcinoma. Oncotarget,2021, vol.12(No.6) pp:534-548

[17] Yao Yao, Zhongyi Yan, Senlin Lian: Prognostic Value of novel immune related genomic biomarkers identified

in head and neck squamous cell carcinoma. J Immunother Cancer 2020;8:e000444. Doi:10.1136/jitc-2019-000444

[18] Y.-P. Chen, Y.-Q. Wang, J.-W. Lv : Identification and validation of novel microenvironment-based immune molecular subgroups of head and neck squamous cell carcinoma: implications for immunotherapy. Annals of Oncology 30: 68-75, 2019 doi:10.1093/annonc/mdy470

[19] Bohai Feng and Jochen Hess : Immune-related mutational landscape and gene signatures: Prognostic value and therapeutic impact for head and neck cancer. Cancers2021,18,1162. DOI.org/10.3390/cancers13051162

[20] Hyung Kwon Byeon, Minhee Ku, Jaemoon Yang : Beyond EGFR Inhibition: multilateral combat strategies to stop the progression of head and neck cancer. Experimental & Molecular Medicine 2019, 51:8 doi: 10.1038/s12276-018-0202-2

[21] James A. Bonner, Paul M. Harari, Jordi Giralt: Radiotherapy plus Cetuximab for Squamous-Cell Carcinoma of the Head and Neck N Engl J Med 2006; 354:567-578. DOI: 10.1056/NEJMoa053422)10.1056/NEJMoa053422)

[22] Jean-Pascal H Machiels, Robert I Haddad, Jérôme Fayette : Afatinib versus methotrexate as second-line treatment in patients with recurrent or metastatic squamous-cell carcinoma of the head and neck progressing on or after platinum-based therapy (LUX-Head & Neck 1): an open-label, randomised phase 3 trial. Lancet Oncol 2015; 16: 583-94. doi.org/10.1016/S1470-2045(15)70124-5

[23] Ha PK, Benoit NE, Yochem R : A transcriptional progression model for head and neck cancer. Clin Cancer Res 2003;9:3058-3064

[24] Cromer A, Carles A, Millon R : Identification of genes associated with tumorigenesis and metastatic potential of hypopharyngeal cancer by microarray analysis. Oncogene 2004;23: 2484-2498

[25] Roepman P, Wessels LF, Kettelarij N: An expression profile for diagnosis of lymph node metastases from primary head and neck squamous cell carcinomas. Nat Genet 2005;37:182-186.

[26] Georgia Karpothiou, Marie-Laurie Stachowitz, Jean Marc Dumollard: Gene Expression comparison between the primary tumor and it's lymph node metastases in Head Neck Squmous cell carcinoma, a pilot Study. Cancer Genomics and Proteomics 16:155-161 (2019)

[27] Jose P. Zevallos, Angela L. Mazul Vonn Walter: Gene Expression Subtype predicts nodal metastases and survival in HPV negative head neck cancer. Laryngoscope 2019 January; 129(1): 154-161

[28] Ilda Patrícia Ribeiro, Francisco Caramelo, Luísa Esteves : Genomic predictive model for recurrence and metastasis development in head and neck squamous cell carcinoma patients Scientific reports | 7: 13897 | DOI:10.1038/s41598-017-14377-x

[29] Juncheng Wang, Xun Chen, Yuxi Tian : Six-gene signature for predicting survival in patients with head and neck squamous cell carcinoma January 2020 Aging 12(1) DOI:10.18632/aging.102655

[30] Ram Bhupal Reddy, Samanta S. Khora, Amritha Suresh : Molecular prognosticators in clinically and pathologically distinct cohorts of head and neck squamous cell carcinoma—A meta-analysis approach PLoS ONE 14(7): e0218989

[31] Antoine Galmiche, Zuzana Saidak, Jebrane Bouaoud : Genomics and

Precision Surgery for head neck squamous cell carcinoma. CanLet 481: 1July2020, 45-54

[32] Biswas NK, Das C, Das S, Maitra A, Nair S, Gupta T : Lymph node metastasis in oral cancer is strongly associated with chromosomal instability and DNA repair defects. Int J Cancer 2019;145: 2568-2579.

[33] van Hooff SR, Leusink FK, Roepman P : Validation of a gene expression signature for assessment of lymph node metastasis in oral squamous cell carcinoma. J Clin Oncol. 2012;30: 4104-4110.

[34] Zhang L, Poh CF, Williams M, Laronde DM : Loss of heterozygosity (LOH) profiles--validated risk predictors for progression to oral cancer. Cancer Prev Res (Phil). 2012;5: 1081-1089

[35] Goddard ET, Bozic I, Riddell SR, Ghajar CM. Dormant tumour cells, their niches and the influence of immunity. Nat Cell Biol. 2018;20:1240-1249.

[36] Wang W, Lim WK, Leong HS : An eleven gene molecular signature for extra-capsular spread in oral squamous cell carcinoma serves as a prognosticator of outcome in patients without nodal metastases. Oral Oncol. 2015;51:355-362

[37] Saidak Z, Clatot F, Chatelain D, Galmiche A : A gene expression profile associated with perineural invasion identifies a subset of HNSCC at risk of post-surgical recurrence. Oral Oncol. 2018;86:53-60.

[38] Saidak Z, Pascual C, Bouaoud J : A three-gene expression signature associated with positive surgical margins in tongue squamous cell carcinomas: Predicting surgical resectability from tumour biology? Oral Oncol. 2019;94:115-120

[39] Hayashi M, Wu G, Roh JL, Chang X : Correlation of gene methylation in surgical margin imprints with locoregional recurrence in head and neck squamous cell carcinoma. Cancer 2015;121:1957-1965.

[40] Liu SA, Wang CC, Jiang RS, Wang WY, Lin JC : Genetic analysis of surgical margins in oral cavity cancer. Br J Surg. 2018;105:e142-e149

[41] Ogbureke KU, Weinberger PM, Looney SW, Li L, Fisher LW : Expressions of matrix metalloproteinase-9 (MMP-9), dentin sialophosphoprotein (DSPP), and osteopontin (OPN) at histologically negative surgical margins may predict recurrence of oral squamous cell carcinoma. Oncotarget 2012;3:286-298

[42] Park J, Kim HJ, Kim KR, Lee SK, Kim H, Park KK, Chung WY : Loss of RUNX3 expression inhibits bone invasion of oral squamous cell carcinoma. Oncotarget 2017;8: 9079-9092

[43] Hanna GJ, Adkins DR, Zolkind P, Uppaluri R : Rationale for neoadjuvant immunotherapy in head and neck squamous cell carcinoma. Oral Oncol. 2017;73:65-69

[44] Uppaluri R, Zolkind P, Lin T, Nussenbaum B, Jackson RS : Neoadjuvant pembrolizumab in surgically resectable, locally advanced HPV negative head and neck squamous cell carcinoma (HNSCC). J Clin Oncol 2017;35(suppl.):6012.

[45] Horton JD, Knochelmann H, Kent Armeson : Neoadjuvant presurgical PD-1 inhibition in oral cavity squamous cell carcinoma. J Clin Oncol 2019; 37(suppl):2574.

[46] Zuur CL, Elbers JBW, Vos JL : Feasibility and toxicity of neoadjuvant nivolumab with or without ipilimumab prior to extensive (salvage) surgery in patients with advanced head and neck cancer (the IMCISION trial,

NCT03003637). J Clin Oncol 2019;37 (Suppl):2575.

[47] Saidak Z, Clatot F, Chatelain D, Galmiche A : A gene expression profile associated with perineural invasion identifies a subset of HNSCC at risk of post-surgical recurrence. Oral Oncol. 2018;86:53-60.

[48] Mroz EA, Patel KB, Rocco JW : Intratumor heterogeneity could inform the use and type of postoperative adjuvant therapy in patients with head and neck squamous cell carcinoma. Cancer 2020

[49] Davide B. Gissi, Achille Tarsitano, Andrea Gabusi : 13-gene DNA Methylation Analysis from Oral Brushing: A Promising Non Invasive Tool in the Follow-up of Oral Cancer Patients. J. Clin. Med. 2019, 8, 2107; doi:10.3390/jcm8122107

[50] Javier F. Torres-Roca, Steven Eschrich Haiyan Zhao : Prediction of Radiation Sensitivity using a gene expression classifier. Cancer Res 2005; 65: (16). August 15, 2005.

[51] Jimmy Pramana, Michiel W M Van Den Brekel, Marie-Louise F van Velthuysen : Gene expression profiling to predict outcome after chemoradiation in head and neck cancer. Inj J Radiat Oncol Biol Phys 2007 Dec 1;69(5):1544-1552 Doi: 10.1016/j.ijrobp.2007.08.032.

[52] Esrich SA, Praana J, Zhang H et : A gene expression model of intrinsic tumor radiosensitivity: prediction of response and prognosis after chemoradiation. Int J Radiat Oncol Biol Phys 2009; 75: 489-496. PubMed: 19735873

[53] Jacob G Scott, Anders Berglund, Michael J Schell : A genome-based model for adjusting radiotherapy dose(GARD): a retrospective, cohort-based study. Lancet Oncol. 2017 Feb: 18(2): 202-211. Doi: 10.1016/S1470-2045 (16)30648-9

[54] Toustrup K, Sorensen BS, Nordsmark M, et al : Development of a hypoxia gene expression classifier with predictive impact for hypoxic modification of radiotherapy in head and neck cancer. Cancer Res 2011; 71: 5923-5931. PubMed: 21846821

[55] Whitney Sumner, Xenia Ray, Leisa Sutton : Gene Alterations as predictors of radiation-induced toxicity in head and neck squamous cell carcinoma. J Transl Med 2021; 19: 212. Doi.10.1186/ s12967-021 -02876-5

[56] M. Giefing, M. Wierzbicka, K. Szyfter : Moving towards personalised therapy in head and neck squamous cell carcinoma through analysis of next generation sequencing data. European Journal of Cancer 55 (2016) 147e157. http://dx.doi.org/10.1016/j.ejca.2015. 10.0700

[57] Sanne R. Martens-de Kemp, Arjen Brink, Ida H. van der Meulen : FA/BRCA pathway identified as the major predictor of cisplatin response in head neck cancer by functional genomics.Mol Cancer Ther; 16(3) March 2017

[58] Goretti Duran, Santiago Aguín, Raquel Cruz : Association of GSTP1 and ERCC1 polymorphisms with toxicity in locally advanced head and neck cancer platinum-based chemoradiotherapy treatment Head & Neck. 2019;1-12 DOI: 10.1002/hed.25754

[59] Hiroyuki Shimomura, Tomonori Sasahira, Chie Nakashima : Non-SMC Condensin I Complex Subunit H (NCAPH) Is Associated with Lymphangiogenesis and Drug Resistance in Oral Squamous Cell Carcinoma. J. Clin. Med. 2020, 9, 72; doi:10.3390/jcm9010072

[60] Barbara Burtness [1], Kevin J Harrington [2], Richard Greil:

Pembrolizumab alone or with chemotherapy versus cetuximab with chemotherapy for recurrent or metastatic squamous cell carcinoma of the head and neck (KEYNOTE-048): a randomised, open-label, phase 3 study. Lancet 2019 Nov 23;394(10212):1915-1928. doi: 10.1016/S0140-6736 (19)32591-7

[61] R.L. Ferris, G. Blumenschein, Jr., J. Fayette: Nivolumab for Recurrent Squamous-Cell Carcinoma of the Head and Neck. N Engl J Med. 2016 Nov 10; 375(19): 1856-1867. PMID: 27718784

[62] Kerstin Zwirner, Franz J. Hilke, German Demidov: Radiogenomics in head and neck cancer: correlation of radiomic heterogeneity and somatic mutations in TP53, FAT1 and KMT2D 2. Strahlentherapie und Onkologie volume 195, pages771-779 (2019)

[63] Grégoire Marret, Ivan Bièche, Célia Dupain : Genomic Alterations in Head and Neck Squamous Cell Carcinoma: Level of Evidence According to ESMO Scale for Clinical Actionability of Molecular Targets (ESCAT) JCO Precision Oncology no. 5 (2021) 215-226.

[64] Carlo Restoghini, Analisa Trama, Elio Borgonovi.: Big Data in head and neck cancer. Curr. Treat. Options in Oncol (2018) 19:62

Chapter 4

Targeting Oncogene Addiction for Cancer Therapy

Sonia Thapa, Rafiq A. Rather, Shashank K. Singh and Madhulika Bhagat

Abstract

Oncogene addiction, a term first coined by Bernard Weinstein in 2000, refers to a condition where a tumor cell, despite harboring a multitude of genetic alterations, depends on a single oncogenic pathway or oncoprotein for sustained proliferation and survival. Several lines of evidence from mammalian cell culture models, genetically modified mice models, and human intervention trials of targeted drugs have revealed that many tumors, if not all, rely on oncogene addiction for sustained proliferation and survival. Oncogene addiction strongly impacts the therapeutic response of tumors to acute oncoprotein inhibition. An important implication of oncogene addiction is that inhibiting this critical pathway, on which cancer cells become dependent, can cause selective and specific cell death in cancer cells while sparing normal surrounding cells that are not oncogene addicted. However, the mechanism by which cancer cells become dependent on a single pathway or activated oncoprotein is not precisely understood in most cases. Thus, a better understanding of oncogene addiction may provide a rationale for improving current cancer therapies and help develop novel therapeutic strategies for the management of cancer.

Keywords: oncogene, oncogene addiction, cancer, targeted drugs, therapy

1. Introduction

Many cellular programs and signaling pathways that are normally used during development are reactivated and modified by cancer cells to acquire sustained proliferative characteristics. During embryogenesis and tissue homeostasis, these programs regulate coordinated actions, such as cell proliferation, cell polarity, migration, differentiation, and apoptosis. Cancer evolves with random mutations and epigenetic modifications in these pathways, followed by clonal selection of genetically altered cells that can survive and reproduce in conditions that would ordinarily be harmful [1]. Although several oncogenes (such as PI3K and RAS) and tumor suppressors (such as p53, PTEN, Rb, and p16INK4a) are typically altered in cancer cells, there appears to be a huge number of low-frequency genetic alterations that can contribute to tumorigenesis. Indeed, evidence from tumor sequencing initiatives reveals a staggering range of mutations in cancers [2]. The malignant phenotype of cancer cells depends significantly on the rewiring of metabolic pathways and survival pathways. As a result, identifying important functional nodes in the oncogenic signaling network whose blockage would result in system failure, that is, the end of the tumorigenic state via apoptosis, necrosis, senescence, or

IntechOpen

differentiation, is critical to successful therapy [3]. Furthermore, therapeutic drugs targeting these nodes must have a big enough therapeutic window to destroy tumor cells while sparing normal surrounding cells from damage. Many tumors are highly dependent on a single oncogenic pathway for sustained proliferation and survival, a condition known as oncogene addiction. The term "oncogene addiction" was first described by Bernard Weinstein to describe the dependence of certain tumor cells on a single activated oncoprotein or signaling pathway, despite harboring multiple gain-of-function mutations and loss-of-function mutations that contribute to the malignant phenotype, to maintain their malignant behavior [4]. Various xenograft models and genetically engineered mice models have revealed that many oncogene-driven tumors, if not all, undergo tumor regression, growth arrest, differentiation, and/or apoptosis in response to acute inhibition of oncoprotein function [5]. The process of oncogene addiction, irrespective of mechanistic basis, contributes significantly to the clinical activity of various drugs that have recently been observed following treatment with so-called "rationally-targeted" agents. The purpose of cancer therapeutics is to specifically target the mutations that initiate and maintain the proliferation and survival of cancer cells. Although the majority of cancers are known to possess multiple oncogenic mutations, many cancers are sensitive to targeted inhibition of a single oncogene, a phenomenon known as oncogene addiction [6]. Oncogene addiction supports the growth of cancer cells, signifying the role of oncogene-targeted therapies in cancer management. However, in many cases, resistance to oncogene-targeted therapies develops which limits the therapeutic targeting of oncogene addiction in clinical settings. Luckily, oncogene addiction offers several opportunities that can be utilized for achieving therapeutically useful outcomes [7]. Oncogene addiction is seen in several cancers. An important example is chronic myelogenous leukemia (CML), a disease driven by the BCR-ABL mutant oncogene. The mutant BCR-ABL fusion gene encodes for a type of enzyme known as tyrosine kinase which stimulates uncontrolled growth of leukemic cells. The addiction of CML to BCR-ABL is apparent from the profound clinical response of patients to imatinib, a drug that targets BCR-ABL. This addiction of CML to BCR-ABL is also noticeable from the reactivation of BCR-ABL kinase activity which imparts drug resistance to CML [8]. Observations of this type furnish proof for the concept of oncogene-targeted cancer therapy. It may appear insignificant that a tumor cell can be dependent on a single protein that contributed to the malignant phenotype at some time in its history. Somatic deletion of the KRAS oncogene in human colorectal cancer cells with a KRAS mutation causes reversion of the transformed phenotype and eliminates the capacity of these cells to develop tumors in nude mice [9]. Drugs targeting the appropriate proto-oncogene should be effective in treating cancers lacking the tumor suppressor in circumstances where a tumor suppressor negatively regulates the activity of a proto-oncogene. PI3K inhibitors are expected to be responsive in cancers that have lost the tumor suppressor and lipid phosphatase (PTEN), which acts to prevent PI3K activation [10]. Loss of Rb, p16, p21, or p27, for example, causes an increase in cyclin-dependent kinase (CDK) activity, which stimulates cell-cycle entrance. In theory, cancers arising from these genetic alterations may be more susceptible to CDK inhibitors. The fact that inactivating the normal counterpart of such oncogenic proteins in normal tissues is frequently tolerated with no apparent consequences underscores the distinct state of addiction that appears to occur in cancer. Switching off this critical pathway, on which cancer cells have become reliant, should have fatal consequences for cancer cells while protecting normal cells that are not similarly reliant. Of course, any effective cancer therapy requires this discriminating activity. There is no obvious positive signaling pathway to target in cases where the tumor suppressors p53 or ARF are lost, thus alternative therapeutic techniques must be investigated [11, 12].

2. Oncogene addiction

It is a process in which cancer cells become dependent on a single activated malignant gene or protein or pathway to maintain their malignant behavior [13]. Cancer cells have multiple genetic and epigenetic abnormalities. Besides this, they may depend on the single activated malignant gene for their sustained growth and proliferation. The concept of oncogene addiction emphasizes that the inactivation of this single gene or protein can provide a rationale for molecular targeted therapy [14]. The phenomenon of oncogene addiction is widely recognized as one of the major factors contributing to the impressive clinical activity observed after treatment with "rationally-targeted" agents [15, 16]. Oncogene addiction has been largely explained by three molecular models at the molecular level.

2.1 Genetic streamlining

This theory postulates that non-essential pathways are inactivated during tumor evolution so that the dominant or addictive pathways are not substituted by any compensatory signals. Therefore, when dominant signals are abrogated, there is a collapse in the whole cellular architecture of cancer cells and undergo cell cycle arrest and apoptosis [17].

2.2 Oncogenic shock model

In the "oncogenic shock" model, addictive oncoproteins (e.g., RTKs) trigger at the same time pro-survival and pro-apoptotic signals. Under normal conditions, the pro-survival signals dominate over the pro-apoptotic signals. Thus, subsequent to blockade of the addictive receptor or oncoprotein, the rapid decline in the activity of survival pathways subverts this balance in favor of death-inducing signals which tend to last longer and eventually lead to apoptotic death [17].

2.3 Synthetic lethality

Two genes are considered to be in a synthetic lethal relationship when loss of one or the other is still compatible with survival but the loss of both is fatal [17]. A majority of drugs used in cancer cure are targeted at genes and pathways that are mutated which limits the range of drugs that can be used for cancer treatment. Synthetic lethality exploits the fact that the presence of a mutation in a cancer gene is often associated with a new vulnerability that can be targeted therapeutically, thus considerably expanding the range of potential drug targets.

3. Activated kinases—The "Achilles' heel" of many cancers

Chronic oncogenic signaling may result in the inactivation of signaling pathways in cancer cells as a result of genetic drift at the biochemical and transcriptional levels. Indeed, a degree of reactive adaptation, such as activation of compensatory pathways and positive or negative feedback loops, is expected to offset the persistent activity of dominant oncogenes [18]. For example, the presence of "sensitive" and "indifferent" pathways addicted to the mesenchymal–epithelial transition factor (MET) oncogene can be observed in several cell lines. This protooncogene encodes the tyrosine kinase receptor for a hepatocyte growth factor (HGF) and is often used as a model addicting oncoprotein to explore potential and pitfalls stemming from the implementation of anticancer strategies targeting oncogene addiction [7]. Once activated, the MET receptor stimulates phosphatidylinositol 3-kinase (PI3K/AKT) and mitogen-activated protein kinase (ERK/MAPK) pathways, RAS, and STAT3. In these circumstances, MET or EGFR suppression causes a selective reduction of RAS- and PI3K-dependent cascades, whereas many other signals known to affect MET and EGFR-driven proliferation in non-addicted cells, such as JNK, p38, STATs, and NF-kB, remain active or show only minor responses [6]. In terms of genetic streamlining, this finding supports the idea that cancer cells have a significant number of inactive and functionally neutral pathways, as well as a small number of functionally active, self-sufficient transducers. The absence of buffering circuits and the existence of only a small number of functioning signaling nodes highlight the susceptibility of oncogene addiction state [8].

3.1 Molecular mechanism of oncogene addiction

The genetic streamlining hypothesis is derived from the well-established concept of natural selection, in which cancer cells undergo constant genetic drift as a result of the selective pressure exerted by the tumor microenvironment during the tumorigenic process [13, 19]. As a result, cancer cells may lose certain functions, which are unnecessary for cell survival or genome organization [20]. More precisely, at the molecular level, the tumor microenvironment may exert selective pressure over non-essential genes and may induce epigenetic modifications and have little effect on cell growth dynamics [13, 17].

Bernard Weinstein had proposed the synthetic lethal relationship concept of oncogene addiction, which states that two genes will be in a synthetically lethal relationship if one of either genes gets inactivated, rather than both, but still is compatible for cell survival [14]. Therefore, in these types of cancer cells, both the oncogene (that is activated and inactivated one) is believed to be in a synthetic lethal relationship with one another. Thus, under these conditions the elimination of the activated oncogene will lead to the death of cancer cell, but the same would not be observed in normal cells, which does not possess a synthetic lethal relationship [20, 21]. More specifically, cancer cells are more dependent on a particular oncogene in comparison with normal cells. Since there are various inactivated genes are found in cancer cells, which make them less adaptable [22, 23]. Even it is reported from *in vitro* studies that elimination of the critical oncogene cause death in cancer cells due to differential attenuation rates in the ratio of prosurvival and proapoptotic signals, a phenomenon known as "oncogene shock" [15].

Oncogene addiction has been recently proposed as "lineage survival oncogenes". Since it is recognized for years that there is a close nexus between cell lineage and cancer phenotype, which during the development govern lineage proliferation and survival, might also underlie tumorigenic mechanisms [24]. Even many somatic genetic alterations express lineage-restricted patterns in cancer cells, which clearly indicates the genetic alteration in cancer might be conditioned by the lineage programs that exist in tumor precursor cells. There are genes termed as lineage-survival oncogenes which comprise master regulatory genes and are presumed to promote tumor progression. For example, transcription factor MITF in melanoma and androgen receptors in prostate cancer are listed as prototype lineage-survival oncogenes [25, 26].

3.2 Oncogenic shock model

Oncogenic shock model is a concept proposed by Settleman and colleagues in order to explain the death of oncogene addicted cancer cells via inhibition of the addicted oncoprotein. *In vitro* studies revealed that there is an imbalance in the duality of pro-survival and pro-apoptotic signals overexposure to kinase inhibitor drugs [27]. MYC oncogene possesses apoptosis-inducing properties and can be inhibited by PI3K/AKT pathway activation or by the overexpression of anti-apoptotic BCL-2 protein but normally, the pro-apoptotic function of MYC is evident during the development, since it causes negative selection of T-lymphocytes upon antigen stimulation [28, 29]. It is believed that c-MYC induces cell death through distinct "death priming" and "death triggering" events in which "death priming" and mitogenic signals are well coordinated.

The oncogenic shock hypothesis relies on the experimental observation that targeted disruption of signal-generating oncoproteins results in differential kinetics of downstream signal decay: anti-apoptotic effectors (such as ERKs, AKT) display rapid diminution of activity; while death-inducing molecules (such as p38) display delayed accumulation [17, 30]. This temporal imbalance has been demonstrated in a variety of cellular systems driven by oncogenically active tyrosine kinases, including BCR-ABL, SRC, and EGFR [31]. The oncogenic shock hypothesis deserves at least two comments. First, it postulates that the apoptotic response observed following the abrogation of addictive oncoproteins is an active process of signal-mediated induction of cell death; this is in contrast to the passive occurrence of signal deprivation predicted in the genetic streamlining model. Second, the "potency" of the oncogenic signal in generating pro-survival and pro-apoptotic outputs seems to be more crucial than the temporal appearance of the dominant genetic lesion [32]. While it can be intuitive to think that an initiating oncogene will be more influential as a dominant alteration than genetic lesions occurring subsequently during tumor evolution, we can also reasonably argue that addictive oncogenes with powerful pro-apoptotic activity are likely to arise late during the tumor's natural history when at least some apoptotic safeguards have been disengaged; otherwise, cells would die, and oncogene hyperactivity would be negatively selected [9, 15].

4. Salient features of oncogene addiction

Malignant cells are thoroughly dependent on a particular protooncogene and/or tumor suppressor gene for their proliferation and survival [21]. The inhibition of addicted oncogenes via RNA interference (RNAi) or chemical inhibitors would cause apoptosis in oncogene-addicted cancer cells, but not in other cells. For example, imatinib (Gleevec, a BCR-ABL1 kinase inhibitor) and gefitinib (Iressa, an EGFR inhibitor) are typical examples of drugs successfully targeted to the appropriate molecules and are effective for the treatment of chronic myeloid leukemia (CML) and non-small cell lung cancer (NSCLC), respectively [21]. Oncogene may play a more essential and qualitatively different role in a given pathway or "module" in cancer cells compared with its role in normal cells [21]. Although with limitations, targeting oncogene addiction is clinically significant in the therapeutics of many cancers. For example, a very high percentage of anaplastic lymphoma kinase (ALK) mutated lung tumors, BRAF mutant melanomas, and EGFR mutant non-small cell lung cancers respond to drugs that selectively inhibit these mutationally activated kinases (**Table 1**) [21]. During a clinical trial investigating the efficacy of imatinib in blast-crisis CML patients, the issue of acquired resistance to targeted anticancer treatments initially surfaced. Following that, substantial rates of mutations in the BCR-ABL gene were discovered in individuals who developed insensitivity to imatinib despite initial remission [38]. T315I, commonly known as the "gatekeeper" mutation, was discovered to obstruct the insertion of the drug into the ATP-binding pocket of the ABL-kinase via steric hindrance while maintaining kinase activity,

Targeted oncogene	Cancer cell line	References
Cyclin D1	Esophagus, colon, pancreas, squamous	[33]
β-Catenin	Colon	[13]
Cyclin E	Liver	[34]
Mutant B-RAF	Melanoma	[35]
Mutant K-RAS	Pancreas	[36]
HER-2	Breast	[37]

Table 1.
Examples of oncogene addiction.

resulting in drug insensitivity [39]. Other mutations that inhibit drug binding by disrupting the conformational changes essential for appropriate interaction between the drug and the kinase active site have also been discovered [40]. Novel drugs targeting the mutant form of the protein, such as dasatinib and nilotinib are the only inhibitors that can block the activity of the T315I BCR-ABL mutation. These drugs have been developed to treat relapsed CML patients who have developed resistance to imatinib [40, 41]. The acquisition of secondary mutations that prevent drug binding to the target kinase catalytic site, which has been shown for a range of oncogene-addicted cancers, including EGFR in NSCLC, has been highlighted as a recurrent theme in the landscape of targeted therapy [42].

5. Acquired drug resistance and oncogene addiction

The primary mechanism of acquired resistance to epidermal growth factor receptor (EGFR) tyrosine kinase inhibitors (TKIs) is the acquisition of a secondary mutation in exon 20 of the EGFR gene which results in threonine to methionine substitution at position 790 and has been found to account for ~50% of tumors with acquired resistance to EGFR TKIs which include afatinib, dacomitinib, erlotinib, gefitinib, and osimertinib. Another mechanism of resistance found in NSCLC tumors resistant to gefitinib is an amplification of the gene encoding the MET receptor [43]. Overall, resistance mechanisms that appear to act either vertically or horizontally can bypass targeting the addictive oncoprotein in cancer cells: in the first scenario, acquired lesions at the level of the inhibited oncoprotein re-stabilize previously inactivated signaling pathways (e.g., T790M mutation within the EGFR gene), while in the latter, parallel signaling axes are active. Importantly, variability across cancer cell populations could indicate the availability of pre-existing insensitive subclones that could be selected by drug treatment, perhaps leading to acquired resistance mechanisms [44, 45].

Some combinatorial techniques that target multiple tumor vulnerabilities at the same time could be useful in preventing or delaying the formation of resistance mechanisms [46]. Indeed, apoptosis may prevail in systems driven by growth inhibitory signals that gradually shut down after specific oncogene activity is disrupted. Resistance mechanisms could emerge in systems with quick removal of pro-apoptotic signals emitted by the targeted oncoprotein, allowing escape from apoptosis and allowing time for survival signaling pathways to re-establish [47]. According to the findings, BRAF-mediated activation of the SPRY family of RTK inhibitory proteins occurs, meaning that targeted suppression of BRAF activity causes survival signaling to decay, which then reduces SPRY-mediated inhibition of RTK activity [48].

The MET signaling pathway has been discovered to have critical roles in a variety of physiological and developmental cellular processes, in addition to its involvement as an oncogene in several human cancers. Indeed, epithelial cells from a range of organs, including the kidney, liver, muscle, pancreas, prostate, and bone marrow, have been shown to express it. Under physiological conditions, the interaction between MET and its ligand HGF, which is secreted by cells of mesenchymal origin, activates the morphogenetic program known as "invasive growth" (also known as "cell scattering"), which is critical for epithelial growth, morphogenesis, and differentiation during embryogenesis, thus acting as a master developmental regulator [49, 50]. MET and its ligand are required for organ protection and regeneration after injury, recruitment in adult hematopoiesis, and regulation of bone remodeling during adulthood, in addition to their crucial involvement during organ development [51]. Regenerating hepatic skeletal muscle and infarcted myocardium are two examples of the aforementioned circumstances. Furthermore, MET has been found to play a critical function in immune system modulation [52]. The principle that some tumors rely on a single oncoprotein for continuous growth and the conclusion that this oncoprotein is the target for therapeutic intervention has emerged as a master rule in translational cancer research over the last decade, providing a rational framework for developing new targeted compounds for the treatment of various cancer types. A series of successful clinical trials demonstrating the efficacy of targeted treatments when administered correctly in selected cohorts of patients with oncogene-addicted tumors attest to this line of action [1].

5.1 BCR-ABL in chronic myeloid leukemia

It was first identified as a cytogenetic abnormality correlated with chronic myelogenous leukemia (CML) by Nowell and Hungerford in 1960. The fusion transcript of the breakpoint cluster region (BCR) and the gene coding for the Abelson tyrosine kinase (ABL) in Philadelphia (Ph) chromosome is produced many years after the chromosome translocation could actually be confirmed [53]. Several subsequent studies reported that BCR-ALB possesses a crucial role in the pathogenesis and maintenance of chronic myelogenous leukemia (CML); indeed, it was the first oncogene that could be considered addictive before the concept of oncogene addiction became popular. Then, as it should be expected, much effort was devoted to research on chemical compounds that could inhibit BCR-ABL. The results of subsequent clinical studies confirmed that almost 100% of patients experienced complete hematologic responses [54]. The magnitude and frequency of clinical responses were remarkably high even when trials were conducted on patients going through blast crisis, indicating that BCR-ABL continued to serve as causative factors in sustaining malignant proliferation throughout the disease. In approximately 90% of gastrointestinal stromal tumors (GISTs), activating mutations in the KIT gene have been identified, whereas 35% have to activate mutations in platelet-derived growth factor receptor alpha (PDGFRA) [55]. Imatinib can be effectively used in advanced solid tumors, where the functional significance of driver mutations does not yet make much sense because the late-stage disease is characterized by an increasingly demystifying landscape of driver mutations [55].

In the context of cancer treatment, imatinib represented a paradigm shift: medical oncologists had to contend with the concept that cancer is partly a genetic disease, both at the molecular level and therapeutically [56]. A small-molecule inhibitor was synthesized and characterized very thoroughly in the development of imatinib. Unlike many traditional chemotherapeutic drugs, imatinib was not discovered by chance. It was designed by collaborating academics and industrialists for years [57, 58].

The overexpression of the HER2 protein in breast cancers is a consequence of gene amplification, which is associated with a poor prognosis in 25–30% of cases. The fact that a genetically altered with a prognostic significance also plays a causal role in sustaining mammary malignant phenotypes was shown to be further evidence that HER2 amplification plays a driving role in tumors development [59, 60].

Humanized monoclonal antibodies targeting the extracellular domain of HER2 were the first agents that inhibited HER2 activity clinically. Breast cancer HER2 amplification and CML BCR-ABL translocation share the same basis (an inherited genetic defect). The characteristic of the disease that predicts response to imatinib is highly prevalent in the patients with CML: almost all patients display the mutation that predicts response to the drug, and almost all of them respond to the drug. Amplification of HER2 defines only a subset of breast cancers, and responses are found only in a fraction of cases in HER2-amplified tumors. Together, these features highlight the addictive power of HER2 amplification in breast cancer [61, 62]. The so-called "primary" or "de novo" resistance of HER2-alternative pathways dominates the hyperactivation of HER2 or blunts the detectability of HER2-dependent signals in trastuzumab-resistant tumors [63]. In addition, parallel activation of PI3K-based transduction cascades and the overexpression of EGF family ligands are examples of parallel activation of IGF1 receptor signaling. In line with these findings, a functional RNAi screen identified PTEN down-regulation as a mechanism for trastuzumab resistance. Mutations in the PIK3CA gene, loss of function of PTEN are responsible for activation of the PI3K pathway [64, 65].

The important revelation that certain EGFR kinase domain-activating mutations were strongly linked with objective response to receptor blockade was made after retrospective genetic analysis of NSCLCs in responders and non-responders. The importance of mutationally activated kinases as anti-cancer therapeutic targets was once again underscored by this association [66, 67]. The major takeaway message from this example is that targeted inhibition of tyrosine kinases is only successful in a small subset of patients in some instances, and kinase mutations are necessary predictors for patient stratification. Furthermore, the rarity of genetically characterized responsive patient subsets raises the concern that a reliable portrayal of genetic variation necessitates a far larger sample of patients within a cancer type than previously anticipated [68, 69]. This could be related to other changes in the EGFR coding sequence, such as minor exon 20 insertions or deletions, or uncommon mutations coexisting with typical activating mutations [70]. The use of crizotinib, a small molecule inhibitor of anaplastic lymphoma kinase (ALK) in NSCLC patients is the most current insight into the successful therapeutic use of the oncogene addiction principle. The fusion protein contains a constitutively active ALK and has tumorigenic potential, according to biochemical and functional tests [71, 72].

When a clinical trial of imatinib in blast-crisis CML patients revealed that some subjects developed clinical insensitivity to the drug after a dramatic but brief remission, the formation of secondary (acquired) resistance at some point during therapy became clear. According to preliminary research, the average chronic-phase patient using imatinib had a 10% chance of relapsing into blast crisis every year [73]. The BCR-ABL gene has a significant incidence of mutations, according to an analysis of BCR-ABL sequences in myeloid clones of patients with the imatinib-resistant, relapsing illness. The prototypical amino-acid change (T315I) causes a steric barrier in the ATP-binding pocket of the ATP-binding pocket of the kinase [74]. Other mutations impede imatinib binding by locking the BCR-ABL kinase domain in an active state [75].

Chemicals that can bind to this conformation should be able to achieve their full inhibitory potential in this circumstance. Dasatinib (Sprycel, Bristol-Myers Squibb)

Target	Disease	Agent	Regimen
HER-2	Breast	Trastuzumab	Combination
BCR/ABL	CML	Imatinib	Monotherapy
C-KIT	Stromal Tumor	Imatinib	Monotherapy
EGFR	NSCLC	Gefitinib Erlotinib	Monotherapy
EGFR	Pancreas	Erlotinib	Combination
VEGF	Breast Kidney	Bevacizumab	Combination

Table 2.
Clinical evidence of oncogene addiction.

and nilotinib (Tasigna, Novartis) are two compounds that have this feature and are being utilized to treat relapse, resistant CML patients [76]. Imatinib resistance is caused by amplification of the BCR-ABL gene, which results in elevated levels of the matching protein product in a minority of cases. Secondary resistance has been described for various targets and in different oncogene-addicted tumors, including mutant EGFR and EML4-ALK in NSCLCs and mutant c-KIT in GISTs, as well as the acquisition of secondary mutations that inhibit drug binding to the kinase catalytic cleft. Alternatively, other oncogenes can be genetically altered to create aberrant signaling in place of the suppressed target's pathways that are no longer maintained [77, 78]. There are several examples that provide clinical evidence for oncogene addiction and the treatment regimen may involve a single agent (monotherapy) or combination of several drug agents (combination) (**Table 2**).

Resistance-inducing mutations have also been found in relapsed patients' tumor tissue. The inactivated target is bypassed in all of these examples by compensating lesions that may act vertically or horizontally: in the former, secondary alterations within the same upstream target re-stimulate the downstream signaling flux along with the same, previously inhibited pathway; in the latter, parallel axes are activated to replace the block [79–81]. Under the selection pressure of medication exposure, genetic instability may fuel the emergence of oncogenic lesions that have been evolutionarily chosen to drive cancer survival and growth [81].

6. Non-oncogene addiction (NOA)

In addition to oncogene addiction, several other examples of non-oncogene addiction have been reported in the literature. The concept of non-oncogene addiction (NOA) is based on the idea that tumorigenicity is dependent on the activity of a wide range of genes and pathways, many of which are not inherently oncogenic [82]. These genes and pathways are essential to maintain the oncogenic phenotype of cancer cells, but not to the same extent for normal cell viability. These dependencies should yield a large number of pharmacological targets that, when inhibited, will cause synthetic lethality with the underlying tumor genotype. Anti-tumor medicines can take use of NOA genes and pathways. Tumor-intrinsic and tumor-extrinsic NOA genes are the two types of NOA genes. Tumor-intrinsic NOA genes support the tumor cell's oncogenic state in a cell-autonomous way, whereas tumor-extrinsic NOA genes function in stromal and vascular cells, providing heterotypic support for the tumor. Targeting these accessory cells has the advantage of being genetically more stable than tumor cells, which means they are less likely to develop drug resistance. However, tumors may be able to evolve a reduced reliance on these accessory cells in some circumstances [82–84].

7. Conclusion

Oncogene addiction is a phenomenon in which tumor cells develop a dependency on a driver oncogenic product that plays a role in nurturing and fueling the malignant phenotype, laying the groundwork for the development of anticancer therapies that target single oncoproteins in specific cancer patient populations. Despite their exceptional translational impact, clinical application of molecularly targeted anticancer treatments demonstrated the establishment of similar resistance mechanisms across most tumor subtypes, which severely reduces the benefit of oncoprotein-targeted therapy. These recurring resistance mechanisms must be thoroughly investigated in order to block disease progression or at least predict the disease progression. Combinations of several drugs may provide greater therapeutic benefit and postpone the establishment of resistance mechanisms in such situations. Cancer cells' ability to quickly adapt to their surroundings and clonal heterogeneity are essential features of human malignancies. The increased ability to understand, and so forecast, cancer evolution in response to therapy in order to accompany it to the intended destination, we believe, will be a major step toward the creation of more successful anticancer therapies. In years to come, the ability of cancer cells to evolve will continue to challenge researchers. Consequently, our approach to cancer therapy will also need to evolve.

Acknowledgements

ST is thankful to University Grants Commission, New Delhi, India for Junior Research Fellowship (UGC-JRF). RAR is grateful to the SERB-National Postdoctoral Fellowship program and *Science and Engineering Research Board*, *Department of Science and Technology*, New Delhi, India (Grant Number: PDF/2016/002730) for financial support.

Author contributions

RAR and ST conceived the idea. ST wrote the chapter with assistance of RAR, SKK, and MB. All authors contributed to the writing of the chapter and approved the final submitted version.

Conflict of interest

The authors have declared that there are no conflicts of interest.

Author details

Sonia Thapa[1,2], Rafiq A. Rather[3]*, Shashank K. Singh[1,2] and Madhulika Bhagat[3]

1 Cancer Pharmacology Division, CSIR-Indian Institute of Integrative Medicine, Jammu, Jammu and Kashmir, India

2 Academy of Scientific and Innovative Research (AcSIR), Ghaziabad, Uttar Pradesh, India

3 School of Biotechnology, University of Jammu, Jammu, Jammu and Kashmir, India

*Address all correspondence to: rafiqueahmadd@gmail.com

References

[1] Pagliarini R, Shao W, Sellers WR. Oncogene addiction: Pathways of therapeutic response, resistance, and road maps toward a cure. EMBO Reports. 2015;**16**(3):280-296

[2] Gutierrez A, Look AT. NOTCH and PI3K-AKT pathways intertwined. Cancer Cell. 2007;**12**(5):411-413

[3] Yuan T, Cantley L. PI3K pathway alterations in cancer: Variations on a theme. Oncogene. 2008;**27**(41): 5497-5510

[4] Grant S. Cotargeting survival signaling pathways in cancer. The Journal of Clinical Investigation. 2008; **118**(9):3003-3006

[5] Palomero T et al. Mutational loss of PTEN induces resistance to NOTCH1 inhibition in T-cell leukemia. Nature Medicine. 2007;**13**(10):1203-1210

[6] Suda K et al. Conversion from the "oncogene addiction" to "drug addiction" by intensive inhibition of the EGFR and MET in lung cancer with activating EGFR mutation. Lung Cancer. 2012;**76**(3):292-299

[7] Comoglio PM, Giordano S, Trusolino L. Drug development of MET inhibitors: Targeting oncogene addiction and expedience. Nature Reviews Drug Discovery. 2008;**7**(6): 504-516

[8] Pellicano F, Mukherjee L, Holyoake TL. Concise review: Cancer cells escape from oncogene addiction: Understanding the mechanisms behind treatment failure for more effective targeting. Stem Cells. 2014;**32**(6): 1373-1379

[9] Garber K. New Insights Into Oncogene Addiction Found. JNCI: Journal of the National Cancer Institute. 2007;**99**(4):263-269

[10] Gallipoli P, Abraham SA, Holyoake TL. Hurdles toward a cure for CML: The CML stem cell. Hematology/ Oncology Clinics. 2011;**25**(5):951-966

[11] Harper JW, Elledge SJ. Cdk inhibitors in development and cancer. Current Opinion in Genetics & Development. 1996;**6**(1):56-64

[12] Malumbres M et al. CDK inhibitors in cancer therapy: What is next? Trends in Pharmacological Sciences. 2008; **29**(1):16-21

[13] Weinstein IB, Joe AK. Mechanisms of disease: Oncogene addiction—A rationale for molecular targeting in cancer therapy. Nature Clinical Practice Oncology. 2006;**3**(8):448-457

[14] Weinstein IB, Joe A. Oncogene addiction. Cancer Research. 2008; **68**(9):3077-3080

[15] Sharma SV, Settleman J. Oncogene addiction: Setting the stage for molecularly targeted cancer therapy. Genes & Development. 2007;**21**(24): 3214-3231

[16] Sawyers CL. Shifting paradigms: The seeds of oncogene addiction. Nature Medicine. 2009;**15**(10):1158-1161

[17] Torti D, Trusolino L. Oncogene addiction as a foundational rationale for targeted anti-cancer therapy: Promises and perils. EMBO Molecular Medicine. 2011;**3**(11):623-636

[18] Tsai C-J, Nussinov R. The molecular basis of targeting protein kinases in cancer therapeutics. Seminars in Cancer Biology. 2013;**23**:235-242

[19] Salgueiro L et al. Acquisition of chromosome instability is a mechanism to evade oncogene addiction. EMBO Molecular Medicine. 2020;**12**(3):e10941

[20] Luo J, Solimini NL, Elledge SJ. Principles of cancer therapy: Oncogene and non-oncogene addiction. Cell. 2009;**136**(5):823-837

[21] Bellovin DI, Das B, Felsher DW. Tumor dormancy, oncogene addiction, cellular senescence, and self-renewal programs. Advances in Experimental Medicine and Biology. 2013;**734**:91-107

[22] Hübner A, Jaeschke A, Davis RJ. Oncogene addiction: Role of signal attenuation. Developmental Cell. 2006;**11**(6):752-754

[23] McCormick F. Cancer therapy based on oncogene addiction. Journal of Surgical Oncology. 2011;**103**(6):464-467

[24] Garraway LA, Sellers WR. Lineage dependency and lineage-survival oncogenes in human cancer. Nature Reviews Cancer. 2006;**6**(8):593-602

[25] Garraway L et al. "Lineage addiction" in human cancer: Lessons from integrated genomics. Cold Spring Harbor Symposia on Quantitative Biology. 2005;**70**:25-34

[26] Jonkers J, Berns A. Oncogene addiction: Sometimes a temporary slavery. Cancer Cell. 2004;**6**(6):535-538

[27] Sharma SV et al. "Oncogenic shock": Explaining oncogene addiction through differential signal attenuation. Clinical Cancer Research. 2006;**12**(14): 4392s-4395s

[28] Hatzi E et al. N-myc oncogene overexpression down-regulates IL-6; evidence that IL-6 inhibits angiogenesis and suppresses neuroblastoma tumor growth. Oncogene. 2002;**21**(22): 3552-3561

[29] Hawksworth D et al. Overexpression of C-MYC oncogene in prostate cancer predicts biochemical recurrence. Prostate Cancer and Prostatic Diseases. 2010;**13**(4):311-315

[30] Sharma SV, Settleman J. Exploiting the balance between life and death: Targeted cancer therapy and "oncogenic shock". Biochemical Pharmacology. 2010;**80**(5):666-673

[31] Wang Y, McAlpine S. C-terminal heat shock protein 90 modulators produce desirable oncogenic properties. Organic & Biomolecular Chemistry. 2015;**13**(16):4627-4631

[32] Jubair L, McMillan NA. The therapeutic potential of CRISPR/Cas9 systems in oncogene-addicted cancer types: Virally driven cancers as a model system. Molecular Therapy-Nucleic Acids. 2017;**8**:56-63

[33] Musgrove EA et al. Cyclin D as a therapeutic target in cancer. Nature Reviews Cancer. 2011;**11**(8):558-572

[34] Liang Y et al. siRNA-based targeting of cyclin E overexpression inhibits breast cancer cell growth and suppresses tumor development in breast cancer mouse model. PLoS One. 2010;**5**(9): e12860

[35] Hall A et al. Dysfunctional oxidative phosphorylation makes malignant melanoma cells addicted to glycolysis driven by the V600EBRAF oncogene. Oncotarget. 2013;**4**(4):584

[36] O'Leary K. Tracing the origins of KRAS oncogene addiction. Nature Reviews Cancer. 2021;**21**(2):69-69

[37] Savas P et al. Oncogene addiction and immunity: Clinical implications of tumour infiltrating lymphocytes in breast cancers overexpressing the HER2/neu oncogene. Current Opinion in Oncology. 2014;**26**(6):562-567

[38] Engelman JA, Settleman J. Acquired resistance to tyrosine kinase inhibitors during cancer therapy. Current Opinion in Genetics & Development. 2008; **18**(1):73-79

[39] Choi HG et al. A type-II kinase inhibitor capable of inhibiting the T315I "gatekeeper" mutant of Bcr-Abl. Journal of Medicinal Chemistry. 2010;**53**(15): 5439-5448

[40] Gibbons DL et al. The rise and fall of gatekeeper mutations? The BCR-ABL1 T315I paradigm. Cancer. 2012; **118**:293-299

[41] Liu J et al. Recent advances in Bcr-Abl tyrosine kinase inhibitors for overriding T315I mutation. Chemical Biology & Drug Design. 2021;**97**(3): 649-664

[42] Ichihara E et al. Clinical significance of repeat rebiopsy in detecting the EGFR T790M secondary mutation in patients with non-small cell lung cancer. Oncotarget. 2018;**9**(50):29525

[43] Sasaki T et al. A novel ALK secondary mutation and EGFR signaling cause resistance to ALK kinase inhibitors. Cancer Research. 2011; **71**(18):6051-6060

[44] Xia H, Hui KM. Mechanism of cancer drug resistance and the involvement of noncoding RNAs. Current Medicinal Chemistry. 2014;**21**(26):3029-3041

[45] Ramos P, Bentires-Alj M. Mechanism-based cancer therapy: Resistance to therapy, therapy for resistance. Oncogene. 2015;**34**(28): 3617-3626

[46] Pauwels E et al. Multidrug resistance in cancer: Its mechanism and its modulation. Drug News & Perspectives. 2007;**20**(6):371-377

[47] Housman G et al. Drug resistance in cancer: An overview. Cancers. 2014; **6**(3):1769-1792

[48] Zaman A, Wu W, Bivona TG. Targeting oncogenic BRAF: Past, present, and future. Cancers. 2019; **11**(8):1197

[49] Organ SL, Tsao M-S. An overview of the c-MET signaling pathway. Therapeutic Advances in Medical Oncology. 2011;**3**(1_suppl):S7-S19

[50] Peruzzi B, Bottaro DP. Targeting the c-Met signaling pathway in cancer. Clinical Cancer Research. 2006;**12**(12): 3657-3660

[51] Eder JP et al. Novel therapeutic inhibitors of the c-Met signaling pathway in cancer. Clinical Cancer Research. 2009;**15**(7):2207-2214

[52] Jung KH, Park BH, Hong S-S. Progress in cancer therapy targeting c-Met signaling pathway. Archives of Pharmacal Research. 2012;**35**(4): 595-604

[53] Hughes T, Branford S. Molecular monitoring of BCR–ABL as a guide to clinical management in chronic myeloid leukaemia. Blood Reviews. 2006; **20**(1):29-41

[54] Weisberg E et al. Second generation inhibitors of BCR-ABL for the treatment of imatinib-resistant chronic myeloid leukaemia. Nature Reviews Cancer. 2007;7(5):345-356

[55] Jeffs AR et al. The BCR gene recombines preferentially with Alu elements in complex BCR-ABL translocations of chronic myeloid leukaemia. Human Molecular Genetics. 1998;7(5):767-776

[56] Shekarian T et al. Paradigm shift in oncology: Targeting the immune system rather than cancer cells. Mutagenesis. 2015;**30**(2):205-211

[57] La Thangue NB, Kerr DJ. Predictive biomarkers: A paradigm shift towards personalized cancer medicine. Nature reviews Clinical oncology. 2011; **8**(10):587-596

[58] Madden DL. From a patient advocate's perspective: Does cancer immunotherapy represent a paradigm shift? Current Oncology Reports. 2018;**20**(1):1-7

[59] Neve R, Lane H, Hynes N. The role of overexpressed HER2 in transformation. Annals of Oncology. 2001;**12**:S9-S13

[60] Yano T et al. Comparison of HER2 gene amplification assessed by fluorescence in situ hybridization and HER2 protein expression assessed by immunohistochemistry in gastric cancer. Oncology Reports. 2006; **15**(1):65-71

[61] Kurebayashi J. Biological and clinical significance of HER2 overexpression in breast cancer. Breast Cancer. 2001;**8**(1):45-51

[62] Ménard S et al. Role of HER2 gene overexpression in breast carcinoma. Journal of Cellular Physiology. 2000;**182**(2):150-162

[63] Baselga J, Albanell J. Mechanism of action of anti-HER2 monoclonal antibodies. Annals of Oncology. 2001;**12**:S35-S41

[64] Samuels Y et al. High frequency of mutations of the PIK3CA gene in human cancers. Science. 2004;**304**:554

[65] Bachman KE et al. The PIK3CA gene is mutated with high frequency in human breast cancers. Cancer Biology & Therapy. 2004;**3**(8):772-775

[66] Zhou W et al. Novel mutant-selective EGFR kinase inhibitors against EGFR T790M. Nature. 2009;**462**(7276):1070-1074

[67] Pao W et al. Acquired resistance of lung adenocarcinomas to gefitinib or erlotinib is associated with a second mutation in the EGFR kinase domain. PLoS Medicine. 2005;**2**(3):e73

[68] Krause DS, Van Etten RA. Tyrosine kinases as targets for cancer therapy. New England Journal of Medicine. 2005;**353**(2):172-187

[69] Schlessinger J. Cell signaling by receptor tyrosine kinases. Cell. 2000;**103**(2):211-225

[70] Hubbard SR. Juxtamembrane autoinhibition in receptor tyrosine kinases. Nature Reviews Molecular Cell Biology. 2004;**5**(6):464-471

[71] Webb TR et al. Anaplastic lymphoma kinase: Role in cancer pathogenesis and small-molecule inhibitor development for therapy. Expert Review of Anticancer Therapy. 2009;**9**(3):331-356

[72] Ai X et al. An interaction map of small-molecule kinase inhibitors with anaplastic lymphoma kinase (ALK) mutants in ALK-positive non-small cell lung cancer. Biochimie. 2015; **112**:111-120

[73] Lübbert C et al. Rapid emergence of secondary resistance to gentamicin and colistin following selective digestive decontamination in patients with KPC-2-producing *Klebsiella pneumoniae*: A single-centre experience. International Journal of Antimicrobial Agents. 2013;**42**(6):565-570

[74] Gorre ME et al. Clinical resistance to STI-571 cancer therapy caused by BCR-ABL gene mutation or amplification. Science. 2001; **293**(5531):876-880

[75] Nardi V, Azam M, Daley GQ. Mechanisms and implications of imatinib resistance mutations in BCR-ABL. Current Opinion in Hematology. 2004;**11**(1):35-43

[76] Quintás-Cardama A, Kantarjian H, Cortes J. Flying under the radar: The new wave of BCR–ABL inhibitors. Nature Reviews Drug Discovery. 2007;**6**(10):834-848

[77] Quintas-Cardama A et al. Dasatinib (BMS-354825) is active in Philadelphia chromosome–positive chronic myelogenous leukemia after imatinib and nilotinib (AMN107) therapy failure. Blood. 2007;**109**(2):497-499

[78] Baccarani M, Pane F, Saglio G. Monitoring treatment of chronic myeloid leukemia. Haematologica. 2008;**93**(2):161-169

[79] Shi W et al. CKS1B as drug resistance-inducing gene—A potential target to improve cancer therapy. Frontiers in Oncology. 2020;**10**:1978

[80] Sabnis AJ, Bivona TG. Principles of resistance to targeted cancer therapy: Lessons from basic and translational cancer biology. Trends in Molecular Medicine. 2019;**25**(3):185-197

[81] Duso BA et al. Secondary mechanisms of anti-HER2 resistance in breast cancer: NF1 as an actionable target. Annals of Oncology. 2019; **30**:iii6-iii7

[82] Solimini NL, Luo J, Elledge SJ. Non-oncogene addiction and the stress phenotype of cancer cells. Cell. 2007;**130**(6):986-988

[83] Nagel R, Semenova EA, Berns A. Drugging the addict: Non-oncogene addiction as a target for cancer therapy. EMBO Reports. 2016;**17**(11):1516-1531

[84] Chang HR et al. Targeting non-oncogene addiction for cancer therapy. Biomolecules. 2021;**11**(2):129

Section 2

Tumor Suppressor Genes

Chapter 5

Cancer Genes and Breast Cancers

Metin Budak and Hatice Segmen

Abstract

Cancer is the name given to all malignant tumors, the main reason for which is uncontrolled growth, and the tumor, which has become a mass as a result of uncontrolled cell proliferation, also attacks the surrounding cells and envelops the whole body (metastasis) in the later stages of the disease. Although cancer is an important health problem, it is not a common disease in childhood. On the other hand, statistics show that cancer affects one in three adults, causes up to 20% of all deaths, and covers about 10% of treatment costs in developed countries. Although it is known that cancer develops under the influence of genetic and environmental factors, environmental factors are more prominent in the formation of some types of cancer. Breast cancer is one of the cancer types known to have tumor suppressor genes in its etiology. These tumor suppressor genes are BRCA1 and BRCA2 genes. Studies have shown that these two genes are particularly effective in the development of familial breast cancers. These types of cancers occur much earlier than non-familial cancers. The research, two genes; It has shown that it is especially effective in the development of familial breast cancers.

Keywords: BRCA1, BRCA2, tumor suppressor, oncogenes, cancer

1. Introduction

The term cancer is not the name of a single disease, but the name was given to all malignant tumors, the main reason for which is uncontrolled growth. The tumor, which becomes a mass as a result of uncontrolled cell proliferation, also attacks the surrounding cells and tends to spread throughout the body in the later stages of the disease (metastasis). Although cancer is an important health problem, it is not a common disease in childhood. On the other hand, statistics show that cancer affects one in three adults, causes up to 20% of all deaths, and covers about 10% of treatment costs in developed countries [1]. Cancer, which develops as a result of uncontrolled cell growth and development, is a phenomenon that occurs as a result of a complex series of cellular mechanisms working differently from normal. It is known that cancer occurs as a result of mutations in somatic cells and these mutations affect the expression of a series of genes. Cancers can develop in each tissue group depending on age, gender, and environmental factors [2–4]. Although it is known that cancer develops under the influence of genetic and environmental factors, environmental factors are more prominent in the formation of some types of cancer. It is now known to affect [5, 6]. There are two gene groups known to be involved in cancer formation. These are (1) Tumor suppressor genes and (2) proto-oncogenes [7, 8]. Breast cancers are the leading cancer types known to have tumor suppressor genes in their etiology. BRCA1 and BRCA2 genes are the leading tumor suppressor genes specific to breast cancers [9]. Studies have shown that these

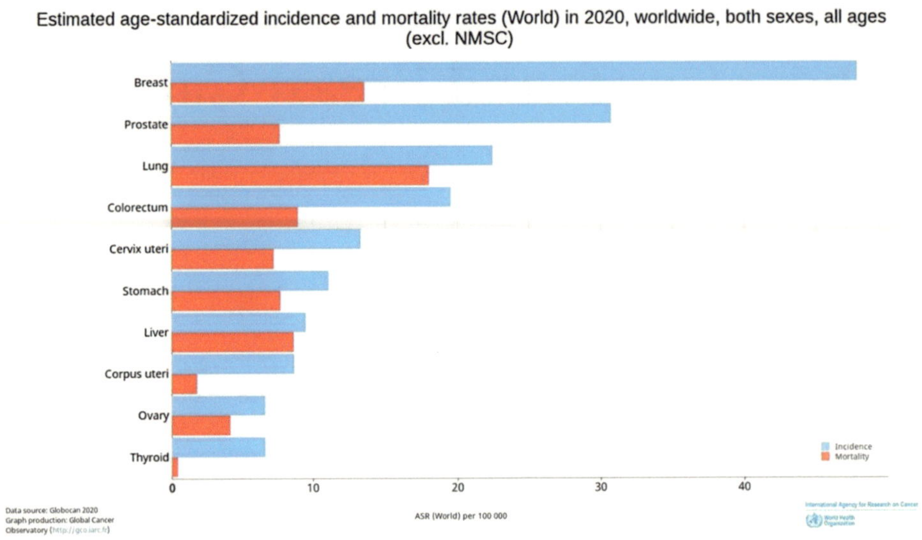

Figure 1.
Estimated age-standardized incidence and mortality rates (world) in 2020, worldwide, for both sexes, all ages [17].

two genes are particularly effective in the development of familial breast cancers. While the majority of cancers are sporadic, a small percentage can be hereditary, that is, familial. While the first mutation in the genes involved in hereditary cancers is inherited familial, the fact that the second mutation occurs in a limited number of somatic cells after birth is sufficient for cancerization. These types of cancers occur much earlier than non-familial cancers [9–16]. According to World Health Organization; When cancer-related deaths in women were investigated between 2019 and 2020 worldwide, the most common type of cancer in all ages and genders is breast cancer, followed by prostate cancer and lung cancer, the least common cancer is thyroid cancer. However, the most common cause of death is lung cancer and breast cancer is the second most common type of cancer. According to International Agency for Research on Cancer of the World Health Organization; new cases and death rates of cancer the worldwide for 2020 are given below (**Figure 1**) [17–20], https://gco.iarc.fr/.

2. Causes of cancer

Although a lot of important information about the etiology of cancer has been obtained in recent years, the molecular mechanisms that cause cancer formation, that is, the excessive proliferation of a normal cell out of control, are still not fully clarified, and a new mechanism may emerge every year and hereditary factors are known to play a role together. Environmental factors include some chemical agents (nicotine), nutrition, radiation, viruses, living environmental conditions, and lifestyle [16, 21, 22].

2.1 Environmental factors

2.1.1 Chemical carcinogens

There is a threshold value for many carcinogens, amounts that do not exceed this threshold value are harmless. One-third of cancers seen in the USA and Europe are cancers that develop due to the use of cigarettes and other tobacco products. Working conditions and some occupational chemicals are among the other environmental factors that cause cancer. It is known that chemical agents such as asbestos and nicotine cause cancer formation [23–26].

2.1.2 Physical carcinogens

Ionizing Radiation. Skin cancers were common in the hands of radiologists in the periods when primitive devices were used and prevention methods were not well known. In studies conducted in the following years, it has been shown that bone, thyroid, lung, breast cancer, leukemia, and lymphoma develop with the effect of radiation [27–29]. Ultraviolet Rays (U.V). U.V rays have been shown to be associated with skin cancers. These include basal cell skin cancer, squamous (stratified squamous epithelium) skin cancer, and skin cancers such as melanoma [30–34].

2.1.3 Hereditary and genetic factors

Although cancer is a genetic disease, very few cancer cases show hereditary characteristics. Among all cancer types, the rate of hereditary cancers is less than 1%. In families with hereditary cancer cases, cancer occurs more frequently than in the normal population. In families where cancer is inherited; The probability of passing the cancer gene from mother or father to child is 50%. Cancer cases in individuals in such families occur at an earlier age than in the general population. The tissues with the most familial cancer cases are colon, endometrium, ovary, and breast [35–37]. Two groups are very important in the formation of cancer. These; proto-oncogenes are tumor suppressor genes.

2.1.3.1 Proto-oncogenes and oncogenes

It is known that proto-oncogenes that regulate cell growth and differentiation have important roles in normal cell physiology (30). If a proto-oncogene differentiates or starts to be expressed more than normal as a result of mutation or change in external stimulus; These changes cause uncontrolled growth and therefore malignant formations in the cell. With the mutation of proto-oncogenes, they turn into genes called oncogenes that stimulate continuous cell division [38, 39]. Proto-oncogenes can be grouped into 4 groups according to the biochemical properties of protein products [40, 41].

a. **Growth Factors:** Growth factors are signal molecules in polypeptide structure that are secreted out of the cell and stimulate differentiation in the target cell. They recognize the target cell with special receptors on the cell surface and stimulate differentiation in the cell. The best-known growth factor is the platelet-derived growth factor (PDGF) (9). Growth factors are proteins that weigh between 4000 and 60,000 daltons and can affect cellular activities even in small amounts. 6 Growth factors are substances that enable growth and proliferation in various cell types. Many growth factors such as epidermal growth factor (EGF), mesodermal growth factor (MGF), platelet-derived growth factor (PDGF), granulocyte colony-stimulating factor (G-KUF), granulocyte macrophage colony-stimulating factor (GM-KUF) are isolated 7. As a result of studies with antioxidants, it has been explained that antioxidants may have a common function with growth factors and also have effects on factors [42, 43].

b. **Epidermal Growth Factor (Epidermal growth factor, EGF):** It is a 53 amino acid polypeptide that is identical to Urogastron. It is found in many tissues and is released during platelet degranulation. Most cells have receptors for EGF. The most numerous receptors are found on epithelial cells; however, there are also receptors on endothelial cells, fibroblasts, and smooth muscle cells. It has chemotactic properties for epithelial cells, endothelium, and fibroblasts. It has the feature of stimulating angiogenesis and collagenase activity [44, 45].

FGF has also been studied in various animal models; After topical application to the wound in the guinea pig ear, basic FGF has been shown to accelerate epithelialization. Cell number and collagen content increased with subcutaneous injection in guinea pigs. Topical basic FGF has a positive effect on wound healing problems that can be caused by infection and diabetes in mice [46–49].

c. **Growth Factor receptors:** Differentiated forms of some viral oncogenes produce normal growth factors with tyrosine kinase activity. Therefore, by binding to normal cells, they stimulate cell division and cause cancer development. The most well-known growth factor receptors are erb B, erb B-2, and fms. GHR, the specific transmembrane receptor of growth hormone (GH), belongs to the class I hematopoietic cytokine receptor superfamily and is widely found in peripheral tissues. This group of receptors is associated with adapter tyrosine kinases such as Janus kinase 2. GHR; consists of three parts: extracellular, transmembrane, and intracellular. The extracellular portion of the GH receptor forms the high-affinity binding protein. GH binds to its receptor by the extracellular binding site of the receptor protein; The receptor is then activated by dimerization. Activation of the receptor is followed by activation of the JAK–STAT pathway, followed by increased expression of IGF-1 and other growth hormone-related genes. After all, GHR; It regulates the effect of GH by removing it from the circulation [50–53].

d. **Transcription Factors**: Core proteins encoded by many genes form transcription factors. Transcriptional control is done by binding these proteins to specific DNA sequences or DNA motifs. Transcription factors provide the expression of the target gene with positive or negative control. Gene activity is mainly regulated at the transcriptional level. As is known, many genes in prokaryotes are clustered in units called operons. Regulation of transcription of genes in operons is provided by activating by activator proteins and inhibiting by repressor proteins. Gene activity in eukaryotes is basically controlled at the transcriptional level. However, eukaryotic chromosomes have both a larger structure and a higher degree of structural organization than prokaryotic chromosomes. Yeast, fruit fly, and human genomes contain 4, 40, and 1000 times more DNA than Escherichia coli genomes, respectively. This redundancy not only gives eukaryotes potentials that are not found in prokaryotes, but also brings new dimensions to the replication and gene activity events in them. The activity of some specific genes in eukaryotic chromosomes depends on transcription factors. For example, transcription of 5S ribosomal RNA genes may depend on the binding of proteins with multiple metal-binding stretches that fit into grooves in DNA to these genes [53–56].

e. **Programmed Cell Death controls:** Normal tissue structure; is achieved by the balance between differentiating cells and dying cells. Programmed cell death is crucial in normal embryogenesis and organ development. It has been shown that the programmed cell death mechanism is lost in cancer cells. This mechanism is specifically controlled by the bcl 2 proto-oncogene. As a result of chromosomal translocations of this gene, it can be activated especially in lymphomas [57–59].

f. **Oncogene activation mechanisms:** Oncogenes can be activated in three ways: 1, Mutations; 2, Gene amplification; 3, Chromosomal rearrangements.

1. **Mutations:** Changes occur in the structure of proteins encoded by oncogenes activated as a result of mutations such as point mutations and frameshifts. As a result of these, changes occur in the critical binding sites of the protein, and they lose their protein binding properties and cause cancer development by failing to fulfill their duties.

2. **Gene Amplification:** Gene amplification occurs when the number of copies of a gene in the cell genome increases. The increase in gene copy number occurs especially with karyotype duplications. These formations are only seen quite frequently in tumor tissues.

3. **Chromosomal Rearrangements:** Chromosomal rearrangements are mostly changes that occur in hematological malignant tumors. Chromosomal translocations, and inversions are the most common rearrangements [60–64]. The best example of chromosomal rearrangements of human proto-oncogenes is the (9;22) translocation. In approximately 95% of patients with chronic myeloid leukemia (CML), a reciprocal translocation occurs in bone marrow cells between chromosomes 9 and 22. As a result of this translocation, the Philadelphia chromosome, which is smaller than the normal 22 chromosome number, is formed [65–67]. As a result of this translocation, the abl proto-oncogene is transferred from its normal location 9q34.1 to chromosome 22. The abl gene joins in its new location ("Breakpoint cluster region") with a special sequence called bcr. The hybrid gene resulting from this fusion causes the synthesis of a new protein believed to be responsible for tumor formation in bone marrow cells. This new protein has tyrosine kinase activity and activates cell division to form tumors [8, 66, 67].

2.1.3.2 Tumor suppressor genes

Tumor suppressor genes were found for the first time as a result of studies on retinoblastoma, one of the very rare hereditary cancer types. Retinoblastoma is the most common type of cancer among childhood eye cancers and occurs bilaterally in 20–30% of cases [68, 69]. All bilateral cases and 15% of unilateral cases show autosomal dominant inheritance. The gene responsible for this disease is the Rb1 gene located proximal to the long arm of chromosome 13 [70, 71]. As a result of chromosomal changes or point mutations, the functional protein related to this gene is either absent or unable to function in cells in tumor tissue. In such cases, hereditary mutation; is found in only one of the gene pairs and is therefore in a heterozygous state. In order for a tumor to develop in a person carrying the mutant gene, a new mutation must also occur in the normal partner of the mutant gene in the retinal cell(9). As a result of a second mutation, a tumor occurs when the other intact allele is changed or lost. This situation is also called loss of heterozygosity [72, 73], (**Figure 2**).

In hereditary retinoblastoma cancers, the first mutation occurred in the person either as a result of germline mutations or inherited from one of the

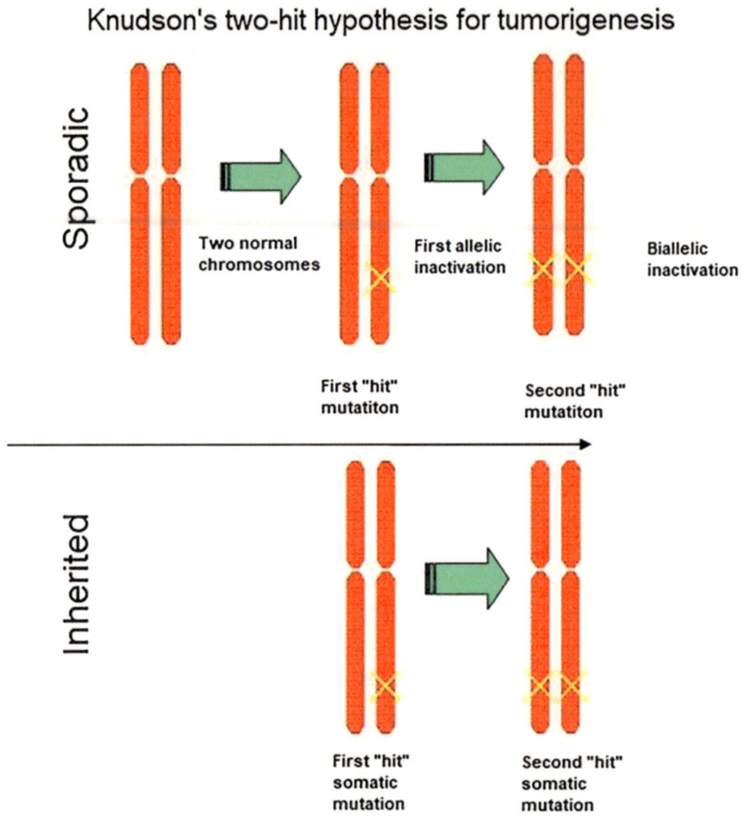

Figure 2.
Cancer formation model.

parents. In people carrying this gene, retinoblastoma occurs at a very early age [74]. As a result of studies on the localization of many tumor types that show oss of heterozygosity for chromosome 13 and the localization of other tumor suppressor genes, more than 20 tumor suppressor gene regions were identified, the main ones being p53, retinoblastoma, BRCA 1, BRCA 2 (**Table 1**) [76–80].

2.1.3.2.1 p53 gene

The p53 gene is located in band 13 of the short arm of human chromosome 17. This gene, which is about 20 kb long; encodes a 2.8 kb mRNA and its product is a core phosphoprotein of 393 amino acids of 53 kD (10). Nucleotide and amino acid sequence analyzes have shown that; The p53 gene contains 5 conserved regions from neopus to human during evolution. This region includes exons 1, 4, 5, 7, and 8. These conserved regions are thought to be essential sites for the p53 wild-type protein. Specifically, the DNA binding region of the p53 gene contains 2 SV40 tumor antigen binding (T-ag), a nuclear localization signal, and multiple phosphorylation sites (**Figure 3**). The p53 protein controls gene expression positively or negatively by stopping the cell cycle in the G1 phase and binding to specific sequences and transcription factors. Normal p53 protein stops the cell cycle and leads the cell to programmed cell death in the absence of appropriate differentiation or proliferation factors [81–85].

Gene	Cancer	Localization	Function	Hereditary Syndrome
APC	Colon cancer	Cytoplasm	Cellular adhesion	Familial
DCC	Colon cancer	Cell membrane	Cell adhesion molecule	—
NF1	Neurofibromas	Cytoplasm	GTPase activator	Neurofibromatosis Type 1
NF2	Schwannomas and Meningioma	Cell membrane	Cell membrane	Neurofibromatosis Type 2
p53	Colon cancer and many other cancers	Nucleus	Transcription factor	Li-Fraumeni syndrome
RB	Retinoblastoma	Nucleus	Transcription factor	Retinoblastoma
RET	Thyroid cancer pheochromocytom	Cell membrane	Tyrosine kinase receptor	Multiple endocrine neoplasm Type 2
VHL	Kidney cancer	Cell membrane	Transcription factor	Von Hippel–Lindau disease
WT-1	Nephroblastoma	Nucleus	Transcription factor	Wilms tumor
BRCA1	Breast cancer	Breast tissue	DNA repair, mismatch repair	Familial breast cancers
BRCA2	Breast cancer	Breast tissue epithelium	DNA repair, mismatch repair	Familial breast cancers

Table 1.
Some tumor suppressor genes and the types of cancer they cause [75].

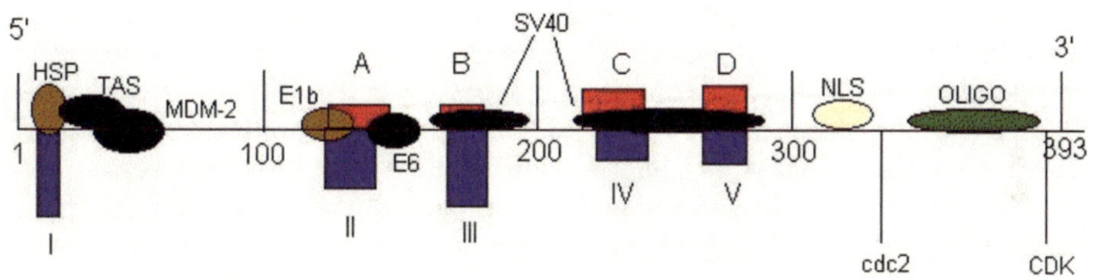

Figure 3.
Schematic structure of the p53 gene; TAS: Transcription activation region, protein binding region (HSP), SV40 wide T-antigen region, adenovirus E1b and papillomavirus E6 binding region, cellular Mdm2 binding region, nuclear localization signal (NLS), oligomerization region (OLIGO) and phosphorylation region (cdc2 and CDK). The 5 conserved regions in evolution are indicated by the letters I, II, III, IV, and V, and the hot spot regions are indicated by the letters A, B, C, D.

2.1.3.2.2 BRCA1 gene

The chromosomal location of the BRCA 1 gene (Breast cancer susceptibility gene) was first identified in 1990 and cloned in 1994 [86]. The BRCA1 gene has 24 exons (20) with approximately 100,000 base pairs, occupying 4 cM, located in the q12–21 region of chromosome 17; It is a gene that encodes a tumor suppressor protein. The 11th exon of the BRCA1 gene, which is very large, constitutes 61% of the entire gene. The BRCA1 gene encodes a tumor-suppressing protein with DNA binding properties that negatively affect cancer formation [87]. Recent studies have shown that the product of the BRCA1 gene; It has been shown to be a zing-finger protein with a zinc-binding site at the amino end [87–89].

2.1.3.2.3 Mutation distribution

Breast tumors occur with the loss of both the wild-type allele of the BRCA1 gene at 17q [90]. Since there are 500 different types and the BRCA 1 gene is a large gene, the frequency of mutation is quite high. Several clinically important mutations have been found in this gene. While approximately 90% of these mutations are frameshift or nonsense mutations, the rest are mutations that cause changes in the stop codon and cause the immature protein to be made at the translation stage [35, 91–94]. Studies have been ongoing since the gene was cloned to develop a test that could detect familial cancer risk by detecting BRCA 1 mutations. The second most common group of mutations in the BRCA1 gene are 185delAG and 5382insG mutations [95, 96]. These constitute 10% of all mutations in the BRCA1 gene. These two mutations are seen with a frequency of approximately 10% in Ashkenazi and non-Ashkenazi Jews. The carrier rate of these mutations in the same group is 1%. Mutations 185delAG and 5382insG have also been shown to be found in Moroccan and non-Jewish families. The high incidence of deletions in the AG sequence at position 185 of BRCA1 has caused this region to be called the 'Hotspot' region. In germ-line mutation studies in all women, the incidence of breast cancer before the age of 40 was found to be 20% in 185delAG carriers [95, 97–99]. While the 5832insC mutation is most common in Russians and Jews of European origin, it is very low in Israeli Jews [100, 101]. The most common mutation in the Russian population is 4153delA4 (**Figure 4**) [102].

2.1.3.2.4 The function of BRCA1

The BRCA 1 protein is a ring-finger protein of 1863′ amino acids (45, 46, 47). BRCA 1 is made in the differentiated epithelial cells of developing organs during embryonic development and puberty development. A significant increase in the mRNA level of BRCA 1 has been observed in breast epithelial cells during pregnancy in women without cancer. BRCA 1 expression in humans is stimulated by estrogen and decreases after birth (38,48). Suppression of BRCA 1 expression increases growth in both normal cells and malignant mammary epithelial cells [86, 90, 93]. Since the BRCA1 gene was isolated, its functions have been thought to play a role in

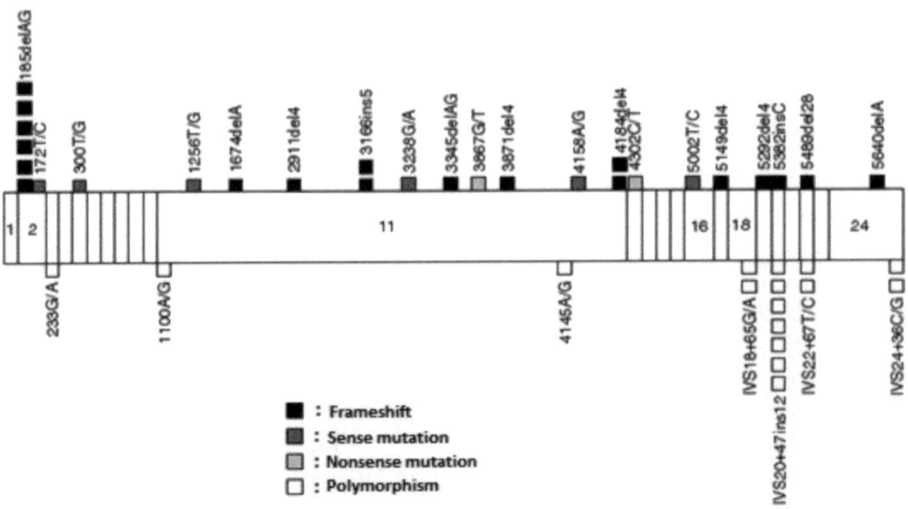

Figure 4.
Mutation distribution in the BRCA1 gene.

transcription, control the cell cycle, and be associated with DNA repair mechanisms. It is a gene that participates in DNA repair mechanisms by interacting with basic transcriptional mechanisms (with RNA polymerase II, Transcription factors TFIIH, TFIIE, and RNA helicase A). BRCA1 and BRCA2 proteins together provide a repair of DNA double-strand breaks in mitotic cells [103, 104] BRCA1 protein interacts with the gamma-tubulin subunits of the centrosome during mitosis, stopping the cell cycle and providing damage control in DNA [105].

2.1.3.2.5 BRCA2 gene

BRCA2 is another tumor suppressor gene that was mapped to the long arm of the 13th chromosome by Wooster et al. in 1994 (7). The 13q12-13 region containing BRCA2 is also a region close to the retinoblastoma gene (36, 39). The BRCA2 gene is a 70 kb gene with 27 exons, occupies 6 cM, and the product of the gene is a protein consisting of 3418 amino acids(36). The fact that exon 3 is similar to transcription factors indicates that it may have a function in this direction (33,). BRCA2 has a large 11th exon just like BRCA1(50). This exon makes up about 58% of the whole gene [86, 106–108]. While the risk of breast cancer and ovarian cancer is higher in patients with germline mutations in this gene, 30–40% loss of heterozygosity is observed in patients with sporadic breast and ovarian cancer [109, 110]. Interestingly, almost all BRCA2 mutations are familial [111]. This theorizes that BRCA mutations can theoretically be traced back to an initial sporadic case and may indicate the presence of a 'founder effect'. The majority of mutations in the BRCA 2 gene cause a frameshift condition. The most common frameshift mutation is the 999del5 mutation, which is also seen in Iceland. Other than that, the mutations seen in other populations are as follows. Ashkenazi Jewish-6174delT, Dutch-5579insA, Finns- 8555 T > G, 999del5, IVS23-2A > G, French Canadians 8765delAG, 3398delAAAAG, Hungarians-9326insA, Pakistanis-3337C > T, Slovenians-IVS16-2A > G [112]. People with certain mutations of the BRCA2 gene increase the risk of breast cancer by causing hereditary breast-ovarian cancer syndrome. As a result of research, hundreds of mutations in the BRCA2 gene, many of which cause an increased risk of cancer, have been identified. BRCA2 mutations are usually the addition or loss of a small number of DNA base pairs in the gene. As a result of these mutations, the protein product of the BRCA2 gene is abnormal and does not work properly. Research emerges as a result of the inability of the dysfunctional BRCA2 protein to repair the damages in the DNA that make up the genome. As a result, there is an increase in mutations due to this faulty synthesis after unrepaired DNA damages, and some of these mutations can lead to uncontrolled division of cells and the formation of a tumor [107, 113, 114].

3. Conclusion

By revealing the environmental and genetic factors that are effective in the development of breast cancer, which is a very important social problem, studies to prevent breast cancer gain hope. The incidence of breast cancer differs from country to country in the world. While Hawaii, California, and Canada are in the first place with an incidence of 80–90 per hundred thousand per year, the same value is only between 12 and 15 per hundred thousand in Japan. Although the majority of breast cancers are sporadic cases, 5–10% of all cases are hereditary. BRCA1 and BRCA2 genes are known to be effective in the development of breast cancer. The BRCA1 gene is thought to be responsible for 4–5% of all breast cancers and 45% of hereditary breast cancers. The risk of developing breast cancer up to the age of 70 in BRCA1 gene carriers is 94%. The rate of breast cancer cases occurring before the age of 30 is 25%. The BRCA 1 gene is responsible for half of all familial breast cancer cases and 80–90% of multiple breast and ovarian cancer cases. This shows that due to the importance of BRCA1 and BRCA2 genes in the etiology of breast cancer, detecting both BRCA1 and BRCA2 genes, especially in familial breast cancer cases, is important for public health. As a result, routine applications with rapid, reliable, and inexpensive methods to detect BRCA1 and BRCA2 gene mutations are known to be involved in the etiology of breast cancer in patients and families with multiple breast cancer or ovarian cancer or diagnosed with breast cancer at an early age may need to be seen as potential chemotherapy targets.

Conflict of interest

There is no conflict of interest.

Author details

Metin Budak[1]* and Hatice Segmen[2]

1 Faculty of Medicine, Department of Biophysics, Trakya University, Edirne, Turkey

2 Department of Neurology, Kanuni Sultan Suleyman Training and Research Hospital, Saglik Bilimleri University, Turkey

*Address all correspondence to: genomicdna2@yahoo.com; metinbudak@trakya.edu.tr

References

[1] Bailar JC, Gornik HL. Cancer undefeated. New England Journal of Medicine. 1997;**336**(22):1569-1574

[2] Zhang W-j, Wang X-h, Gao S-t, Chen C, Xu X-y, Zhou Z-h, et al. Tumor-associated macrophages correlate with phenomenon of epithelial-mesenchymal transition and contribute to poor prognosis in triple-negative breast cancer patients. Journal of Surgical Research. 2018;**222**:93-101

[3] Conteduca V, Poti G, Caroli P, Russi S, Brighi N, Lolli C, et al. Flare phenomenon in prostate cancer: Recent evidence on new drugs and next generation imaging. Therapeutic Advances in Medical Oncology. 2021;**13**:1758835920987654

[4] Delgado-López PD, CorralesGarcía EM. Influence of internet and social media in the promotion of alternative oncology, cancer quackery, and the predatory publishing phenomenon. DOI: 10.7759/cureus.2617

[5] Coyle YM. The effect of environment on breast cancer risk. Breast Cancer Research and Treatment. 2004;**84**(3): 273-288

[6] Gray J, Evans N, Taylor B, Rizzo J, Walker M. State of the evidence: The connection between breast cancer and the environment. International Journal of Occupational and Environmental Health. 2009;**15**(1):43-78

[7] Martínez-Jiménez F, Muiños F, Sentís I, Deu-Pons J, Reyes-Salazar I, Arnedo-Pac C, et al. A compendium of mutational cancer driver genes. Nature Reviews Cancer. 2020;**20**(10):555-572

[8] Chiu H-S, Somvanshi S, Patel E, Chen T-W, Singh VP, Zorman B, et al. Pan-cancer analysis of lnc RNA regulation supports their targeting of cancer genes in each tumor context. Cell Reports. 2018;**23**(1):297-312. e12

[9] Waks AG, Winer EP. Breast cancer treatment: A review. JAMA. 2019;**321**(3):288-300

[10] Momenimovahed Z, Salehiniya H. Epidemiological characteristics of and risk factors for breast cancer in the world. Breast Cancer: Targets and Therapy. 2019;**11**:151

[11] Britt KL, Cuzick J, Phillips K-A. Key steps for effective breast cancer prevention. Nature Reviews Cancer. 2020;**20**(8):417-436

[12] Tutt AN, Garber JE, Kaufman B, Viale G, Fumagalli D, Rastogi P, et al. Adjuvant olaparib for patients with BRCA1-or BRCA2-mutated breast cancer. New England Journal of Medicine. 2021;**384**(25):2394-2405

[13] Samstein RM, Krishna C, Ma X, Pei X, Lee K-W, Makarov V, et al. Mutations in BRCA1 and BRCA2 differentially affect the tumor microenvironment and response to checkpoint blockade immunotherapy. Nature Cancer. 2020;**1**(12):1188-1203

[14] Cline MS, Liao RG, Parsons MT, Paten B, Alquaddoomi F, Antoniou A, et al. BRCA challenge: BRCA exchange as a global resouce for variants in BRCA1 and BRCA2. PLoS Genetics. 2018;**14**(12):e1007752

[15] Choi Y-H, Terry MB, Daly MB, Mac Innis RJ, Hopper JL, Colonna S, et al. Association of risk-reducing salpingo-oophorectomy with breast cancer risk in women with BRCA1 and BRCA2 pathogenic variants. JAMA Oncology. 2021;7(4):585-592

[16] Rebbeck TR, Friebel TM, Friedman E, Hamann U, Huo D, Kwong A, et al. Mutational spectrum in a worldwide study of 29, 700 families with BRCA1 or BRCA2 mutations. Human Mutation. 2018;**39**(5):593-620

[17] Available from: https://gco.iarc.fr/

[18] Miller KD, Ortiz AP, Pinheiro PS, Bandi P, Minihan A, Fuchs HE, et al. Cancer statistics for the US Hispanic/Latino population, 2021. CA: A Cancer Journal for Clinicians. 2021;**71**(6): 466-487

[19] Ferlay J, Colombet M, Soerjomataram I, Parkin DM, Piñeros M, Znaor A, et al. Cancer statistics for the year 2020: An overview. International Journal of Cancer. 2021;**149**(4):778-789

[20] Cao W, Chen H-D, Yu Y-W, Li N, Chen W-Q. Changing profiles of cancer burden worldwide and in China: A secondary analysis of the global cancer statistics 2020. Chinese Medical Journal. 2021;**134**(07):783-791

[21] Tron L, Belot A, Fauvernier M, Remontet L, Bossard N, Launay L, et al. Socioeconomic environment and disparities in cancer survival for 19 solid tumor sites: An analysis of the French network of cancer registries (FRANCIM) data. International Journal of Cancer. 2019;**144**(6):1262-1274

[22] da Costa Araújo AP, Mesak C, Montalvão MF, Freitas ÍN, Chagas TQ, Malafaia G. Anti-cancer drugs in aquatic environment can cause cancer: Insight about mutagenicity in tadpoles. Science of the Total Environment. 2019;**650**: 2284-2293

[23] Kobets T, Williams GM. Review of the evidence for thresholds for DNA-reactive and epigenetic experimental chemical carcinogens. Chemico-Biological Interactions. 2019;**301**:88-111

[24] Grunberger D, Weinstein I. Conformational changes in nucleic acids modified by chemical carcinogens. Chemical Carcinogens and DNA. 2019;**62**:59-94

[25] Peter Guengerich F, Avadhani NG. Roles of cytochrome P450 in metabolism of ethanol and carcinogens. Alcohol and Cancer. 2018;**1032**:15-35

[26] Hartwig A, Arand M, Epe B, Guth S, Jahnke G, Lampen A, et al. Mode of action-based risk assessment of genotoxic carcinogens. Archives of Toxicology. 2020;**94**(6):1787-1877

[27] Hauptmann M, Daniels RD, Cardis E, Cullings HM, Kendall G, Laurier D, et al. Epidemiological studies of low-dose ionizing radiation and cancer: Summary bias assessment and meta-analysis. JNCI Monographs. 2020;**2020**(56):188-200

[28] Hong J-Y, Han K, Jung J-H, Kim JS. Association of exposure to diagnostic low-dose ionizing radiation with risk of cancer among youths in South Korea. JAMA Network Open. 2019;**2**(9): e1910584-e1910584

[29] Richardson DB, Cardis E, Daniels RD, Gillies M, Haylock R, Leuraud K, et al. Site-specific solid cancer mortality after exposure to ionizing radiation: a cohort study of workers (INWORKS). Epidemiology (Cambridge, Mass.). 2018;**29**(1):31

[30] Laikova KV, Oberemok VV, Krasnodubets AM, Gal'chinsky NV, Useinov RZ, Novikov IA, et al. Advances in the understanding of skin cancer: Ultraviolet radiation, mutations, and antisense oligonucleotides as anticancer drugs. Molecules. 2019;**24**(8):1516

[31] Paulo MS, Adam B, Akagwu C, Akparibo I, Al-Rifai RH, Bazrafshan S, et al. WHO/ILO work-related burden of disease and injury: Protocol for systematic reviews of occupational exposure to solar ultraviolet radiation and of the effect of occupational exposure to solar ultraviolet radiation on melanoma and non-melanoma skin cancer. Environment International. 2019;**126**:804-815

[32] Grant WB, Moukayed M. Vitamin D3 from ultraviolet-B exposure or oral intake in relation to cancer incidence

and mortality. Current Nutrition Reports. 2019;**8**(3):203-211

[33] Hacker E, Horsham C, Vagenas D, Jones L, Lowe J, Janda M. A mobile technology intervention with ultraviolet radiation dosimeters and smartphone apps for skin cancer prevention in young adults: Randomized controlled trial. JMIR mHealth and uHealth. 2018;**6**(11):e9854

[34] Solak SS, Yondem H, Urun YG, Cezik M, Can N. High prevalence of high-risk cutaneous squamous cell carcinoma in the thrace region of Turkey. Turk Dermatoloji Dergisi-Turkish Journal of Dermatology. 2020;**14**(4):83-89

[35] Samadder NJ, Giridhar KV, Baffy N, Riegert-Johnson D, Couch FJ. Hereditary cancer Syndromesd-a primer on diagnosis and management, part 1: Breast-ovarian cancer syndromes. Mayo Clinic Proceedings. 2019;**94**(6): 1084-1098

[36] Nagy R, Sweet K, Eng C. Highly penetrant hereditary cancer syndromes. Oncogene. 2004;**23**(38):6445-6470

[37] Frank TS. Hereditary cancer syndromes. Archives of Pathology & Laboratory Medicine. 2001;**125**(1):85-90

[38] Malebary SJ, Khan R, Khan YD. ProtoPred: Advancing oncological research through identification of proto-oncogene proteins. IEEE Access. 2021;**9**:68788-68797

[39] Grible JM, Zot P, Olex AL, Hedrick SE, Harrell JC, Woock AE, et al. The human intermediate prolactin receptor is a mammary proto-oncogene. NPJ Breast Cancer. 2021;**7**(1):1-11

[40] Rong S, Bodescot M, Blair D, Dunn J, Nakamura T, Mizuno K, et al. Tumorigenicity of the met proto-oncogene and the gene for hepatocyte growth factor. Molecular and Cellular Biology. 1992;**12**(11):5152-5158

[41] Velu TJ, Beguinot L, Vass WC, Willingham MC, Merlino GT, Pastan I, et al. Epidermal-growth-factor-dependent transformation by a human EGF receptor proto-oncogene. Science. 1987;**238**(4832):1408-1410

[42] Stromberg K, Pigott DA, Ranchalis JE, Twardzik DR. Human term placenta contains transforming growth factors. Biochemical and Biophysical Research Communications. 1982;**106**(2):354-361

[43] Berg DK. New neuronal growth factors. Annual Review of Neuroscience. 1984;**7**(1):149-170

[44] Carpenter G, Cohen S. Epidermal growth factor. Journal of Biological Chemistry. 1990;**265**(14):7709-7712

[45] Boonstra J, Rijken P, Humbel B, Cremers F, Verkleij A, Henegouwen PVB e. The epidermal growth factor. Cell Biology International. 1995;**19**(5):413-430

[46] LeGrand EK. Preclinical promise of becaplermin (rhPDGF-BB) in wound healing. The American Journal of Surgery. 1998;**176**(2):48S-54S

[47] Amento EP, Beck LS. TGFb and wound healing. Clinical Applications of TGFb. 2008;**157**:115-129

[48] Ab Ghani N. The Effect of Insulin and Growth Hormone on Full Thickness Wound of Guinea Pigs. Kuantan, Pahang: Kulliyyah of Medicine, International Islamic University; 2011

[49] Wimmer C, Mees K, Stumpf P, Welsch U, Reichel O, Suckfüll M. Round window application of D-methionine, sodium thiosulfate, brain-derived neurotrophic factor, and fibroblast growth factor-2 in cisplatin-induced ototoxicity. Otology & Neurotology. 2004;**25**(1):33-40

[50] Kontomanolis EN, Koutras A, Syllaios A, Schizas D, Mastoraki A,

Garmpis N, et al. Role of oncogenes and tumor-suppressor genes in carcinogenesis: A review. Anticancer Research. 2020;**40**(11):6009-6015

[51] Sainsbury J, Sherbet G, Farndon J, Harris A. Epidermal-growth-factor receptors and oestrogen receptors in human breast cancer. The Lancet. 1985;**325**(8425):364-366

[52] Singleton KR, Kim J, Hinz TK, Marek LA, Casás-Selves M, Hatheway C, et al. A receptor tyrosine kinase network composed of fibroblast growth factor receptors, epidermal growth factor receptor, v-erb-b2 erythroblastic leukemia viral oncogene homolog 2, and hepatocyte growth factor receptor drives growth and survival of head and neck squamous carcinoma cell lines. Molecular Pharmacology. 2013;**83**(4):882-893

[53] Sirkisoon SR, Carpenter RL, Rimkus T, Anderson A, Harrison A, Lange AM, et al. Interaction between STAT3 and GLI1/tGLI1 oncogenic transcription factors promotes the aggressiveness of triple-negative breast cancers and HER2-enriched breast cancer. Oncogene. 2018;**37**(19): 2502-2514

[54] Rajagopal C, Lankadasari MB, Aranjani JM, Harikumar K. Targeting oncogenic transcription factors by polyphenols: A novel approach for cancer therapy. Pharmacological Research. 2018;**130**:273-291

[55] Hasanpourghadi M, Pandurangan AK, Mustafa MR. Modulation of oncogenic transcription factors by bioactive natural products in breast cancer. Pharmacological Research. 2018;**128**:376-388

[56] Wu S, Turner KM, Nguyen N, Raviram R, Erb M, Santini J, et al. Circular ecDNA promotes accessible chromatin and high oncogene expression. Nature. 2019;**575**(7784): 699-703

[57] Carneiro BA, El-Deiry WS. Targeting apoptosis in cancer therapy. Nature Reviews Clinical Oncology. 2020;**17**(7):395-417

[58] Matsushima M, Kobayashi K, Eml M, Saito J, Suzumori K, Nakamura Y. Mutation analysis of the BRCA1 gene in 76 Japanese ovarian cancer patients: Four germline mutations, but no evidence of somatic mutation. Human Molecular Genetics. 1995;**4**(10):1953-1956

[59] Thomadaki H, Scorilas A. BCL2 family of apoptosis-related genes: Functions and clinical implications in cancer. Critical Reviews in Clinical Laboratory Sciences. 2006;**43**(1):1-67

[60] Kotsantis P, Petermann E, Boulton SJ. Mechanisms of oncogene-induced replication stress: Jigsaw falling into place. Cancer Discovery. 2018;**8**(5):537-555

[61] Park M, Dean M, Cooper CS, Schmidt M, O'Brien SJ, Blair DG, et al. Mechanism of met oncogene activation. Cell. 1986;**45**(6):895-904

[62] Wilmes S, Hafer M, Vuorio J, Tucker JA, Winkelmann H, Löchte S, et al. Mechanism of homodimeric cytokine receptor activation and dysregulation by oncogenic mutations. Science. 2020;**367**(6478):643-652

[63] Tanaka H, Watanabe T. Mechanisms underlying recurrent genomic amplification in human cancers. Trends in Cancer. 2020;**6**(6):462-477

[64] Jia Q, Chen S, Tan Y, Li Y, Tang F. Oncogenic super-enhancer formation in tumorigenesis and its molecular mechanisms. Experimental & Molecular Medicine. 2020;**52**(5):713-723

[65] Chereda B, Melo JV. Natural course and biology of CML. Annals of Hematology. 2015;**94**(2):107-121

[66] Griesinger F, Hennig H, Hillmer F, Podleschny M, Steffens R, Pies A, et al. A BCR–JAK2 fusion gene as the result of at (9, 22)(p24; q11. 2) translocation in a patient with a clinically typical chronic myeloid leukemia. Genes, Chromosomes and Cancer. 2005;**44**(3):329-333

[67] Singh P, Kumar V, Gupta SK, Kumari G, Verma M. Combating TKI resistance in CML by inhibiting the PI3K/Akt/mTOR pathway in combination with TKIs: A review. Medical Oncology. 2021;**38**(1):1-16

[68] Marshall CJ. Tumor suppressor genes. Cell. 1991;**64**(2):313-326

[69] Knudson AG Jr. Retinoblastoma and, Essentials of Ophthalmic Oncology. Vol. 323. Berlin/Heidelberg, Germany: Springer; 2009. p. 168

[70] Dyson NJ. RB1: A prototype tumor suppressor and an enigma. Genes & Development. 2016;**30**(13):1492-1502

[71] Berry JL, Polski A, Cavenee WK, Dryja TP, Murphree AL, Gallie BL. The RB1 story: Characterization and cloning of the first tumor suppressor gene. Genes. 2019;**10**(11):879

[72] Ryland GL, Doyle MA, Goode D, Boyle SE, Choong DY, Rowley SM, et al. Loss of heterozygosity: What is it good for? BMC Medical Genomics. 2015;**8**(1):1-12

[73] Tomlinson IP, Lambros MB, Roylance RR, Cleton-Jansen AM. Loss of heterozygosity analysis: Practically and conceptually flawed? Genes, Chromosomes and Cancer. 2002;**34**(4):349-353

[74] Polski A, Xu L, Prabakar RK, Gai X, Kim JW, Shah R, et al. Variability in retinoblastoma genome stability is driven by age and not heritability. Genes, Chromosomes and Cancer. 2020;**59**(10):584-590

[75] Karp G. Cell and Molecular Biology, Concepts and Experiments 4. Hoboken, New Jersey, United States: John Wiley & Sons; 2005

[76] Dunham A, Matthews L, Burton J, Ashurst J, Howe K, Ashcroft K, et al. The DNA sequence and analysis of human chromosome 13. Nature. 2004;**428**(6982):522-528

[77] Hu N, Goldstein AM, Albert PS, Giffen C, Tang Z-Z, Ding T, et al. Evidence for a familial esophageal cancer susceptibility gene on chromosome 13. Cancer Epidemiology and Prevention Biomarkers. 2003;**12**(10):1112-1115

[78] Dahlén A, Debiec-Rychter M, Pedeutour F, Domanski HA, Höglund M, Bauer HC, et al. Clustering of deletions on chromosome 13 in benign and low-malignant lipomatous tumors. International Journal of Cancer. 2003;**103**(5):616-623

[79] Hosoki S, Ota S, Ichikawa Y, Suzuki H, Ueda T, Naya Y, et al. Suppression of metastasis of rat prostate cancer by introduction of human chromosome 13. Asian Journal of Andrology. 2002;**4**(2):131-136

[80] Topyalin N, Budak M, Ozbay N, Yildiz M, Kaner T, Aydin A, et al. A comparative histopathological and immunohistochemical study of Survivin and Ki-67 proteins in glial tumours. Biotechnology & Biotechnological Equipment. 2019;**33**(1):504-509

[81] Bourdon J-C. p53 and its isoforms in cancer. British Journal of Cancer. 2007;**97**(3):277-282

[82] Xu Y. Regulation of p53 responses by post-translational modifications. Cell Death & Differentiation. 2003;**10**(4)

[83] Oren M. Relationship of p53 to the control of apoptotic cell death. Seminars in Cancer Biology. 1994;**5**:221-227

[84] Sigal A, Rotter V. Oncogenic mutations of the p53 tumor suppressor: The demons of the guardian of the genome. Cancer Research. 2000;**60**(24):6788-6793

[85] Sayhan N, Yazici H, Budak M, Bitisik O, Dalay N. P53 codon 72 genotypes in colon cancer. Association with Human Papillomavirus Infection, Research Communications in Molecular Pathology and Pharmacology. 2001;**109**(1-2):25-34

[86] Blackwood MA, Weber BL. BRCA1 and BRCA2: From molecular genetics to clinical medicine. Journal of Clinical Oncology. 1998;**16**(5):1969-1977

[87] Paull TT, Cortez D, Bowers B, Elledge SJ, Gellert M. Direct DNA binding by Brca1. Proceedings of the National Academy of Sciences. 2001;**98**(11):6086-6091

[88] Parvin JD. Overview of history and progress in BRCA1 research: The first BRCA1 decade. Cancer Biology & Therapy. 2004;**3**(6):505-508

[89] Foulkes WD, Shuen AY. In brief: BRCA1 and BRCA2. The Journal of Pathology. 2013;**230**(4):347-349

[90] Neuhausen SL, Marshall CJ. Loss of heterozygosity in familial tumors from three BRCA1-linked kindreds. Cancer Research. 1994;**54**(23):6069-6072

[91] Futreal PA, Liu Q, Shattuck-Eidens D, Cochran C, Harshman K, Tavtigian S, et al. BRCA1 mutations in primary breast and ovarian carcinomas. Science. 1994;**266**(5182): 120-122

[92] Stratton JF, Gayther SA, Russell P, Dearden J, Gore M, Blake P, et al. Contribution of BRCA1 mutations to ovarian cancer. New England Journal of Medicine. 1997;**336**(16):1125-1130

[93] Couch FJ, DeShano ML, Blackwood MA, Calzone K, Stopfer J, Campeau L, et al. BRCA1 mutations in women attending clinics that evaluate the risk of breast cancer. New England Journal of Medicine. 1997;**336**(20): 1409-1415

[94] Rajendran P, Alzahrani AM, Rengarajan T, Veeraraghavan VP, Krishna Mohan S. Consumption of reused vegetable oil intensifies BRCA1 mutations. Critical Reviews in Food Science and Nutrition. 2021;**62**:1-8

[95] Durr-e-Samin MS-U, Rehman MS-U-R. Association of BRCA1 185 del AG with early age onset of breast cancer patients in selected cohort from Pakistani population. Pakistan Journal of Medical Sciences. 2018;**34**(5):1158

[96] Schlosser S, Rabinovitch R, Shatz Z, Galper S, Shahadi-Dromi I, Finkel S, et al. Radiation-associated secondary malignancies in BRCA mutation carriers treated for breast cancer. International Journal of Radiation Oncology* Biology* Physics. 2020;**107**(2):353-359

[97] Salmi F, Maachi F, Tazzite A, Aboutaib R, Fekkak J, Azeddoug H, et al. Next-generation sequencing of BRCA1 and BRCA2 genes in Moroccan prostate cancer patients with positive family history. PLoS One. 2021;**16**(7):e0254101

[98] Laraqui A, Cavaillé M, Uhrhammer N, ElBiad O, Bidet Y, El Rhaffouli H, et al. Identification of a novel pathogenic variant in PALB2 and BARD1 genes by a multigene sequencing panel in triple negative breast cancer in Morocco. Journal of Genomics. 2021;**9**:43

[99] Algebaly A, Suliman R, Al-Qahtani W. Comprehensive study for BRCA1 and BRCA2 entire coding regions in breast cancer. Clinical and Translational Oncology. 2021;**23**(1): 74-81

[100] Rizk MM, El-etreby NM, El-Attar LM, Elzyat EA, Saied MH. A case–control study of BRCA1 founder

mutations 185delAG and 5382insC in a cohort of Egyptian ovarian cancer patients using pyrosequencing technique. Egyptian Journal of Medical Human Genetics. 2022;**23**(1):1-9

[101] Anisimenko M, Paul G, Kozyakov A, Gutkina N, Berdyugina D, Garanin AY, et al. The spectrum of BRCA1 gene mutations in early onset breast cancer patients from Russia. Сибирский онкологический журнал. 2018;**17**(4):53-58

[102] Gayther SA, Harrington P, Russell P, Kharkevich G, Garkavtseva R, Ponder B. Rapid detection of regionally clustered germ-line BRCA1 mutations by multiplex heteroduplex analysis. UKCCCR Familial Ovarian Cancer Study Group. American Journal of Human Genetics. 1996;**58**(3):451

[103] Caestecker KW, Van de Walle GR. The role of BRCA1 in DNA double-strand repair: Past and present. Experimental Cell Research. 2013;**319**(5):575-587

[104] Scully R, Anderson SF, Chao DM, Wei W, Ye L, Young RA, et al. BRCA1 is a component of the RNA polymerase II holoenzyme. Proceedings of the National Academy of Sciences. 1997;**94**(11):5605-5610

[105] Weber A, Chung H-J, Springer E, Heitzmann D, Warth R. The TFIIH subunit p89 (XPB) localizes to the centrosome during mitosis. Analytical Cellular Pathology. 2010;**32**(1-2): 121-130

[106] Narod SA, Foulkes WD. BRCA1 and BRCA2: 1994 and beyond. Nature Reviews Cancer. 2004;**4**(9):665-676

[107] Yang H, Jeffrey PD, Miller J, Kinnucan E, Sun Y, Thoma NH, et al. BRCA2 function in DNA binding and recombination from a BRCA2-DSS1-ssDNA structure. Science. 2002; **297**(5588):1837-1848

[108] Patel KJ, Veronica P, Lee H, Corcoran A, Thistlethwaite FC, Evans MJ, et al. Involvement of Brca2 in DNA repair. Molecular Cell. 1998;**1**(3):347-357

[109] Consortium BCL. Cancer risks in BRCA2 mutation carriers. Journal of the National Cancer Institute. 1999;**91**(15): 1310-1316

[110] Wooster R, Bignell G, Lancaster J, Swift S, Seal S, Mangion J, et al. Identification of the breast cancer susceptibility gene BRCA2. Nature. 1995;**378**(6559):789-792

[111] Sarantaus L, Huusko P, Eerola H, Launonen V, Vehmanen P, Rapakko K, et al. Multiple founder effects and geographical clustering of BRCA1 and BRCA2 families in Finland. European Journal of Human Genetics. 2000;**8**(10):757-763

[112] Karami F, Mehdipour P. A comprehensive focus on global spectrum of BRCA1 and BRCA2 mutations in breast cancer. BioMed Research International. 2013; **2013**:928562

[113] Friebel TM, Domchek SM, Rebbeck TR. Modifiers of cancer risk in BRCA1 and BRCA2 mutation carriers: a systematic review and meta-analysis. Journal of the National Cancer Institute. 2014;**106**(6):dju091

[114] Holloman WK. Unraveling the mechanism of BRCA2 in homologous recombination. Nature Structural & Molecular Biology. 2011;**18**(7):748-754

Chapter 6

Two Faces of Nrf2 in Cancer

Mustafa Yildiz and Hatice Segmen

Abstract

Nuclear factor erythroid 2–related factor 2 (Nrf2) serves as a "main regulator" in response to internal or external cell stressors through coordinated induction of a wide range of cytoprotective genes. In cancer cells, Nrf2 increases expression of cytoprotective genes and, as a result, promotes proliferation through inhibition of apoptosis and metabolic reprogramming. Therefore, the activation of Nrf2 is an important regulator for prevention of cancer triggered by stresses and toxins. Defense system is activated by cellular pathways to ensure that response to stresses and toxins is sufficient for needs of the body. Nrf2 is a regulator of genes mediated by antioxidant response elements. Nrf2 is a pleiotropic gene that represents highly researched strategy in cancers. During recent decades, emerging evidence shows that Nrf2 is generally activated in many types of cancer by many mechanisms. Nrf2 has been showed to contribute to chemoresistance of cancer cells, as well as carcinogenesis due to inflammation, in recent studies. This review provides an overview of current mechanisms of regulation of Nrf2 in normal cells and its dual effects in cancer. This chapter aims to rationalize these double roles by criticizing dependence of Nrf2 functions and methods behind these contradictory data.

Keywords: cancer, Nrf2, Keap1, oxidative stress, ARE

1. Introduction

Nrf2 is a central regulator of antioxidant response element (ARE)-related gene expression and immune response. This gene encodes a transcription factor that is a member of basic leucine zipper (bZIP) protein family. The encoded transcription factor regulates genes containing antioxidant response elements (ARE) that many of these genes involve the generation of free radicals. Nrf2 is expressed in the kidney, liver, and intestine where detoxification occurs routinely. Nrf2 is located in cytoskeleton attached to Keap1. Nrf2, encoded by the nuclear factor (erythroid derived 2)-like 2 (Nfe2l2) gene, is a leucine zipper protein and a polypeptide. It has a molecular weight of 66 kDa and is widely expressed [1, 2]. Nfe2l2 gene contains a xenobiotic responsive element (XRE) at −712(XREL1) position of promoter region and two additional XRE-like elements found in +755(XREL2) and + 850(XREL3) positions, which are directly modulated by aryl hydrocarbon receptor (AHR) activation [3]. Nrf2, which is found in the cytoplasm in normal or stress-free conditions, migrates to the nucleus in case of oxidative stress and attaches to DNA. Mutations and changes in Nrf2 expression have been described in many cancer types [4–9]. Upregulation of Nrf2 is linked with many types of cancer, including the lung, skin, prostate, breast, and head–neck [6, 8, 10, 11]. Many mechanisms have been reported for the increased activity of Nrf2 in cancer cells. Some of them, (1) somatic mutations in Kelch-like ECH-related protein 1 (Keap1), Cullin 3 (CUL3) or

Nrf2 [12]; (2) epigenetic silencing of Keap1 [13]; (3) abnormal protein accumulation that disrupts the interaction between Nrf2 and Keap1 [14]; (4) transcriptional upregulation of Nrf2 through oncogene-dependent signaling [15]; and modification of Keap1 by metabolic programming [16]. Increasing studies show that Nrf2 activation may not be beneficial in all types and stages of cancer over the past few years. In fact, Nrf2 can ensure survival of not only normal cells, but also cancer cells, and supports the process by which Nrf2 activation in malignant cells can sustain development of the disease. The roles of the bad or good side of Nrf2 [7, 8] have caused debates because it is still not clear whether Nrf2 acts as a tumor suppressor or oncogene [7, 9]. Nrf2 hyperactivity in tumors creates a protective environment that promotes survival by protecting cancer cells from radiotherapy, oxidative stress, and chemotherapeutic agents. Therefore, there is a growing range of research aimed at identifying the boundaries between Nrf2 positive and negative responses in cancer and targeting Nrf2 therapeutically [17–19]. It is clear that Nrf2 exactly plays its protective role without distinguishing for cancer and normal cells. Current studies acknowledge the double roles of Nrf2 in carcinogenesis: protective in the early stages and harmful in the later stages.

2. Basal state induction and cellular positions

Nrf2 is inactivated transcriptionally by binding to its regulator Keap1, which targets Nrf2 for proteasomal degradation in basal conditions. CUL3 ubiquitin ligase, which governs the degradation, is a third protein. Under stable conditions, ubiquitous Nrf2 is rapidly disrupted by 26S proteasome (**Figure 1**). Nrf2 has a very short half-life of less than 30 minutes. Therefore, Nrf2 is not abundant under basal conditions and, in light of current studies, supports the claim that Nrf2 is found at a relatively low level in most organs or tissues [20–22]. Nrf2-Keap1 is of first importance in balancing homeostatic environment since cells need to respond by adapting to different stresses. Cells can use highly toxic molecules to be used in the physiological signal. These molecules contain reactive oxygen species (ROS) and reactive nitrogen types (RNSs) such as hydrogen peroxide (H_2O_2) and nitric oxide (NO). Low concentrations of these molecules are used for adaptive intracellular signaling, and high concentrations are used for defense mechanisms against microorganisms [23, 24]. But, physiological concentrations of these molecules need to be precisely regulated, and Nrf2-Keap1 play important role in this signaling.

Nrf2 is a transcription factor that regulates cellular stress signals and reacts by directing different transcriptional programs. Limited number of researchers were working only on inhibiting its protective role and carcinogenesis in suppressing oxidative or electrophilic stress till a little more than a decade ago [25, 26], but recently, Nrf2 has become a topic of widespread interest and research area. Kelch-like ECH-related protein 1 (Keap1) is a negative regulator, has encouraged many publications, and has become an important topic of discussion. The debate focuses on whether Nrf2 is tumor suppressor or reverse oncogenic, leading to the question of whether Nrf2 should be targeted for anticancer therapeutic agents [27].

Genetic analysis has shown mutations in Nrf2 and Keap1 in some cancers. These mutations increase Nrf2 expression and are related with resistance to chemotherapy and poor survival rate from cancer [18, 28]. Sequence analyses of Nrf2 and Keap1 have identified many mutations within Kelch domain and in the Neh2 domain of Keap1-Nrf2; this causes Nrf2 to unstable due to Keap1's inability to target Nrf2 for degradation and ubiquitination (**Figure 1a**). Whether activation or inhibition of Nrf2 is a good strategy for treatment or prevention of cancer is still unclear. In vivo studies have shown that basal Nrf2 protein levels decrease with age and associate

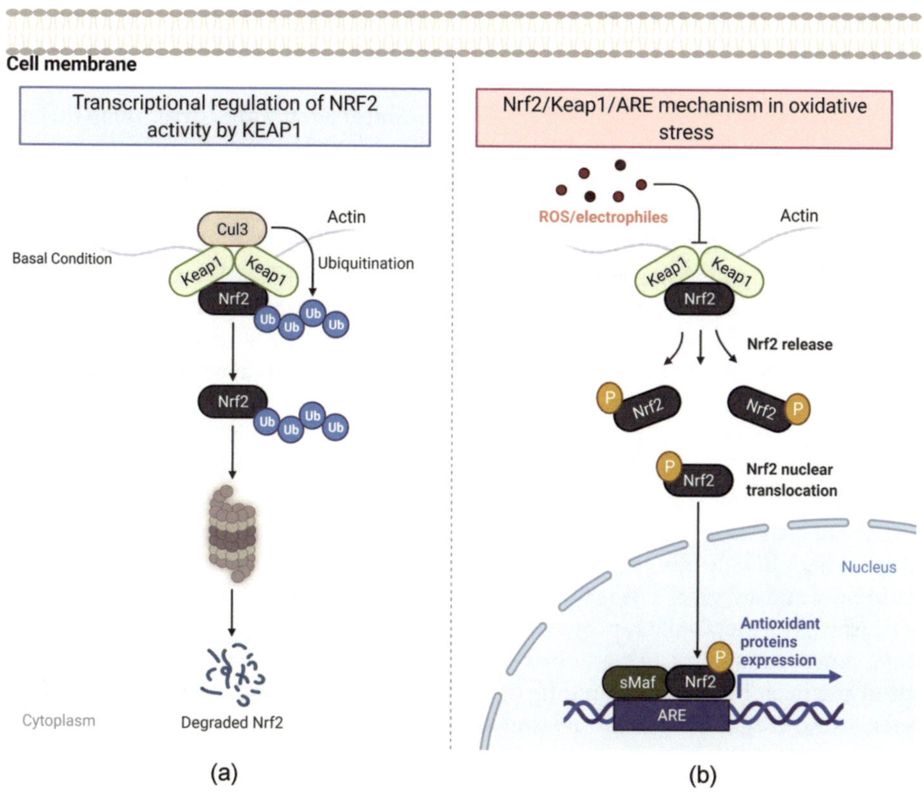

Figure 1.
Schematic of Nrf2 pathway. a) under normal conditions, Nrf2 is structurally bound to Keap1 protein in the cytoplasm. Keap1 regulates Nrf2. Keap1 targets Nrf2 for ubiquitination and then degradation via proteasomal pathway. b) ROS/electrophiles can cause sequestration of the Nrf2/Keap1 complex and subsequent phosphorylation of Nrf2, which is transferred to the nucleus. Nrf2 regulates transcriptional activation of antioxidant and detoxifying enzymes by binding target genes to antioxidant-sensitive elements (ARE) in promoter regions.

with lower expression target genes of Nrf2 [29, 30]. Therefore, it is more probable that Nrf2 acts as a defense against the aging process caused by free radicals, which gradually decreases over time, leading to accumulation of free radicals that can cause cancer progression [31, 32].

3. Keap1-Nrf2-ARE signaling

Keap1 has more than 20 groups of free sulfhydryl (-SH) in the cysteine residues. These highly reactive molecules for stress act as sensitive sensors. Reactive cysteine thiols are present as (S-) under physiological pH and are more reactive to ROS/RNS than sulfhydryl groups [33]. Keap1 alters cysteine residues, giving a response to oxidative or electrophilic stresses [34, 35]. Tert-butylhydroquinone (tBHQ), an electrophile, reacts with reactive cysteine residues in Keap1 to activate Nrf2 [36]. Binding of tBHQ to Keap1 does not impair binding of Nrf2 to Keap1; this indicates that sequestration of Nrf2 from Keap1 homodimer cannot explain electrophilic mediated induction of Nrf2 accumulation within cells [37]. These modifications result in conformational changes of Keap1 and reverse degradation of Nrf2, which is then transcriptionally activated.

Different types of stressors react differently with the cysteine residues in Keap1, suggesting that the residues of cysteine in some way contribute to activity of Keap1 individually or in combination (23,24). This indicates that Nrf2-Keap1 mechanism is not a simple "on" or "off" button mechanism but can instead respond with different mechanisms by various stress factors [23, 35].

Some of the promising Nrf2 activator or inhibitor agents are currently in different phases of clinical trials [38–40]. Human clinical trials were kept assessing the effects of inducers [41, 42]. These include: (1) approved and other purpose agents such as dimethyl fumarate (DMF) and Oltipraz; (2) compounds purified from natural sources such as broccoli sprouts, curcumin, resveratrol, and sulforaphane; and (3) highly potent triterpenoid derivatives, e.g., RTA 402-408 and CXA-10 [43].

Nrf2 protein, which forms a heterodimer structure with MA or Jun protein in the nucleus (**Figure 1b**), binds to ARE (Antioxidant Response Element) sequence on DNA and provides regulation of related gene expressions in favor of activation of antioxidant mechanisms [44]. PI3-kinase is responsible for nuclear translocation of Nrf2 and binding of Nrf2 to ARE to induce enzymes such as GST, HO-1, and NQO1. It is essentially a common DNA sequence called an antioxidant response element (ARE) similar to Nrf2-binding motif for induction [45].

Cancer cells have higher ROS levels than normal cells. Nevertheless, they can adapt to high ROS levels with the activating of certain ways that allow them to proliferate and survive. These ways include the activation of antioxidants to reduce ROS, as well as metabolic reprogramming pathways that can produce more ROS and make cancer cells more vulnerable to future stress [46, 47]. Keap1-Nrf2 pathway is one of the most important signaling pathways that play a role in the survival and defense of cell against xenobiotics and oxidative stress.

4. Keap1-dependent regulation of Nrf2

Keap1 contains 27 cysteines, which account for 4.33% of all amino acids, whereas the average cysteines content in human proteins is 2.26% [48]. Proteomic analyses have found that several of the 27 cysteines in Keap1 have been modified to respond to different electrophiles [49]. However, only three of the Keap1 cysteines, Cys151, Cys273, and Cys288, were found to be functionally important for Keap1-Nrf2 regulation [50]. Cys273 and Cys288 target Cys151, which is a subset of Nrf2 activators, although they are essentials for Keap1 to inhibit Nrf2 under basal conditions. During oxidative stress, ROS reacts with cysteine residues of Keap1, including C151, C273, and C288, allowing Nrf2 to escape Keap1-mediated degradation [51].

Human Nrf2 protein has 605 amino acids and seven highly preserved Neh (Nrf2-ECH homology) domains from Neh1 to Neh7 (**Figure 2**). Neh1 domain contains small musculoaponeurotic fibrosarcoma homologous proteins (MafF, MafG or MafK) and a basic leucine zipper (bZIP) motif that is heterodimerized for DNA binding and transcriptional activation [52]. Neh2 regulatory domain of N-terminal contains DLG and ETGE motifs critical to Keap1 binding and resulting in Nrf2 degradation [53].

Neh3 domain is located in C-terminal of Nrf2 contains VFLVPK motif, which is critical for binding to CHD6 helicase [54]. Nrf2's N-terminal includes two transactivation domains, Neh4 and Neh5, and both domains were found to be necessary for Nrf2's maximum transactivation activity [55]. Neh6 domain contains a degron containing a DSG motif embedded in a set of serine-rich residues. This binding region is a docking site for adaptor protein β-TrCP, which mediates ubiquitin ligase of Nrf2 by a Cullin1-Rbx1 complex [56]. Neh7 domain interacts with the retinoic acid receptor a (RARa) and suppresses Nrf2 transcriptional activity in the nucleus [57].

Nrf2 degradation can be stopped when exposed to electrophiles and ROS. Reactive cysteines are a small set of protein cysteines with pKa values relatively low

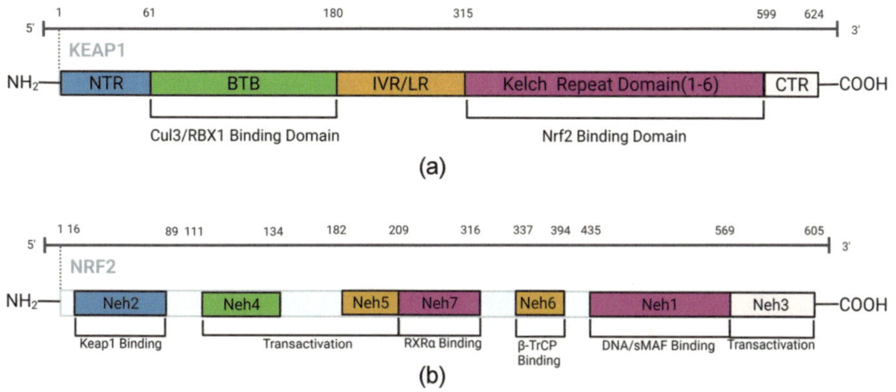

Figure 2.
Domain structure of Keap1 and Nrf2. a) Keap1 is sectioned into five domains. These are N-terminal region (NTR), Tramtrack, and Bric-à-Brac (BTB) domain, an intervening region (IVR), six Kelch repeats, and a C-terminal region (CTR). The BTB domain mediates homodimerization of Keap1 monomers as well as Cul3 binding. The IVR contains several important cysteines for regulating Keap1 activity by forming a complex with CUL3 and RBX1 to form a component of E3 ubiquitin ligase. Both IVR and CTR are responsible for Keap1 to retain Nrf2 in the cytoplasm. The NTR contains 60 amino acids. The Kelch domain in Keap1 consists of six repeat sequences (K1–K6) and interacts with DLG and ETGE of Nrf2 domain. The Kelch domain also contains double glycine repeats (DGR). b) Nrf2 comprises seven Nrf2-ECH(Neh1-7) homology domains. The Neh6 domain, which is serine-rich region, and Neh2 are important for binding because they are negative regulatory domains of Keap1 and β-TrCP, respectively, resulting in Nrf2 ubiquitination and proteasomal degradation. Neh3, Neh4, and Neh5 domains are necessary for binding to transcriptional activity. The Neh1 domain is a basic leucin zipper motif, which is responsible for its stability, ARE sequence to bind in DNA, and dimerization with sMaf proteins. The Neh7 domain interacts with the retinoid X receptor alpha (RXRα), which is a repressor of Nrf2.

around 4 and 5 due to the effect of surrounding amino acid microenvironment, unlike most protein cysteine thiols with pKa values of about 8.5. Reactive thiols are perfectly targets for electrophiles, and indeed, several electrophilic reagents have been shown to directly alter thiols. The modification of Keap1 is thought to impair structural integrity of Keap1-Cul3 E3 ligase complex, causing a decrease in ubiquitination activity, thereby facilitating accumulation of Nrf2 [58, 59]. In recent studies, presence of unrestricted Keap1 has recognized deleterious effects to cellular homeostasis and highlighted Nrf2's role as Keap1's suppressor that implies that Nrf2 and Keap1 are mutually blocking each other [60]. Under normal conditions, Keap1 plays an important role in limiting Nrf2 activity by binding to DLG/ETGE motifs in the Neh2 domain and inducing ubiquitination and proteasomal degradation of Nrf2 (**Figure 1a**) [61].

Permanent activation of Nrf2 in tumor cells is activation of p62, that is, a multifunctional protein involved in selective autophagy that is often overexpressed in tumors [6]. p62 in phosphoryl form can bind with Keap1 in the same binding domain for Nrf2, thereby competitively inhibiting Keap1/Nrf2 interaction resulting in Nrf2 stabilization and translocated into the nucleus. Nrf2 can consecutively upregulate p62 gene expression, thereby upregulation of a pro-survival circuit that can support tumor formation. The accumulation of proteins and metabolites that disrupt Keap1-Nrf2 can activate Nrf2 in cancer. p62 is the best-known disruptor that competes with Nrf2 for direct attachment to Keap1 through an SQSTM1 motif similar to ETGE motif in Nrf2 [62]. After p62 is bound to Keap1, it causes Keap1 to go into autophagic degradation [63]. Recent studies have shown that p62 gene expression is upregulated in hepatocellular carcinoma and that the activation of Nrf2 induced by p62 is critical for HCC development [64, 65].

Kelch domain of Keap1 interacts with two different sequences of amino acids found in the N-terminal of Nrf2: ETGE and DLG [66]. Based on a series of critical observations, "Hinge-Latch model" (**Figure 3**) that is Keap1-Nrf2 interactive two-site binding model was proposed [66]. ETGE motif has a higher affinity for Kelch-repetition domain than DLG motif. Therefore, Keap1 captures Nrf2 through ETGE motif before DLG motif is attached to adjacent unoccupied Kelch-repeat domains; this is called the "hinge and latch" mechanism [67, 68]. The modes of binding DLG and ETGE to Keap1 are quite different [69]. Keap1-DLG binding is

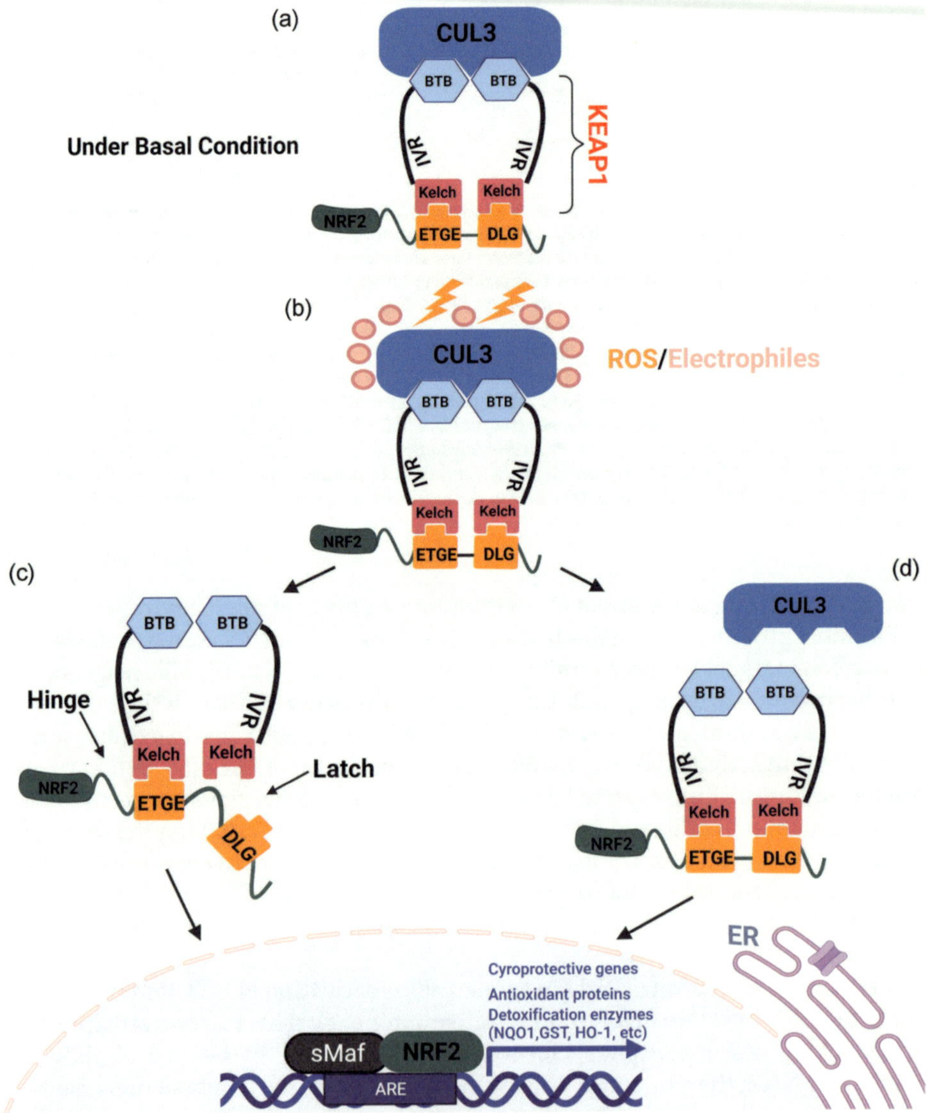

Figure 3.
*The regulation of Nrf2 via the Nrf2-Keap1-ARE mechanism under basal and stress conditions, as explained with the "hinge and latch" model. a) under basal condition, two Keap1 molecules and one Nrf2 molecule form a trimer structure and Nrf2 is polyubiquitylated by the Keap1-Cul3 E3 ubiquitin ligases and then disrupted by 26S proteasome (**Figure 1a**). b) under induced conditions, inducers(ROS/electrophiles) modify Keap1 cysteine thiols and inhibit Nrf2 ubiquitination, causing Nrf2 activation and induction. c) the binding of Nrf2 to Keap1 is disrupted by the modifications of cysteine residues of Keap1, which contains what is known as the "cysteine code." these modifications lead to conformational changes that enable Nrf2 to escape from degradation and lead to Nrf2 upregulation. It occurred via the loss of binding of the low-affinity interaction with DLG(latch) motif to Keap1 and binding with the ETGE(hinge) motif remains. d) Stress-induced modification of Keap1 cysteines disrupted Keap1's ability to serve as an adapter for the Cul3-Keap1 ubiquitin ligase complex, thereby causing stabilization and transcriptional activation of Nrf2. On both models shown in C and D, Nrf2 translocates to the nucleus, binds to the ARE, and activates gene expression such as NQO1, HO-1, and GST.*

characterized as kinetically a "fast-on-fast-off," which is thermodynamically guided by both enthalpy and entropy. In contrast, ETGE-Keap1 binding is characterized by completely enthalpy guided and involves a two-state reaction that leads to more stable conformation [70, 71]. These findings support the claim that DLG motif serves as a converter that transmits environmental stress to Nrf2 induction as a latch (**Figure 3**).

5. Nrf2-regulated cytoprotective genes

Nrf2 plays a major role in the protective mechanism against xenobiotics, which can initiate carcinogenesis by damaging DNA [72]. Nrf2 increases expression of antioxidant enzymes. Gene transcription profiles showed that not all genes around Nrf2 are transcriptionally regulated by Nrf2 binding. These genes require transcription factors, cofactors, and intermediaries for complete activation [73]. Antioxidant molecules such as glutathione (GSH), vitamin C and E, bilirubin, and antioxidant proteins such as thioredoxin (Trx), Superoxide Dismutase (SOD), catalase, peroxiredoxin, glutathione peroxidase (GPx) are major antioxidant molecules that play a role in balancing oxidative stress. Nrf2 and its downregulatory effectors have been shown to be critically important regulators in the regulation of intracellular redox state and in protecting cells from oxidative stress and chemical damage in the lungs and liver [74, 75]. Nrf2 loss has been associated with advanced metastasis. For example, loss of Nrf2 initiates a harmful cascading of decreased GST expression and raises ROS level, ultimately leading to DNA damage and tumor formation [76]. The role of Nrf2 signaling as a tumor suppressor is due to a lot of in vivo studies comparing susceptibility to carcinogenicity chemically induced in Nrf2-knockout mice (Nfe2l2−/−) and wild-type mice. In this context, Nrf2-null mice were found to be more prone to developing bladder, stomach, and skin cancer when exposed to carcinogen substances compared with wild-type mice. This gene has a deficiency and susceptibility to oxidative damage, and chemical carcinogenesis increases in Nrf2-knockout mice [75]. Expression of antioxidant and phase II enzymes was found to be eliminated in mice with Nrf2 deficiency. Heavy quinone-induced made mice with Nrf2 deficiency more prone to skin cancer, while NQO1 and GST expression regulated by Nrf2 decreased compared with wild mice [77]. In addition, expression levels of ARE-mediated genes such as glutathione-*S*-transferases (GSTs) isozymes, NADP(H): quinone oxidoreductase (NQO1), stress response proteins such as heme oxygenase (HO-1), glutamate cysteine ligase (GCL), and UDP-glucuronosyltransferase (UGT) were found to be significantly repressed in mice with Nrf2 deficiency compared with their wild types [25, 78, 79]. Nrf2 transcriptional targets are not only a well-known antioxidant enzyme such as glutathione peroxidase (GPX) and superoxide dismutase (SOD) to clean ROS, but also two other genes related to detoxification and anabolic reprogramming.

Nrf2 downstream targets are separated into three main groups: phase I and phase II drug metabolizing enzymes (DMEs) and phase III drug carriers. Phase I enzymes oxidize drugs or xenobiotics such as aldo-ketoreductases (AKRs) and cytochrome P450s (CYPs) encoded by genes regulated by Nrf2; Phase II enzymes conjugate products of phase I reactions, while phase III enzymes carry final metabolites out of cells in collaboration to implement a cytoprotective function. Several phase I enzymes also play important roles in removal of xenobiotics through hydrolysis, reduction, and oxidation. Phase I, cytochrome P450 (CYP) family, aldehyde oxidase (ACO) contain modification of xenobiotics by enzymes such as aldehyde dehydrogenases (ALDHs), aldo-ketoreductases (AKRs), alcohol dehydrogenases (ADHs), esterase, flavins-containing monooxygenases (FMOs), and cyclooxygenases (COXs) [80]; (ii) phase II enzymes such as GST, UGT, Sulfotransferases (SULTs), N-acetyltransferases (NATs), and methyltransferases (MTs) add polar groups to phase I products to prepare them from excretion [81]; and (iii) carriers, ATP-binding cassette (ABC), and dissolved solute-carrier (SLC) export metabolites (modified) out of the cell [82].

Phase II drug metabolism or conjugation reactions involve a different group of enzymes, which often lead to water-soluble products that can be excreted with bile or urine. Conjugation reactions include: glucuronidation, acetylation, sulfation, methylation, amino acid and glutathione conjugation.

The protective effects of upregulation of Nrf2 signaling can be in various forms. Protection can be instantaneous by stimulation of genes that are directly regulated through Nrf2 binding to AREs in the target genes [83, 84]. Protective effects can be secondary through stimulation of macromolecular damage removal/repair mechanisms [84, 85]. Protective effects can be tertial through induction of tissue repair/regeneration pathways [86]. p53, which is a tumor suppressor, reduces Nrf2 activity, stopping cell growth and inducing apoptosis [87].

Regulation of Nrf2 can be unstable against the loss of inducible nature of Nrf2 signaling and acquisition of a structurally active phenotype. The constructive signal for expression of cytoprotective enzymes would give cells surviving chance under stress conditions. This seemingly positive condition would become a serious disadvantage in progression of cancer pathogenesis and treatment. Therefore, structural activation or increased signaling of Nrf2 pathway can be determined for destiny of cell during tumorigenesis and affect response to radiotherapy and chemotherapy. Under these circumstances, Nrf2 can be described as an oncogene [32, 88].

6. Tumor suppressor and oncogenic roles of Nrf2

Nrf2 protects cells from oxidative stress, in vivo studies with rats have shown that basal Nrf2 protein levels decrease with age and correlate with lower expression of Nrf2 target genes [89]. Increasing Nrf2 activity, which facilitates tumor formation and proliferation of K-Ras, B-Raf, and Myc in cancer cells, helps reduce intracellular ROS levels. Overexpression of Nrf2 also regulates cell proliferation by directing glucose and glutamine to anabolic pathways, increasing purine synthesis and affecting pentose phosphate pathway to promote cell proliferation [90]. In addition, under hypoxia/reoxygenation, Keap1 reduced expression and increased expression of Prx1, Nrf2, and peroxiredoxin-1 (Prx1) proteins, which reduce ROS levels and ultimately protect cancer cell [91]. In a study of Nrf2+/− mice exposed to diesel exhaust and N-nitroso butyl (4-hydroxybutyl) amine, increased pulmonary DNA adducts and bladder tumors were shown [92, 93].

Mutations that cause Keap1 loss of function and Nrf2 function gain and gene mutations that lead to electrophilic metabolite accumulation can also trigger continuous Nrf2 activity in cancer [94]. Nrf2 and its target gene expression levels can serve as biomarkers for diagnosis of lung cancers. Large-scale multi-tumor sequencing efforts by The Cancer Genome Atlas (TCGA) project found that CUL3 and Keap1 function loss and Nrf2 functional gain mutations were significantly enriched in lung adenocarcinoma, pulmonary squamous cell carcinoma and lung squamous cell carcinoma, and bladder cancer [95–97].

Oncogene activation, including oncogenic mutants of K-Ras, B-Raf, and c-Myc, may cause upregulated expression of Nfe2l2 gene [98]. K-Ras and B-Raf activations induce transcription of Nrf2 through activation of Jun and Myc transcription factors. This activation of Nrf2 has been shown to be critical for increased chemoresistance and tumor growth of Ras mutant cancer cells [15, 99].

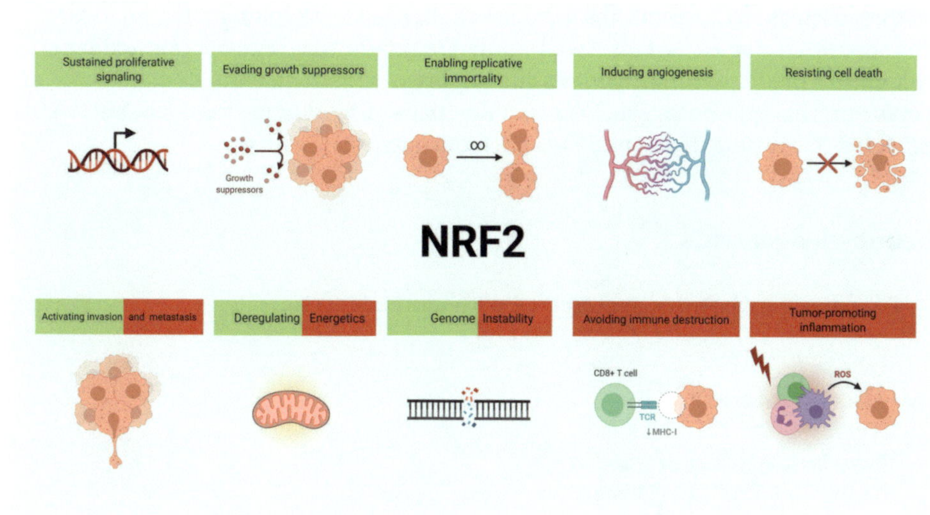

Figure 4.
Involvement of Nrf2 in the hallmarks of cancer contributes directly or indirectly. (red is blocker and green is activator roles to promote tumorigenesis).

mRNA and protein levels of AKRs have been shown to be biomarkers for diagnosis of cancers activated by Nrf2 [100]. AKRs are detected with greater precision than Nrf2. Several studies have shown that cancer cells with high levels of Nrf2 are less susceptible to common chemotherapeutic agents such as etoposide, carboplatin, cisplatin, 5-fluorouracil, and doxorubicin [10, 11, 101, 102].

Nrf2-targeting agents with advanced specificity are needed to increase effectiveness of cancer treatment. In addition, controversial roles of Nrf2 in cancer prevention and progression suggest that more issues need to be addressed to determine optimal use of Nrf2 activators or inhibitors in the clinic [103]. Nrf2 may have both tumor-suppressive and -promoting effects (**Figure 4**). Nrf2 target genes regulate autophagy, mitochondrial physiology, redox homeostasis, proteasomal degradation, energy metabolism, iron metabolism, amino acid metabolism, survival, reproduction, DNA repair, and drug metabolism and excretion [104–106].

Overexpression of sMaf proteins results in a decrease in transcriptional activity of Nrf2. However, there are no studies that identify different gene expressions or mutations of sMaf family proteins in tumors [107].

Dysregulation of epigenetic mechanism is hallmark of cancer. It is shown that acetylation conditions resulted in promoting nuclear localization of Nrf2, while deacetylation promoting cytoplasmic rather than nuclear localization of Nrf2. Hypermethylation of Keap1 promoter has been detected in the breast, lung, brain, and colorectal [108–110] and causes a decrease in Keap1 mRNA production and therefore Nrf2 activation [111–113].

7. Conclusions

In general, the question of whether Nrf2 activation is bilateral role is explained via several contexts, levels, and mechanisms. The above data strongly suggest that inhibition or activation of Nrf2 alone or in combination can be a promising therapeutic strategy for cancer treatment. In numerous in vitro and in vivo studies, multiple genomic, transcriptional, and proteomic mechanisms related to Nrf2 activation in cancer have been explained in detail. Targeting one of redox signaling factors, such as Nrf2, seems like a crucial challenge for designing efficient cancer therapeutic strategies. Nrf2 is a well-known regulator that regulates antioxidant system and mediates tumorigenesis and suppression. Nrf2 should be considered an important therapeutic target. Nrf2 is in the focus of worldwide research, and we are expected to continue to see more research outputs in the future.

Acknowledgements

All figures are licensed and created with biorender.com.

Conflict of interest

There is no conflict of interest.

Author details

Mustafa Yildiz[1*] and Hatice Segmen[2]

1 Faculty of Medicine, Department of Biophysics, Trakya University, Edirne, Turkey

2 Kanuni Sultan Suleyman Training and Research Hospital, Department of Neurology, Saglik Bilimleri University, Istanbul, Turkey

*Address all correspondence to: myildiz@live.com

References

[1] Chanas SA, Jiang Q, McMahon M, McWalter GK, McLellan LI, Elcombe CR, et al. Loss of the Nrf2 transcription factor causes a marked reduction in constitutive and inducible expression of the glutathione S-transferase Gsta1, Gsta2, Gstm1, Gstm2, Gstm3 and Gstm4 genes in the livers of male and female mice. The Biochemical Journal. 2002;**365**(Pt 2): 405-416

[2] Kwak MK, Wakabayashi N, Itoh K, Motohashi H, Yamamoto M, Kensler TW. Modulation of gene expression by cancer chemopreventive dithiolethiones through the Keap1-Nrf2 pathway. Identification of novel gene clusters for cell survival. The Journal of Biological Chemistry. 2003;**278**(10): 8135-8145

[3] Miao W, Hu L, Scrivens PJ, Batist G. Transcriptional regulation of NF-E2 p45-related factor (NRF2) expression by the aryl hydrocarbon receptor-xenobiotic response element signaling pathway: Direct cross-talk between phase I and II drug-metabolizing enzymes. The Journal of Biological Chemistry. 2005;**280**(21):20340-20348

[4] Nioi P, Nguyen T. A mutation of Keap1 found in breast cancer impairs its ability to repress Nrf2 activity. Biochemical and Biophysical Research Communications. 2007;**362**(4): 816-821

[5] Jiang T, Chen N, Zhao F, Wang XJ, Kong B, Zheng W, et al. High levels of Nrf2 determine chemoresistance in type II endometrial cancer. Cancer Research. 2010;**70**(13):5486-5496

[6] Padmanabhan B, Tong KI, Ohta T, Nakamura Y, Scharlock M, Ohtsuji M, et al. Structural basis for defects of Keap1 activity provoked by its point mutations in lung cancer. Molecular Cell. 2006;**21**(5):689-700

[7] Singh A, Misra V, Thimmulappa RK, Lee H, Ames S, Hoque MO, et al. Dysfunctional KEAP1-NRF2 interaction in non-small-cell lung cancer. PLoS Medicine. 2006;**3**(10):1865-1876

[8] Kim YR, Oh JE, Kim MS, Kang MR, Park SW, Han JY, et al. Oncogenic NRF2 mutations in squamous cell carcinomas of oesophagus and skin. The Journal of Pathology. 2010;**220**(4):446-451

[9] He F, Ru X, Wen T. NRF2, a transcription factor for stress response and beyond. International Journal of Molecular Sciences. 2020;**21**(13):4777

[10] Ohta T, Iijima K, Miyamoto M, Nakahara I, Tanaka H, Ohtsuji M, et al. Loss of Keap1 function activates Nrf2 and provides advantages for lung cancer cell growth. Cancer Research. 2008;**68**(5):1303-1309

[11] Shibata T, Kokubu A, Gotoh M, Ojima H, Ohta T, Yamamoto M, et al. Genetic alteration of Keap1 confers constitutive Nrf2 activation and resistance to chemotherapy in gallbladder cancer. Gastroenterology. 2008;**135**(4):1358-1368. 1368 e1-4

[12] Yoo NJ, Kim HR, Kim YR, An CH, Lee SH. Somatic mutations of the KEAP1 gene in common solid cancers. Histopathology. 2012;**60**(6):943-952

[13] Cheng D, Wu R, Guo Y, Kong AN. Regulation of Keap1-Nrf2 signaling: The role of epigenetics. Curr Opin Toxicol. 2016;**1**:134-138

[14] Motohashi H, Yamamoto M. Nrf2-Keap1 defines a physiologically important stress response mechanism. Trends in Molecular Medicine. 2004; **10**(11):549-557

[15] DeNicola GM, Karreth FA, Humpton TJ, Gopinathan A, Wei C, Frese K, et al. Oncogene-induced Nrf2

transcription promotes ROS detoxification and tumorigenesis. Nature. 2011;**475**(7354):106-109

[16] Leinonen HM, Kansanen E, Polonen P, Heinaniemi M, Levonen AL. Dysregulation of the Keap1-Nrf2 pathway in cancer. Biochemical Society Transactions. 2015;**43**(4):645-649

[17] Lau A, Villeneuve NF, Sun Z, Wong PK, Zhang DD. Dual roles of Nrf2 in cancer. Pharmacological Research. 2008;**58**(5-6):262-270

[18] Wang XJ, Sun Z, Villeneuve NF, Zhang S, Zhao F, Li Y, et al. Nrf2 enhances resistance of cancer cells to chemotherapeutic drugs, the dark side of Nrf2. Carcinogenesis. 2008;**29**(6):1235-1243

[19] Sporn MB, Liby KT. NRF2 and cancer: The good, the bad and the importance of context. Nature Reviews. Cancer. 2012;**12**(8):564-571

[20] Kobayashi A, Kang MI, Okawa H, Ohtsuji M, Zenke Y, Chiba T, et al. Oxidative stress sensor Keap1 functions as an adaptor for Cul3-based E3 ligase to regulate proteasomal degradation of Nrf2. Molecular and Cellular Biology. 2004;**24**(16):7130-7139

[21] Taguchi K, Yamamoto M. The KEAP1-NRF2 system as a molecular target of cancer treatment. Cancers (Basel). 2020;**13**(1):46

[22] Itoh K, Wakabayashi N, Katoh Y, Ishii T, O'Connor T, Yamamoto M. Keap1 regulates both cytoplasmic-nuclear shuttling and degradation of Nrf2 in response to electrophiles. Genes to Cells. 2003;**8**(4):379-391

[23] Yamamoto T, Suzuki T, Kobayashi A, Wakabayashi J, Maher J, Motohashi H, et al. Physiological significance of reactive cysteine residues of Keap1 in determining Nrf2 activity. Molecular and Cellular Biology. 2008;**28**(8):2758-2770

[24] Budak M. Radiation and DNA Methylation Mechanisms, DNA Methylation Mechanism. Rijeka: IntechOpen; 2020. pp. 3-17

[25] Itoh K, Chiba T, Takahashi S, Ishii T, Igarashi K, Katoh Y, et al. An Nrf2/small Maf heterodimer mediates the induction of phase II detoxifying enzyme genes through antioxidant response elements. Biochemical and Biophysical Research Communications. 1997;**236**(2):313-322

[26] Ramos-Gomez M, Kwak MK, Dolan PM, Itoh K, Yamamoto M, Talalay P, et al. Sensitivity to carcinogenesis is increased and chemoprotective efficacy of enzyme inducers is lost in nrf2 transcription factor-deficient mice. Proceedings of the National Academy of Sciences of the United States of America. 2001;**98**(6): 3410-3415

[27] Kensler TW, Wakabayashi N. Nrf2: Friend or foe for chemoprevention? Carcinogenesis. 2010;**31**(1):90-99

[28] Taguchi K, Motohashi H, Yamamoto M. Molecular mechanisms of the Keap1-Nrf2 pathway in stress response and cancer evolution. Genes to Cells. 2011;**16**(2):123-140

[29] Zhang H, Davies KJA, Forman HJ. Oxidative stress response and Nrf2 signaling in aging. Free Radical Biology & Medicine. 2015;**88**(Pt B):314-336

[30] Schmidlin CJ, Dodson MB, Madhavan L, Zhang DD. Redox regulation by NRF2 in aging and disease. Free Radical Biology & Medicine. 2019;**134**:702-707

[31] Sykiotis GP, Bohmann D. Stress-activated cap'n'collar transcription factors in aging and human disease. Science Signaling. 2010;**3**(112):re3

[32] Shelton P, Jaiswal AK. The transcription factor NF-E2-related factor 2 (Nrf2): A protooncogene? The FASEB Journal. 2013;**27**(2):414-423

[33] Janssen-Heininger YM, Mossman BT, Heintz NH, Forman HJ, Kalyanaraman B, Finkel T, et al. Redox-based regulation of signal transduction: Principles, pitfalls, and promises. Free Radical Biology & Medicine. 2008; **45**(1):1-17

[34] Hayes JD, McMahon M, Chowdhry S, Dinkova-Kostova AT. Cancer chemoprevention mechanisms mediated through the Keap1-Nrf2 pathway. Antioxidants & Redox Signaling. 2010;**13**(11):1713-1748

[35] Kobayashi M, Li L, Iwamoto N, Nakajima-Takagi Y, Kaneko H, Nakayama Y, et al. The antioxidant defense system Keap1-Nrf2 comprises a multiple sensing mechanism for responding to a wide range of chemical compounds. Molecular and Cellular Biology. 2009;**29**(2):493-502

[36] Abiko Y, Miura T, Phuc BH, Shinkai Y, Kumagai Y. Participation of covalent modification of Keap1 in the activation of Nrf2 by tert-butylbenzoquinone, an electrophilic metabolite of butylated hydroxyanisole. Toxicol Appl Pharm. 2011;**255**(1):32-39

[37] Taguchi K, Yamamoto M. The KEAP1-NRF2 system in cancer. Frontiers in Oncology. 2017;**7**:85

[38] Magesh S, Chen Y, Hu L. Small molecule modulators of K eap1-N rf2-ARE pathway as potential preventive and therapeutic agents. Medicinal Research Reviews. 2012;**32**(4): 687-726

[39] Jimenez-Osorio AS, Gonzalez-Reyes S, Pedraza-Chaverri J. Natural Nrf2 activators in diabetes. Clinica Chimica Acta. 2015;**448**:182-192

[40] Houghton CA, Fassett RG, Coombes JS. Sulforaphane and other nutrigenomic Nrf2 activators: Can the Clinician's expectation Be matched by the reality? Oxidative Medicine and Cellular Longevity. 2016;**2016**:7857186

[41] Kensler TW, Chen JG, Egner PA, Fahey JW, Jacobson LP, Stephenson KK, et al. Effects of glucosinolate-rich broccoli sprouts on urinary levels of aflatoxin-DNA adducts and phenanthrene tetraols in a randomized clinical trial in He Zuo township, Qidong, People's Republic of China. Cancer Epidemiology, Biomarkers & Prevention. 2005;**14**(11 Pt 1):2605-2613

[42] Wang JS, Shen X, He X, Zhu YR, Zhang BC, Wang JB, et al. Protective alterations in phase 1 and 2 metabolism of aflatoxin B1 by oltipraz in residents of Qidong, People's Republic of China. Journal of the National Cancer Institute. 1999;**91**(4):347-354

[43] Tebay LE, Robertson H, Durant ST, Vitale SR, Penning TM, Dinkova-Kostova AT, et al. Mechanisms of activation of the transcription factor Nrf2 by redox stressors, nutrient cues, and energy status and the pathways through which it attenuates degenerative disease. Free Radical Biology & Medicine. 2015;**88**(Pt B): 108-146

[44] Nguyen T, Sherratt PJ, Pickett CB. Regulatory mechanisms controlling gene expression mediated by the antioxidant response element. Annual Review of Pharmacology and Toxicology. 2003;**43**(1):233-260

[45] Ma Q. Role of nrf2 in oxidative stress and toxicity. Annual Review of Pharmacology and Toxicology. 2013;**53**:401-426

[46] Harris IS, Treloar AE, Inoue S, Sasaki M, Gorrini C, Lee KC, et al. Glutathione and thioredoxin

antioxidant pathways synergize to drive cancer initiation and progression. Cancer Cell. 2015;**27**(2):211-222

[47] Schumacker PT. Reactive oxygen species in cancer: A dance with the devil. Cancer Cell. 2015;**27**(2):156-157

[48] Kopacz A, Kloska D, Forman HJ, Jozkowicz A, Grochot-Przeczek A. Beyond repression of Nrf2: An update on Keap1. Free Radical Biology & Medicine. 2020;**157**:63-74

[49] Kansanen E, Jyrkkanen HK, Levonen AL. Activation of stress signaling pathways by electrophilic oxidized and nitrated lipids. Free Radical Biology & Medicine. 2012;**52**(6):973-982

[50] Shibata T, Ohta T, Tong KI, Kokubu A, Odogawa R, Tsuta K, et al. Cancer related mutations in NRF2 impair its recognition by Keap1-Cul3 E3 ligase and promote malignancy. Proceedings of the National Academy of Sciences. 2008;**105**(36):13568-13573

[51] Baird L, Lleres D, Swift S, Dinkova-Kostova AT. Regulatory flexibility in the Nrf2-mediated stress response is conferred by conformational cycling of the Keap1-Nrf2 protein complex. Proceedings of the National Academy of Sciences of the United States of America. 2013;**110**(38): 15259-15264

[52] Chen QM. Nrf2 for cardiac protection: Pharmacological options against oxidative stress. Trends in Pharmacological Sciences. 2021; **42**(9):729-744

[53] Tong KI, Katoh Y, Kusunoki H, Itoh K, Tanaka T, Yamamoto M. Keap1 recruits Neh2 through binding to ETGE and DLG motifs: Characterization of the two-site molecular recognition model. Molecular and Cellular Biology. 2006;**26**(8):2887-2900

[54] Nam LB, Keum YS. Binding partners of NRF2: Functions and regulatory mechanisms. Archives of Biochemistry and Biophysics. 2019;**678**:108184

[55] Katoh Y, Itoh K, Yoshida E, Miyagishi M, Fukamizu A, Yamamoto M. Two domains of Nrf2 cooperatively bind CBP, a CREB binding protein, and synergistically activate transcription. Genes to Cells. 2001;**6**(10):857-868

[56] Rojo AI, Medina-Campos ON, Rada P, Zuniga-Toala A, Lopez-Gazcon A, Espada S, et al. Signaling pathways activated by the phytochemical nordihydroguaiaretic acid contribute to a Keap1-independent regulation of Nrf2 stability: Role of glycogen synthase kinase-3. Free Radical Biology & Medicine. 2012;**52**(2):473-487

[57] Keum YS, Choi BY. Molecular and chemical regulation of the Keap1-Nrf2 signaling pathway. Molecules. 2014;**19**(7):10074-10089

[58] Holland R, Hawkins AE, Eggler AL, Mesecar AD, Fabris D, Fishbein JC. Prospective type 1 and type 2 disulfides of Keap1 protein. Chemical Research in Toxicology. 2008;**21**(10):2051-2060

[59] Sekhar KR, Rachakonda G, Freeman ML. Cysteine-based regulation of the CUL3 adaptor protein Keap1. Toxicol Appl Pharm. 2010;**244**(1):21-26

[60] Bono S, Feligioni M, Corbo M. Impaired antioxidant KEAP1-NRF2 system in amyotrophic lateral sclerosis: NRF2 activation as a potential therapeutic strategy. Molecular Neurodegeneration. 2021;**16**(1):71

[61] Itoh K, Mimura J, Yamamoto M. Discovery of the negative regulator of Nrf2, Keap1: A historical overview. Antioxidants & Redox Signaling. 2010;**13**(11):1665-1678

[62] Copple IM, Lister A, Obeng AD, Kitteringham NR, Jenkins RE, Layfield R, et al. Physical and functional

interaction of sequestosome 1 with Keap1 regulates the Keap1-Nrf2 cell defense pathway. The Journal of Biological Chemistry. 2010;**285**(22): 16782-16788

[63] Jung BJ, Yoo HS, Shin S, Park YJ, Jeon SM. Dysregulation of NRF2 in cancer: From molecular mechanisms to therapeutic opportunities. Biomol Ther (Seoul). 2018;**26**(1):57-68

[64] Komatsu M, Kurokawa H, Waguri S, Taguchi K, Kobayashi A, Ichimura Y, et al. The selective autophagy substrate p62 activates the stress responsive transcription factor Nrf2 through inactivation of Keap1. Nature Cell Biology. 2010;**12**(3):213-223

[65] Umemura A, He F, Taniguchi K, Nakagawa H, Yamachika S, Font-Burgada J, et al. p62, upregulated during Preneoplasia, induces hepatocellular carcinogenesis by maintaining survival of stressed HCC-initiating cells. Cancer Cell. 2016;**29**(6):935-948

[66] Tong KI, Kobayashi A, Katsuoka F, Yamamoto M. Two-site substrate recognition model for the Keap1-Nrf2 system: A hinge and latch mechanism. Biological Chemistry. 2006;**387**(10-11): 1311-1320

[67] Hayes JD, McMahon M. NRF2 and KEAP1 mutations: Permanent activation of an adaptive response in cancer. Trends in Biochemical Sciences. 2009;**34**(4):176-188

[68] Martin-Montalvo A, Villalba JM, Navas P, de Cabo R. NRF2, cancer and calorie restriction. Oncogene. 2011; **30**(5):505-520

[69] Suzuki T, Yamamoto M. Molecular basis of the Keap1-Nrf2 system. Free Radical Biology & Medicine. 2015;**88** (Pt B):93-100

[70] Fukutomi T, Takagi K, Mizushima T, Ohuchi N, Yamamoto M. Kinetic, thermodynamic, and structural characterizations of the association between Nrf2-DLGex degron and Keap1. Molecular and Cellular Biology. 2014;**34**(5):832-846

[71] Baird L, Swift S, Lleres D, Dinkova-Kostova AT. Monitoring Keap1-Nrf2 interactions in single live cells. Biotechnology Advances. 2014;**32**(6):1133-1144

[72] Giudice A, Montella M. Activation of the Nrf2-ARE signaling pathway: A promising strategy in cancer prevention. BioEssays. 2006;**28**(2):169-181

[73] Chorley BN, Campbell MR, Wang X, Karaca M, Sambandan D, Bangura F, et al. Identification of novel NRF2-regulated genes by ChIP-Seq: Influence on retinoid X receptor alpha. Nucleic Acids Research. 2012;**40**(15):7416-7429

[74] Chan K, Han XD, Kan YW. An important function of Nrf2 in combating oxidative stress: Detoxification of acetaminophen. Proceedings of the National Academy of Sciences of the United States of America. 2001;**98**(8):4611-4616

[75] Chan K, Kan YW. Nrf2 is essential for protection against acute pulmonary injury in mice. Proceedings of the National Academy of Sciences of the United States of America. 1999;**96**(22):12731-12736

[76] Frohlich DA, McCabe MT, Arnold RS, Day ML. The role of Nrf2 in increased reactive oxygen species and DNA damage in prostate tumorigenesis. Oncogene. 2008;**27**(31):4353-4362

[77] Long DJ 2nd, Waikel RL, Wang XJ, Perlaky L, Roop DR, Jaiswal AK. NAD(P)H:Quinone oxidoreductase 1 deficiency increases susceptibility to benzo(a)pyrene-induced mouse skin carcinogenesis. Cancer Research. 2000;**60**(21):5913-5915

[78] Wakabayashi N, Dinkova-Kostova AT, Holtzclaw WD, Kang MI, Kobayashi A, Yamamoto M, et al. Protection against electrophile and oxidant stress by induction of the phase 2 response: Fate of cysteines of the Keap1 sensor modified by inducers. Proceedings of the National Academy of Sciences of the United States of America. 2004;**101**(7): 2040-2045

[79] Telkoparan-Akillilar P, Suzen S, Saso L. Pharmacological applications of Nrf2 inhibitors as potential antineoplastic drugs. International Journal of Molecular Sciences. 2019;**20**(8):2025

[80] Fan PW, Zhang D, Halladay JS, Driscoll JP, Khojasteh SC. Going beyond common drug metabolizing enzymes: Case studies of biotransformation involving aldehyde oxidase, gamma-Glutamyl Transpeptidase, Cathepsin B, Flavin-containing monooxygenase, and ADP-Ribosyltransferase. Drug Metabolism and Disposition. 2016; **44**(8):1253-1261

[81] Stanley LA. Drug metabolism. In: Badal S, Delgoda R, editors. Pharmacognosy. London, UK: Elsevier; 2017. pp. 527-545. DOI: 10.1016/B978-0-12-802104-0.00027-5

[82] I.T. Consortium. Membrane transporters in drug development, Nature reviews. Drug discovery. 2010;**9**(3):215

[83] Kim YC, Masutani H, Yamaguchi Y, Itoh K, Yamamoto M, Yodoi J. Hemin-induced activation of the thioredoxin gene by Nrf2. A differential regulation of the antioxidant responsive element by a switch of its binding factors. The Journal of Biological Chemistry. 2001;**276**(21):18399-18406

[84] Wakabayashi N, Slocum SL, Skoko JJ, Shin S, Kensler TW. When NRF2 talks, who's listening? Antioxidants & Redox Signaling. 2010;**13**(11):1649-1663

[85] Kwak MK, Wakabayashi N, Greenlaw JL, Yamamoto M, Kensler TW. Antioxidants enhance mammalian proteasome expression through the Keap1-Nrf2 signaling pathway. Molecular and Cellular Biology. 2003;**23**(23):8786-8794

[86] Gorrini C, Harris IS, Mak TW. Modulation of oxidative stress as an anticancer strategy. Nature Reviews. Drug Discovery. 2013;**12**(12):931-947

[87] Wild AC, Moinova HR, Mulcahy RT. Regulation of gamma-glutamylcysteine synthetase subunit gene expression by the transcription factor Nrf2. The Journal of Biological Chemistry. 1999;**274**(47):33627-33636

[88] Ganan-Gomez I, Wei Y, Yang H, Boyano-Adanez MC, Garcia-Manero G. Oncogenic functions of the transcription factor Nrf2. Free Radical Biology & Medicine. 2013;**65**:750-764

[89] Wang R, Liu L, Liu H, Wu K, Liu Y, Bai L, et al. Reduced NRF2 expression suppresses endothelial progenitor cell function and induces senescence during aging. Aging (Albany NY). 2019;**11**(17):7021

[90] Mitsuishi Y, Taguchi K, Kawatani Y, Shibata T, Nukiwa T, Aburatani H, et al. Nrf2 redirects glucose and glutamine into anabolic pathways in metabolic reprogramming. Cancer Cell. 2012;**22**(1):66-79

[91] Kim YJ, Ahn JY, Liang P, Ip C, Zhang Y, Park YM. Human prx1 gene is a target of Nrf2 and is up-regulated by hypoxia/reoxygenation: Implication to tumor biology. Cancer Research. 2007;**67**(2):546-554

[92] Aoki Y, Sato H, Nishimura N, Takahashi S, Itoh K, Yamamoto M. Accelerated DNA adduct formation in

the lung of the Nrf2 knockout mouse exposed to diesel exhaust. Toxicol Appl Pharm. 2001;**173**(3):154-160

[93] Iida K, Itoh K, Kumagai Y, Oyasu R, Hattori K, Kawai K, et al. Nrf2 is essential for the chemopreventive efficacy of oltipraz against urinary bladder carcinogenesis. Cancer Research. 2004;**64**(18):6424-6431

[94] Ooi A, Dykema K, Ansari A, Petillo D, Snider J, Kahnoski R, et al. CUL3 and NRF2 mutations confer an NRF2 activation phenotype in a sporadic form of papillary renal cell carcinoma. Cancer Research. 2013;**73**(7):2044-2051

[95] Collisson E, Campbell J, Brooks A, Berger A, Lee W, Chmielecki J, et al. Comprehensive molecular profiling of lung adenocarcinoma: The cancer genome atlas research network. Nature. 2014;**511**(7511):543-550

[96] Network CGAR. Comprehensive molecular characterization of urothelial bladder carcinoma. Nature. 2014;**507**(7492):315

[97] Network CGAR. Comprehensive genomic characterization of squamous cell lung cancers. Nature. 2012;**489**(7417):519

[98] Praslicka BJ, Kerins MJ, Ooi A. The complex role of NRF2 in cancer: A genomic view. Current Opinion in Toxicology. 2016;**1**:37-45

[99] Tao S, Wang S, Moghaddam SJ, Ooi A, Chapman E, Wong PK, et al. Oncogenic KRAS confers chemoresistance by upregulating NRF2. Cancer Research. 2014;**74**(24):7430-7441

[100] MacLeod AK, Acosta-Jimenez L, Coates PJ, McMahon M, Carey FA, Honda T, et al. Aldo-keto reductases are biomarkers of NRF2 activity and are co-ordinately overexpressed in non-small cell lung cancer. British Journal of Cancer. 2016;**115**(12):1530-1539

[101] Singh A, Misra V, Thimmulappa RK, Lee H, Ames S, Hoque MO, et al. Dysfunctional KEAP1-NRF2 interaction in non-small-cell lung cancer. PLoS Medicine. 2006;**3**(10):e420

[102] Jaramillo MC, Zhang DD. The emerging role of the Nrf2-Keap1 signaling pathway in cancer. Genes & Development. 2013;**27**(20):2179-2191

[103] Moon EJ, Giaccia A. Dual roles of NRF2 in tumor prevention and progression: Possible implications in cancer treatment. Free Radical Biology & Medicine. 2015;**79**:292-299

[104] Hayes JD, Dinkova-Kostova AT. The Nrf2 regulatory network provides an interface between redox and intermediary metabolism. Trends in Biochemical Sciences. 2014;**39**(4): 199-218

[105] Lee SB, Sellers BN, DeNicola GM. The regulation of NRF2 by nutrient-responsive Signaling and its role in anabolic cancer metabolism. Antioxidants & Redox Signaling. 2018;**29**(17):1774-1791

[106] de la Vega MR, Chapman E, Zhang DD. NRF2 and the hallmarks of cancer. Cancer Cell. 2018;**34**(1):21-43

[107] Katsuoka F, Yamamoto M. Small Maf proteins (MafF, MafG, MafK): History, structure and function. Gene. 2016;**586**(2):197-205

[108] Muscarella LA, Barbano R, D'Angelo V, Copetti M, Coco M, Balsamo T, et al. Regulation of KEAP1 expression by promoter methylation in malignant gliomas and association with patient's outcome. Epigenetics. 2011;**6**(3):317-325

[109] Kovac M, Navas C, Horswell S, Salm M, Bardella C, Rowan A, et al. Recurrent chromosomal gains and heterogeneous driver mutations characterise papillary renal cancer

evolution. Nature Communications. 2015;**6**(1):6336

[110] Budak M, Yildiz M. Epigenetic Modifications and Potential Treatment Approaches in Lung Cancers, Lung Cancer-Strategies for Diagnosis and Treatment. Rijeka: IntechOpen; 2018. pp. 115-135

[111] Wang R, An J, Ji F, Jiao H, Sun H, Zhou D. Hypermethylation of the Keap1 gene in human lung cancer cell lines and lung cancer tissues. Biochemical and Biophysical Research Communications. 2008;**373**(1):151-154

[112] Hanada N, Takahata T, Zhou Q, Ye X, Sun R, Itoh J, et al. Methylation of the KEAP1 gene promoter region in human colorectal cancer. BMC Cancer. 2012;**12**(1):66

[113] Barbano R, Muscarella LA, Pasculli B, Valori VM, Fontana A, Coco M, et al. Aberrant Keap1 methylation in breast cancer and association with clinicopathological features. Epigenetics. 2013;**8**(1):105-112

Chapter 7

Benign Prostatic Hyperplasia: Epidemiology, Pathophysiology, and Clinical Manifestations

Luz Irene Pascual Mathey

Abstract

The prostate secretes 20% of the seminal fluid. One of its main pathologies is benign prostatic hyperplasia (BPH), the most common benign disease in older men. It has an 8–10% prevalence in men 40 years of age and older, increasing to more than 90% in men over 90 years, with lower urinary tract symptoms being one of its main complications. Although the etiology of BPH is not still fully known, testosterone and estradiol have shown a permissive role. Likewise, other factors have emerged, such as inflammation, growth factors, and prolactin, which influence the development of BPH. These factors act through binding to specific receptors, intervening in BPH and prostate cancer development. Existing treatments significantly reduce clinical symptoms, including lower urinary tract symptoms. However, it is a nonpreventable disease; some factors can reduce its incidence: diet, physical activity, and moderate consumption of alcohol and tobacco, some of which have been proposed to have a protective role. Therefore, this chapter aims to update the preclinical and clinical evidence on the etiology of this disease, briefly describing the epidemiology, clinical manifestations, and therapeutic and preventive modalities in managing BPH.

Keywords: BPH, age, LUTS, QOL, risk factors, diagnosis, treatments, prevention

1. Introduction

The prostate is an accessory gland whose primary function is to provide 20% of seminal fluid [1, 2]. Therefore, its location is decisive for developing benign prostatic hyperplasia (BPH), the most common disease in older men. Furthermore, its prevalence increases proportionally with the increasing age of the individual [3], the main complication being lower urinary tract symptoms, which directly impacts patients' quality of life (QOL), producing sadness and depression [4].

Although it is an age-related etiology, multiple factors intervene in its development, such as metabolic syndrome, inflammation, hormonal changes, and growth factors, which influence and regulate the development of this pathology [3, 5–7]. BPH is not a condition with a high mortality rate; its high prevalence is related to complications of severe lower urinary symptoms, including sexual dysfunction, which notoriously affects the QOL of the elderly [2]. Although it is well characterized, its etiology is poorly understood. It is known that androgens play a permissive role [7]. The imbalance between the levels of androgens and estrogens plays a decisive role in developing BPH and cancer [6]. In addition, other factors have emerged, with growth factors responsible for cell differentiation and proliferation, playing a decisive role in the development of BPH [6]. Furthermore, some studies have suggested the participation of other nonsteroidal hormones and proinflammatory cytokines in stimulating the growth of prostate epithelial tissue, contributing to the hyperproliferative process that accompanies BPH [8, 9].

Due to this, different combined treatments are used to reduce symptoms and improve the patient's health. Although alternative therapies have shown improvements in "*in vivo*" and "*in vitro*" models, they do not offer the same efficacy as existing treatments. In severe cases, it is necessary to accompany the pharmacological treatment with surgical procedures, which significantly improve the symptoms, although they can cause side effects [8, 10].

This disease cannot be prevented. However, it has been reported that the modulation of certain habits can decrease BPH incidence. Among these are obesity, diet, physical activity, and the consumption of alcohol and tobacco, which can directly influence the development of this etiology [4, 11].

Due to the high incidence of this etiology in the elderly, it is essential to provide updated information on this pathology. Therefore, this chapter aims to provide recent information on BPH development in older men.

2. Prostate, the energetic reproductive gland in men

The prostate is an accessory sex gland that has an approximate volume of 20–30 g, which is reached between 18 and 20 years. One of its primary functions is to contribute approximately 20% of the secretions from the seminal fluid, together with those produced by the seminal vesicles and the bulbourethral glands [1, 2].

It has a very particular ubication in the lower pelvis, below the bladder. It is related in front with the pubis and behind with the rectum. It is shaped like an inverted cone, with a base of 4 cm in transverse diameter, 2 cm in the anteroposterior direction, and 3 cm in its vertical diameters. It is crossed in its vertical axis by the urethra and, in a more horizontal and posterior plane, by the ejaculatory ducts [2].

Histologically, three well-defined prostate areas have been reported: the transition zone (5%), located near the urethra surrounding the periurethral space; the central zone (25%), where the main ducts of the seminal vesicles and the prostate are found; and the peripheral zone (70%), the widest, which is palpable during the digitorrectal examination, being the site where 90% of prostate cancers (PC) are generated [3]. The periurethral area of the transition zone consists of two separate glands that lie immediately posterior to the periprostatic sphincter. Furthermore, a characteristic that is unique to the prostate gland in humans is that it is surrounded by the prostate capsule, which is formed by a thin layer of fibromuscular tissue that continues with the stroma, limiting the growth of the gland [5].

3. Benign prostatic hyperplasia: cause or consequence of complications

BPH is a hyperplastic process that results in the growth of epithelial and stromal cells located in the periurethral area of the submucosa and transitional zone of the prostate, the leading site where BPH develops. The elongation of this area is accompanied by changes in the tissue's stromal/muscular characteristics [5]. It has a prevalence of 26.2% worldwide, which has remained constant in the last two decades [6]. It is considered the most common benign tumor in men over 40 years of age, representing the second cause of surgical intervention and the first of consultation with a specialist (urologist) [2].

Although it is an age-related disease, there are other associated risk factors: race, diet, obesity, metabolic syndrome, type 2 diabetes mellitus, cardiovascular diseases, alcohol consumption, urinary tract infections (UTIs), and physical inactivity [3, 5–7].

Moreover, there are hereditary factors associated with BPH. In this sense, a relative risk increase of 3.3 has been demonstrated in monozygotic vs. dizygotic twins, in addition to a higher risk of incidence in siblings with an early onset of the disease. Similarly, some specific genetic risk factors have been evidenced. For example, the loss of the Y chromosome and the presence of variants of type II 5α-reductase gene are included [6, 7].

Interestingly, it has been reported that involution of the prostate is related to an alteration of the immune system; the presence of bacteriuria increases with age in men with a sixfold increase in the number of white blood cells in the prostate secretions of those with BPH than in those without, as well as a presence of bacteria in the 36.7% of the cases [12]. The first symptoms appear in the average 40 years, a period after which growth becomes significant; some reports indicate that the annual growth can be from 40 to 90% between 40 and 50 years. Of the total number of people who develop BPH, approximately between 10 and 41% will present lower urinary tract symptoms (LUTS), which increases in severity with age, being the prostatic capsule, the structure involved in development; limiting the growth of the prostate gland causes an increase in urethral resistance and the symptoms associated with LUTS [5, 6].

Among its main symptoms is the low frequency in urinary flow, the feeling of emptying and filling, in addition to post-void symptoms and those related to voiding volume [13]. Moreover, it has been reported that the severity of discomfort caused by LUTS is related to various sexual problems. It has been reported that the lengthening of the transitional zone is associated with a decrease in sexual desire and function, the ejaculatory process, as well as incontinence (on some occasions), which causes a significant impact on the patients' QOL [5, 6].

4. Lower urinary tract symptoms and BPH

LUTS have been reported to have a combination of voiding, filling, and post-void symptoms. All these are present in different degrees of severity. However, voiding symptoms are the most prevalent, while filling symptoms are the most annoying and interfere with patients' QOL [2, 13].

Filling symptoms include urgency, nocturia, frequency, and urge urinary incontinence; voiding consists of weak stream, urination in drip, intermittent stream, delay, effort, and voiding drip; post-void symptoms include the sensation of incomplete voiding and post-void dribbling [2].

The prevalence of LUTS increases with age, reporting 0–20% in men aged 40–60 years; in 70-year-old men, the frequency of moderate-to-severe symptoms is three times higher than in young men [13]; over 20% of men over 60 years of age will have complications from LUTS, a situation that will exceed 40% in those over 70 years of age, which will significantly affect the QOL [7], being one of the main complications, those related to erectile dysfunction (ED), which is generally associated with severe symptoms of LUTS.

4.1 LUTS and erectile dysfunction (ED)

ED is a chronic condition manifested by the inability to achieve/maintain an erection during sexual behavior to have satisfactory sexual function. This condition is directly related to age. Therefore, it follows a very narrow pattern with the development of BPH and the appearance of LUTS [2].

Different causes associated with ED have been described, including psychological and organic. This last includes anatomical or hormonal defects, degeneration, impaired vasodilation of the penile vessels, and in some instances, a combination of both. Therefore, people with cardiovascular or neurodegenerative diseases are more likely to develop ED [2].

Furthermore, a multicenter study in several countries, including the United States, Italy, Netherlands, Germany, Spain, and England, showed that more than 50% of men suffered from sexual dysfunction due to LUTS. Similarly, the study showed an incidence of erection problems in 49% of men aged 50–80 years, suggesting LUTS as independent risk factors for the appearance of ED [2].

5. Risk factors associated with BPH

5.1 Androgens

The role of androgens in the development of the etiology of BPH has not yet been fully elucidated, so the evidence found shows contrasting results. However, in general, it is known that the normal growth and function of the prostate gland are dependent on the presence of testicular androgens. In this sense, it is known that, in the prostate, testosterone (T) is converted to dihydrotestosterone (DHT) through the action of the enzyme 5α-reductase type II, the primary androgen in this tissue, because it has a 10-fold higher affinity for androgen receptors (AR) than T [6, 8].

Surprisingly, it has been shown that DHT levels remain elevated in the older men (90% of its production being of prostate origin and 10% of adrenal origin), while peripheral circulating levels of T decrease with age [5, 6, 8]. Therefore, the effects associated with BPH are attributed to the autocrine, paracrine, and endocrine actions of DHT rather than T [7].

The action mechanism of androgens is carried out by binding to specific AR, which is expressed mainly within the lumen of epithelial cells and in a low proportion in prostate stromal cells. Interestingly, it has been shown that, like DHT, AR is upregulated in tissue with BPH compared with normal tissues. In addition, it has been shown that a deficiency in type II 5α-reductase enzyme does not produce the elongation associated with BPH, with an effect like that observed in eunuchs or patients with hypogonadism, in which the hyperplastic change characteristic of this pathology did not occur. However, until now, there is insufficient evidence about the importance of elevated DHT and AR in the etiology of BPH [6, 12].

5.2 Estrogens

Estrogens are steroid hormones synthesized mainly in the testes through the biotransformation of T to estradiol (E2) by the action of the aromatase enzyme. Once synthesized, it travels through the circulation to exert its activity in different tissues [1, 6].

They are mainly involved in female physiology; however, in men, one of the most studied estrogenic effects is the negative feedback on the secretion of T. This effect is associated with the inhibition of the secretion of luteinizing hormone (LH) at the pituitary gland, affecting the hypothalamic-pituitary-gonad axis (HPG) in charge of stimulating testicular Leydig cells to produce T. Because of this, there will be a decrease in T levels, as well as its active metabolite, DHT [1].

These effects are mediated by binding to specific estrogen receptors (ER; ER α and β), with direct implications in the pathophysiology of the prostate. Evidence shows that ERα promotes proliferation, in contrast to ERβ, which has a pro-apoptotic effect, behaving as a protective factor in BPH and PC. This effect could be due to the ER location since ERα is mainly within the prostatic stromal tissue, while ERβ is primarily at the basal epithelial cells [1, 6].

However, when estrogen exposure is excessive, it is correlated with susceptibility to both benign and malignant hyperproliferative disorders. This seems to be the result of changes in the expression pattern of steroid hormone receptors in the epithelium, which goes from being a predominantly androgen-dependent tissue to one with greater sensitivity to estrogens and, therefore, more susceptible to the development of the BPH [1, 6].

5.3 Growth factors

Growth factors (GFs) are small peptide molecules that have a central role in regulating growth, differentiation, and programmed cell death. These are released mainly by stromal cells in the prostate, acting through autocrine/paracrine communication mechanisms to regulate prostate cell homeostasis [5, 6]. Among these factors, which DHT stimulates, are transforming growth factor-beta (TGF-β), fibroblast growth factor (FGF), and epidermal growth factor (EGF); On the one hand, TGF-β is an inhibitor of epithelial cell growth, in contrast to FGF and EGF, which stimulates cell growth and differentiation [5, 6].

Interestingly, there is a close relationship between GFs and steroid hormones in the development of BPH; the activation of the AR leads to the increase of the GFs responsible for cell proliferation. Specifically, it has been shown that in AR-expressing fibroblast cells, FGF is overexpressed. Similarly, it has been reported that TGF induces the differentiation of fibroblasts into myofibroblasts in the stroma, regulating the response of epithelial cells to insulin-like growth factor-1 (IGF-1), which increases the stromal cell proliferation observed in BPH [6].

Therefore, insulin also plays a vital role in establishing BPH; the evidence shows a higher incidence in diabetic patients. This effect is related to the previously discussed IGF-1 levels [3]. Similarly, it has been reported that patients with metabolic syndrome (hypertension, dyslipidemia, glucose intolerance, obesity, insulin resistance, etc.) have higher prostate volumes than those without it; a similar situation is observed in obese patients (with a high content of fatty tissue), hypertensive, and in those with low levels of high-density lipoprotein (HDL) [7].

5.4 Prolactin

Prolactin (PRL) is a protein hormone synthesized mainly in the adenohypophysis and whose regulation is carried out by topical inhibition of dopamine. It is synthesized in different tissues, including the mammary gland, the ovary, testes, seminal glands, and the prostate. PRL participates in a wide variety of physiological processes, including the regulation of metabolism, behavior, reproduction cell growth, differentiation, and proliferation [9, 14].

The mechanism by which PRL performs its effects is by binding to a specific membrane receptor, the prolactin receptors (PRLR), which belong to the class I cytokine receptor family, and share homology with the growth hormone receptor (GHR) and the thyrotropin-releasing hormone receptor (TRHR) [14]. Under normal conditions, PRL has been shown to increase androgen production in the prostate and the conversion of T to its metabolite DHT. Similarly, "*in vitro*" studies have demonstrated that PRL stimulates epithelial tissue growth, an effect independent of the presence of androgens, increasing growth, division, and DNA synthesis [9].

On the other hand, some reports indicate that PRL levels increase in patients with BPH, suggesting that it can directly stimulate the development of this pathology [9, 12]. Specifically, it has been shown that prostate androgen receptors and PRL are increased in patients with BPH without finding a direct association with T, highlighting the relationship between PRL and BPH development [15].

5.5 Inflammation and BPH

Recently, evidence has emerged on the participation of inflammatory processes in BPH development. In this sense, at the preclinical level, it has been shown that proinflammatory cytokines can stimulate the growth of prostate epithelial cells. Furthermore, this process is highly associated with leukocyte infiltration observed in patients with this etiology [8].

Although it is not known precisely how the inflammatory process originates, the presence of bacteria (*Escherichia coli*) or certain viruses (human papillomavirus; herpes virus), as well as an autoimmune response, infections, hormonal changes, obesity, and metabolic syndrome, is suggested [7, 16].

The initial stimulus causes the activation of T lymphocytes, as well as the release of cytokines and interleukins (IL) responsible for cell damage, as well as a cascade activation of different factors, among which are the increase in the expression of IL-15 in stromal cells; IL-17 on T cells; interferon-γ in basal and stromal cells and IL-8 in epithelial cells; events that promote a process of chronic inflammation whose consequence is the increase in the volume of the prostate gland. Interestingly, this process can cause the appearance of reactive oxygen species (ROS) and the release of the GFs mentioned previously. Furthermore, IL-8 can induce the production of local growth factors, such as vascular endothelial growth factor (VEGF) involved in tissue angiogenesis, an effect that causes neovascularization to provide the oxygen supply to proliferating cells, which has a determining role in the pathophysiology of BPH [3, 7, 10].

Furthermore, the chronic inflammation observed in BPH has been associated with greater positive regulation of cyclooxygenase 2 in the glandular epithelium, causing the release of proinflammatory prostaglandins responsible for prostate cell proliferation. Similarly, inflammatory cells have been reported in tissue from patients with BPH; T lymphocytes were positive in 81% of the specimens; B lymphocytes were positive in 52%; while macrophages were positive in 82% of these specimen [7, 16]. Therefore, inflammatory processes are decisive in developing BPH.

6. Diagnosis and treatments

6.1 Diagnosis

Diagnosis for BPH requires at least physical examination, laboratory testing, and other testings.

Physical examination. The digitorrectal examination (DRE) can analyze the prostate volume, tone, firmness, and asymmetry. In addition, the ultrasound of the suprapubic region can be examined for bladder distention signs. In some cases, the penile or neurological examination is also included in search of any disorder associated with LUTS [7].

Laboratory testing. Urinalysis can identify glucosuria, pyuria, and hematuria; glycosuria assesses diabetes as a risk factor; pyuria (or bacteriuria), some infectious process; and hematuria, a complication of the genitourinary tract. Serum creatinine increase is indicative of alterations associated with kidney diseases. Prostate-specific antigen (PSA) allows discriminating between BPH and PC. It is not generally used as a biomarker in the initial stages of BPH; however, the increase in PSA values positively correlates with prostate enlargement (greater than 30 cc), being a good predictor in those patients who require surgical treatment. In addition, it has been shown that 88% of patients with PC have histological signs of BPH, so the elevation in PSA levels could be associated with the severity of this condition [8].

Other testing. The International Prosthetic Symptom Score (IPSS) is a validated questionnaire to assess lower urinary tract symptoms associated with BPH. It consists of eight questions, of which seven evaluate the intensity of the symptoms, on a scale of 1–5 depending on its severity; a scale of 1–7 is indicative of mild symptomatic; 8–19 of moderate symptoms; and above 20, severe symptoms [7, 17]. These studies can be accompanied by urinary cytology and transrectal ultrasound, among others, which are beneficial noninvasive methods to discriminate the type of treatment given to the urinary patient cytology recommended for patients who have symptoms secondary to treatment and have risk factors for bladder cancer. In contrast, although not recommended in the initial stages, transrectal ultrasound is necessary before surgical treatment [8].

6.2 Treatments

Due to the high presence of androgens in BPH, the primary therapies used in its treatment are the 5α-reductase enzyme inhibitors (5ARIs), which block T's conversion into DHT. Finasteride, and Dutasteride are the most used at the clinical level. Finasteride blocks the activity of type II 5α-reductase enzyme at the prostate stroma, while Dutasteride blocks type I at the prostate epithelium. These drugs make it possible to improve urinary flow and decrease prostate volume with a reduction of between 20 and 25% in prostate volume and 40 and 60% in PSA levels in approximately 6 months to 1 year [6, 8, 17, 18].

In the specific case of lower urinary tract complications, the treatment will depend on the severity of the symptoms. In mild cases, only follow-up is recommended. In moderate cases, the treatment of choice is alpha-adrenergic antagonists or "alpha-blockers" since these can improve and relieve LUTS and urinary flow. In contrast, in severe cases, treatment may require surgical intervention and pharmacological treatment that includes the combination of alpha-blockers, 5ARIs, antimuscarinics, and phosphodiesterase 5 inhibitors (I-PDE5) [13, 17]. Specifically, muscarinic receptor antagonists (MRAs) have been considered adequate (in combination with alpha-blockers) in patients with filling symptoms. At the same time, I-PDE5 (Sildenafil, Tadalafil, and Vardenafil) is known for its efficacy in treating ED and increasing urinary flow. Similarly, several clinical studies have shown that the combination of alpha-blockers and I-PDE5 has been more effective for ED and improved urinary tract symptoms in patients with BPH [3, 8, 18]. Furthermore, blockers are used in the case of complications caused by the alteration of the IGF-1 axis, with metformin being the effective treatment to reduce cell proliferation in BPH [3].

Although the use of phytotherapy does not have sufficient evidence to be validated, the use of alternatives (supplements) has shown efficacy in reducing prostate volume, being the "saw palmetto," which has demonstrated antiproliferative, antiandrogenic, and anti-inflammatory activity; however, there is not enough evidence to support its use in patients with BPH [8, 18]. Similarly, the use of polyphenols and vitamin D receptor agonists has been suggested to reduce BPH symptoms associated with inflammation [3].

Finally, 20–30% of men who reach the age of 80 require surgical intervention [10]. Also, it is considered for those patients in whom pharmacological treatment has failed or who have severe complications of LUTS. For decades, transurethral prostatic resection (TURP) and transurethral prostatic incision (TUIP) were the most common endoscopic procedures when the prostate measures less than 80 g, and prostatectomy, when the gland exceeds 80 g, effectively improving LUTS symptoms [3, 7, 8, 10].

In addition, new technological tools have emerged to treat urinary flow obstruction (blockage) caused by BPH. Among these are laser therapies; holmium or thulium laser enucleation of the prostate (HoLEP and ThuLEP) is the endoscopic procedure of choice regardless of prostate size; however, HoLEP is the gold standard procedure. Photoselective vaporization of the prostate (PVP) is a minimally invasive procedure that uses lasers to clean excess prostate tissue associated with enlarged prostate, reestablishing urinary flow, and improving BPH symptoms. Other new technologies minimize the sexual side effects. For example, prostatic urethral lift (urolift) is used to insert an implant that compresses the prostate, dilating the urethra. While the steam therapy procedure (rezum), also called water vapor thermal therapy (WVTT), uses steam injections to remove obstructive tissue without damaging the urethra. All these technologies are included in the American Urological Association (AUA) guide for treating BPH [8, 19].

7. Modulable risk factors and BPH incidence

Benign prostatic hyperplasia represents a current challenge in public health, since not only is it a nonpreventable disease, so the treatments mentioned above only arrest the growth of the prostate and reduce its clinical symptoms. However, it has been shown that modifying certain habits can improve the patient's health [11].

Obesity. The elongation and volume of the prostate gland correlate with body mass index (BMI) and waist circumference. In this sense, it has been shown that obese individuals (BMI greater than 35 kg/m^2, according to the WHO classification) have a 3.5 times higher risk of developing BPH. Similarly, there is a 2.4 greater probability of developing this etiology in those with a waist circumference greater than 109 cm. However, the mechanism, by which anthropometric measurements influence the etiology of BPH, has been suggested that the rise in the ratio of fatty tissue could be causing a greater aromatization of circulating testosterone into estrogens, whose effect on the etiology of this pathology has already been discussed. Similarly, it has been shown that people with a higher glucose intake are three times more likely to suffer from BPH, while diabetic patients have a two times higher risk, both being associated with the development of LUTS, reporting that low levels of HDL cholesterol are associated with an increase in prostate volume [4, 11].

Diet. Although the relationship of macro- and micronutrients with the incidence of BPH is not well defined, evidence suggests that the consumption of cereals, eggs, red meat, eicosapentaenoic and docosahexaenoic acids, butter, margarine, and starch (bread, pasta, rice) increases the risk of developing BPH, while the consumption of green peas, beans, lentils, vegetables (including tomato, garlic, and onion as a source of antioxidants), fruits (with high levels of β-carotene, lutein, or vitamin C), polyunsaturated fatty acids (including omega-3 fatty acids included in salmon and sardines) decreases risk and helps to reduce the effect of prostaglandins and leukotrienes on inflammation associated with BPH [4, 10, 20]. Concerning the micronutrients, it has been shown that the presence of high levels of vitamins D and E, zinc, lycopene, and selenium has an inverse relationship with the development of BPH, so they are suggested as protective for the PC; interestingly, high zinc and sodium levels have been related to an increase in the risk of BPH and PC [10, 11].

Physical activity. The increase in physical activity directly correlates with decreased BPH risk compared with those who have a sedentary lifestyle. In this sense, it has been shown that walking 2–3 hours a week produces a 25% lower risk of LUTS and BPH evaluated with the IPSS. Moreover, a lower risk (50%) has been reported in men who exercise 3–5 times a week than those who exercise less than two times a week [4, 11].

Alcohol and smoking. About the consumption of alcoholic beverages, it has been shown that moderate consumption causes a 30–41% decrease in the risk of BPH and associated symptoms (40% fewer LUTS, including nocturia). However, some studies indicate that the risk of BPH increases directly with the increase in alcohol consumption. In this sense, men who consume 6–10 units of alcohol per week (mainly beer, wine, and sake) had a 41% greater probability of developing moderate-to-severe symptoms of LUTS, which strongly indicates that the appearance of these symptoms has a dose-dependent relationship. Interestingly, a similar relationship has been observed with cigarette smoking. In this context, moderate tobacco use was associated with a 30% lower probability of presenting BPH and LUTS clinical symptoms. However, in the same way, as with alcohol, smoking more than 35 cigarettes a day directly impacted BPH development and LUTS severity. However, these results are controversial [4, 10, 21].

8. Conclusions

BPH is the most common disease in older men. Its prevalence increases proportionally with age. The main complication is the lower urinary tract symptoms, directly impacting patients' health. Its etiology is poorly understood, but we know that the increase in the ratio of estrogens/androgens plays a decisive role in developing BPH and cancer. In addition, growth factors, nonsteroidal hormones, and proinflammatory cytokines stimulate the growth and neovascularization of prostate epithelial tissue, contributing to the hyperproliferative process that accompanies BPH. Although it is not a preventive or curative disease, different combined treatments reduce symptoms and improve patients' QOL. Moreover, it has been reported that the modulation of diet, obesity, physical activity, and consumption of alcohol and tobacco can improve the clinical symptoms of BPH acting as protective factors. The knowledge of this topic is essential to reduce the clinical symptoms associated with BPH in men.

Acknowledgements

The author thanks the National Council of Science and Technology (CONACyT) for the supporting and funding.

Conflict of interest

The author declares no conflict of interest.

Acronyms and abbreviations

BPH	benign prostatic hyperplasia
QOL	quality of life
PC	prostate cancer
UTIs	urinary tract infections
LUTS	lower urinary tract symptoms

ED	erectile dysfunction
T	testosterone
DHT	dihydrotestosterone
AR	androgen receptors
E2	estradiol
LH	luteinizing hormone
HPG	hypothalamic-pituitary-gonad axis
ERα/ERβ	estrogen receptors α and β
GFs	growth factors
TGF-β	transforming growth factor-beta
FGF	fibroblast growth factor
EGF	epidermal growth factor
IGF-1	insulin-like growth factor 1
HDL	high-density lipoprotein
PRL	prolactin
PRLR	prolactin receptors
GHR	growth hormone receptors
TRHR	thyrotropin-releasing hormone receptor
IL	interleukins
ROS	reactive oxygen species
VEGF	vascular endothelial growth factor
IPSS	International Prosthetic Symptoms Score
DRE	digotorrectal examination
PSA	prostate-specific antigen
5ARIs	5α-reductase enzyme inhibitors
I-PDE5	phosphodiesterase 5 inhibitors
MRAs	muscarinic receptor antagonist
TURP	transurethral prostatic resection
TUIP	transurethral prostatic incision
HoLEP and ThuLEP	holmium or thulium laser enucleation of the prostate
PVP	photoselective vaporization of the prostate
WVTT	water vapor thermal therapy
AUA	American Urological Association
BMI	body mass index

Author details

Luz Irene Pascual Mathey
Faculty of Biology of Pharmaceutical Chemistry, Veracruzana University, Veracruz, Mexico

*Address all correspondence to: lupascual@uv.mx

References

[1] Espinoza JL, Aguilar MEH, Abreu GEA, Durán FR, Denes JM, Ávila GAC, et al. El papel de los estrógenos y sus receptores en la prevención y promoción de enfermedades proliferativas de la glándula prostática. Eneurobiología: Revista electrónica. 2013;**4**(8):1-23. Available from: Http://www.uv.mx/eneurobiologia/vols/2013/8/Locia/HTML.html

[2] Alcántara-Montero A, Brenes-Bermúdez FJ, Pérez-Feito D. Relación entre los síntomas del tracto urinario inferior en el varón y la disfunción eréctil [Relationship between lower urinary tract symptoms in men and erectile dysfunction]. SEMERGEN. 2016;**42**(3):164-171. Spanish. DOI: 10.1016/j.semerg.2015.07.005

[3] Langan RC. Benign prostatic hyperplasia. Primary Care. 2019;**46**(2):223-232. DOI: 10.1016/j.pop.2019.02.003

[4] Parsons JK, Sarma AV, McVary K, Wei JT. Obesity and benign prostatic hyperplasia: Clinical connections, emerging etiological paradigms and future directions. The Journal of Urology. 2013;**189**(1):S102-S106. DOI: 10.1016/j.juro.2012.11.029

[5] Roehrborn CG. Pathology of benign prostatic hyperplasia. International Journal of Impotence Research. 2008;**20**(Suppl 3):S11-S18. DOI: 10.1038/ijir.2008.55

[6] Devlin CM, Simms MS, Maitland NJ. Benign prostatic hyperplasia - what do we know? BJU International. 2021;**127**(4):389-399. DOI: 10.1111/bju.15229

[7] Chughtai B, Forde JC, Thomas DD, Laor L, Hossack T, Woo HH, et al. Benign prostatic hyperplasia. Nature Reviews. Disease Primers. 2016;**2**:16031. DOI: 10.1038/nrdp.2016.31

[8] Kim EH, Larson JA, Andriole GL. Management of benign prostatic hyperplasia. Annual Review of Medicine. 2016;**67**(1):137-151. DOI: 10.1146/annurev-med-063014-123902

[9] Romero L, Muñoz C, López A, Vilches J. Relación de la prolactina con la hiperplasia nodular y el carcinoma de próstata [Relation of prolactin with nodular hyperplasia and carcinoma of the prostate]. Actas urologicas espanolas. 1991;**15**(6):503-509

[10] Das K, Buchholz N. Benign prostate hyperplasia and nutrition. Clinical Nutrition ESPEN. 2019;**33**:5-11. DOI: 10.1016/j.clnesp.2019.07.015

[11] Parsons JK. Modifiable risk factors for benign prostatic hyperplasia and lower urinary tract symptoms: New approaches to old problems. The Journal of Urology. 2007;**178**(2):395-401. DOI: 10.1016/j.juro.2007.03.103

[12] Roper WG. The prevention of benign prostatic hyperplasia (BPH). Medical Hypotheses. 2017;**100**:4-9. DOI: 10.1016/j.mehy.2016.12.013

[13] Carrero-López VM, Cózar-Olmo JM, Miñana-López B. Benign prostatic hyperplasia and lower urinary tract symptoms. A review of current evidence. Actas Urologicas Españolas. 2016;**40**(5):288-294. DOI: 10.1016/j.acuro.2015.12.008

[14] Pascual MLI, Manzo DJ, Goffi V, Kessal K, Aranda-Abreu GE, Estudillo CA, et al. Prolactina: mecanismos intracelulares involucrados en la función prostática. Revista Médica de la Universidad Veracruzana. 2009;**9**(1):36-40

[15] Odoma S, Chisholm GD, Nicol K, Habib FK. Evidence for the association between blood prolactin and androgen receptors in BPH. The Journal of Urology. 1985;**133**(4):717-720. DOI: 10.1016/s0022-5347(17)49168-3

[16] Chughtai B, Lee R, Te A, Kaplan S. Role of inflammation in benign prostatic hyperplasia. Reviews in Urology. 2011;**13**(3):147-150

[17] Mobley D, Feibus A, Baum N. Benign prostatic hyperplasia and urinary symptoms: Evaluation and treatment. Postgraduate Medicine. 2015;**127**(3):301-307. DOI: 10.1080/00325481.2015.1018799

[18] Rossanese M, Crestani A, Inferrera A, Giannarini G, Bartoletti R, Tubaro A, et al. Medical treatment for benign prostatic hyperplasia: Where do we stand? Urologia. 2019;**86**(3):115-121. DOI: 10.1177/0391560319859785

[19] Das AK. Techniques and innovative technologies for the treatment of BPH. The Canadian Journal of Urology. 2019;**26**(4 Suppl. 1):1

[20] ElJalby M, Thomas D, Elterman D, Chughtai B. The effect of diet on BPH, LUTS and ED. World Journal of Urology. 2019;**37**(6):1001-1005. DOI: 10.1007/s00345-018-2568-0

[21] Platz EA, Rimm EB, Kawachi I, Colditz GA, Stampfer MJ, Willett WC, et al. Alcohol consumption, cigarette smoking, and risk of benign prostatic hyperplasia. American Journal of Epidemiology. 1999;**149**(2):106-115. DOI: 10.1093/oxfordjournals.aje.a0

Section 3

Viral Oncogenes

Chapter 8

Molecular Epidemiology of High-Risk Human Papillomavirus Infection in Burkina Faso

Théodora Mahoukèdè Zohoncon, Rogomenoma Alice Ouedraogo, Florencia Wendkuuni Djigma, Lassina Traore, Teega-Wendé Clarisse Ouedraogo, Maimouna Ilboudo, Regine Ilboudo, Catherine Salambanga, Sindimalgdé Patricia Guigma, Sessi Frida Tovo, Mah Alima Esther Traore, Prosper Bado, Ali Kande, Cyrille Bisseye, Abdoul Karim Ouattara, Ina Marie Angèle Traore, Djeneba Ouermi, Tani Sagna, Albert Théophane Yonli, Wendyam Marie Christelle Nadembega, Dorcas Obiri-Yeboah, Yvette Marie Chantal Gyebre, Olga Mélanie Lompo, Charlemagne Marie Ragnag-Newende Ouedraogo and Jacques Simpore

Abstract

The aim of the present study was to determine the distribution of high-risk human papillomavirus (HR-HPV) genotypes in childbearing age women, teenage girls, HIV-infected women, women with high-grade precancerous lesions and cervical cancer, sex workers, men, and otolaryngology tumor cases in Burkina Faso. This descriptive cross-sectional study with several target groups, consisted of 2386 samples from Burkina Faso. HR-HPV genotypes were characterized using real-time multiplex PCR. The prevalence of HR-HPV ranged from 15.63 to 72.31% depending on the target population and the nature of the samples. The most predominant genotypes in descending order were HPV-56, HPV-52, HPV-39, HPV-59, HPV-51, HPV-35, HPV-31, HPV-18, HPV-68, HPV-16, HPV-66, HPV-58, HPV-45, and HPV-33. The results of the present study show a wide variation in the distribution of HR-HPV genotypes in Burkina Faso. Genotypes 16 and 18 covered by HPV vaccines only accounted for 32.23% of HR-HPV cases.

Keywords: HPV, genotypes, cervical cancer, ENT cancer, Burkina Faso

1. Introduction

Virus-induced cancers represent a huge burden, especially in developing countries. According to recent estimates from the International Agency for Research on Cancer (IARC), 16% of new cases of cancer worldwide are attributable to infections, of which 11% are viral infections. In sub-Saharan Africa, one-third of all cancers are infection-induced cancers [1]. Human papillomaviruses are small non-enveloped viruses (about 55 nm in diameter) of the Papillomaviridae family with a compact structure and a small circular genome (8000 base pairs), encoding 8–9 proteins depending on the genotype (LCR, L1, L2, E1, E2, E4, E5, E6, and E7) [2]. E5, E6, and E7 proteins are involved in cell proliferation and transformation [3, 4]. It is noteworthy that persistent infection with high oncogenic risk human papillomavirus (HR-HPV) can lead to precancerous lesions, which generally begin with slight modification (CIN 1), that can progress to more severe lesions such as CIN 2 then CIN 3 (carcinoma *in situ*). These lesions can regress spontaneously or progress to cancer. HR-HPV infection is recognized as the major risk factor associated with cervix, penis, vulva, vagina, anus, and oropharynx cancers [5]. Globally, cervical cancer remains one of the leading causes of morbidity and mortality with about 569,847 cases and 311,365 deaths occurring in 2018 [6]. Low-income countries have the highest incidence, especially sub-Saharan Africa, where it is the second most common female malignancy [7] and the leading cause of cancer death in women [8].

In West Africa, the annual estimate of cervical cancer burden is 31,955 cases and 23,529 deaths [9]. However, most sexually active men and women can be infected with HR-HPV at some point in their lives, and persistent infection could lead to precancerous lesions and progress into invasive cancer [1, 5]. In addition, HPV infection can affect fertility in men [10, 11]. According to the World Health Organization (WHO), men genital infections with any type of HPV are estimated at least at 19.1% in sub-Saharan Africa [12].

In Burkina Faso, cervical cancer is the most commonly diagnosed cancer with an estimated incidence of 2517 cases and 2081 deaths per year [13]. In addition, otolaryngology and cervico-facial cancers are relatively frequent and account for 24.5% of this entity [14]. Gynecological cancers associated with persistent HR-HPV infection, therefore, threaten many African communities and economies, upsetting the trends of positive societal development. Although HR-HPV is the main causative agent of cervical cancer, other important cofactors (environmental or genetic) such as gene polymorphisms (E6, E7, MMP1, MMP3, TNF-alfa, and IL-18) are involved in the clearance and pathway of carcinogenesis [15].

HIV infection is an additional risk factor [16, 17] as well as some risky behaviors such as multiple sexual partners, especially among sex workers, leading to higher rates of cervical cancer [18] and increasing the risk of penile cancer in men [19]. Nevertheless, preventive measures through behavior modification, screening, and vaccination can significantly control these viral-induced cancers. To efficiently combat this pathology, it is, therefore, necessary to investigate whether the HR-HPV genotypes found in our populations, especially the most common in cancers cases, are covered by the available vaccines. To address this concern, the objective of the present study was to determine the distribution of HR-HPV genotypes in a general population including childbearing age women, teenage girls, HIV-infected women, women with high-grade precancerous lesions and invasive cervical cancer, sex workers, men, and histologically confirmed otolaryngology tumor (ear, nose, and throat) in Burkina Faso.

2. Material and methods

2.1 Type and study population, sample collection

From 2013 to 2017, we carried out a large-scale, descriptive cross-sectional, and multicenter epidemiological study in Burkina Faso along with the retrospective data collection and analysis. The population of the present study consisted of 2386 participants, including eight (8) target groups: childbearing age women, teenage girls, HIV-infected women, sex workers, men, women with high-grade precancerous lesions (CIN 2/3), tissue from invasive cervical cancer, and histologically confirmed otolaryngology tumor (ear, nose, and throat cancers) in Burkina Faso.

The study was conducted in two phases: a descriptive cross-sectional study with 2025 participants made up of 1321 childbearing age women, 200 teenage girls, 183 HIV-infected women, 200 sex workers, and 124 men. We first focused on awareness-raising of HPV infection prevention and the risk of developing cervical cancer at several sites.

The goal after awareness-raising was to include in the target groups, all sexually active women (SAW) regardless of age who were not pregnant and provided informed consent to participate in the study. The exclusion was being in the menstruation period, during the study recruitment, and have had a total hysterectomy.

Prior to the samples collection, socio-demographic data, sexual behavior, HIV serology, level of knowledge about HPV and cervical cancer as well as associated diseases were collected using a standardized questionnaire. An individual collection card was used to collect clinical data of each sex worker in the study population. The privacy and confidentiality were respected through the generation of a unique code for each participant.

Midwives and gynecologists using a single-use speculum and sterile swab performed endocervical samples collection at the squamocolumnar junction. The following samples were taken:

- from May 2009 to January 2010, 183 endocervical samples from women aged 20–53 years of age, who tested positive for anti-HIV antibodies at the stage of asymptomatic infection, were collected in three reference health centers accessible to all inhabitants of Ouagadougou [Saint Camille Hospital of Ouagadougou (HOSCO) and Pietro Annigoni Biomolecular Research Center (CERBA), two reference centers for people living with HIV/AIDS (PLWHIV), and Bogodogo University Hospital]. Participants were monitored at HOSCO and CERBA and were annually screened for cervical cancer.

- from September to December 2013, 200 endocervical samples from teenage girls, aged 15–19, were collected in a youth health center (ABBF) of Ouagadougou. The participants were seen at gynecological consultation for voluntary HIV testing;

- from December 2015 to September 2016, 124 sperm samples were collected in three medical clinics of Ouagadougou (Philadelphia, Sainte Elisabeth, and Sandof) after 3–6 days of abstinence according to the WHO recommendations. These male subjects aged 21–72 came for spermogram and spermocytogramanlyses;

- from December 2015 to March 2017, 1321 endocervical samples from childbearing age women (15–76 years of age, general population), including 520 in

Ouagadougou, 535 in the Hauts-Bassins region (Bobo and Orodara), and 266 in the Center-East region (Tenkodogo and Garango);

- from June to August 2017, 200 endocervical samples from sex workers aged 16–50 years were enrolled in Ouagadougou.

The samples thus collected were frozen in a transport medium at −20°C except those from HIV+ women, which were stored at −80°C. The samples were then sent to the CERBA/LABIOGENE molecular biology and genetics laboratory for molecular biology analyzes. Following sampling in women, screening for precancerous lesions was performed using visual inspection of the cervix with acetic acid (VIA) or with Lugol's iodine (VILI).

The second phase, a cross-sectional study with retrospective data collection, involved 358 samples. Using patients medical register available at the Department of Anatomy and Cytopathology of YalgadoOuedraogo University Hospital Center (CHU-YO), 118 cervical tissue specimens were selected based on high-grade (CIN 2/3) intraepithelial lesions diagnosis between February 2009 and May 2015 along with 112 cervical tissue specimens dated from 2009 to 2015 with a histological diagnosis of invasive cervical cancer.

According to the same protocol, we also included 128 histologically confirmed otolaryngology cancerous tissues dated from 2007 to 2017 in four health centers of Ouagadougou, CHU-YO, Shiphra, Sandof, and Philadelphia clinics. All these biopsy specimens were fixed in formalin and embedded in paraffin.

2.2 Extraction of HR-HPV viral DNA from endocervical samples

HR-HPV viral DNA was extracted using the DNA-Sorb-A kit (Sacace Biotechnologies, Como, Italy) from endocervical and sperm samples following the protocol provided by the manufacturer. Endocervical samples of HIV-positive women, DNA was extracted using bio solutions "INSTANT Virus DNA Kit" Analytkjena® (Italy). The extracted DNA was then quantified using UV spectrophotometry at 260 nm and stored at −20°C until PCR amplification.

2.3 Samples deparaffinization and extraction of HR-HPV viral DNA from tissue specimens

In the cytopathology anatomy laboratory of the CHU-YO, the paraffin blocks containing a piece of biopsy were cut with a microtome to obtain five sections of about 20 μm thick. Tissues thus collected in sterile Eppendorf tubes were sent to the CERBA/LABIOGENE for molecular analyzes. DNA extraction was performed using the FFPE DNA Purification Kit, following the protocol provided by the manufacturer.

2.4 Spermogram and spermocytogram

Each semen sample was assessed according to the following parameters: volume, motility, concentration, morphology, and vitality of spermatozoa, using an optical microscope.

2.5 Molecular characterization of HR-HPV genotypes using real-time multiplex PCR

Extracted DNA was amplified with "HPV Genotypes 14 Real-TM Quant" kit (Sacace Biotechnologies, Como, Italy) using Sacycler-96 Real-time PCR v.7.3

(SACACE Biotechnologies®). Fourteen HR-HPV genotypes (HPV 16, 18, 31, 33, 35, 39, 45, 51, 52, 56, 58, 59, 66, and 68) could be detected in a multiplex PCR procedure with β-globin gene as internal control.

Two different techniques were used to amplify the viral DNA extracted from samples of HIV+ women: PCR/Hybridization for the detection of HPV 6, 11, 16, 18, 45, 30'S and 50'S using the "HPV Blot STAR" kit from Diatech® (Italy), without discrimination of the HPV 30'S and 50'S genotypes, respectively. The second technique using the "HPV High-Risk Typing Real-TM" kit (SACACE biotechnologies®, Italy) allows specific detection of the following high-risk genotypes: 16, 18, 31, 39, 45, 59, 33, 35, 56, 51, 52, and 58. The amplification program was as follows: 1 cycle of 95°C for 15 minutes; 5 cycles of 95°C for 05 s, 60°C for 20s, 72°C for 15 s; 40 cycles of 95°C for 05 s, 60°C for 30s, and 72°C for 15 s.

2.6 Ethical considerations

Each phase of the present study received the approval of the Ethics Committee for Health Research of Burkina Faso (CERS) (n °2009-009/CR/135 of April 22, 2009 (HIV+); N2014-8-099 of August 6, 2014 (CIN2/3); Deliberation No. 2016-2102-0012 of 02/03/2016 (general population); No.2017-1026/MS/RCEN/DRSC (sex workers); No. 2014-8-099 (ICC); Ref.2017/CERBA/II-24/0019 of 24-02-2017 (otolaryngology samples) along with approbation of the regional health directorates (DRS) of the various target collection sites. Free and informed consent, anonymity, and confidentiality were strictly observed.

2.7 Statistical analyzes

Statistical analysis of data was performed using IBM SPSS 21 and Epi Info v7.0 software. The Chi-square test was used for comparisons with a significant difference for $p < 0.05$.

3. Results

3.1 Mean age of target groups in our study population

The present study focused on eight (8) target groups, including childbearing age women, adolescent girls, HIV-infected women, sex workers, men, high-grade precancerous lesions (CIN 2/3) cases, invasive cervical cancer, and histologically confirmed otolaryngology tumors in Burkina Faso. The mean age ranged from 18.7 ± 0.7 to 46.32 ± 12.76 years (**Table 1**).

Target groups	childbearing age women in the general population	Teenage girls	Sex workers	CIN 2/3	ICC	HIV+	Men	Otolaryngology cancers
Mean age (years)	32.0 ± 10.1	18.7 ± 0.7	27.3 ± 0.4	41.5 ± 9.8	46.3 ± 12.8	33.9 ± 6.2	37.1 ± 7.6	41.0 ± 19.0
Range	15–76	15–19	16–50	22–74	21–84	20–53	21–72	5–80

Table 1.
Mean age of target groups in the study population.

3.2 Socio-demographic data and sexual behavior of the study population women

The general female population of the present study consisted of 1321 childbearing age women and 200 adolescent girls. Among them, only 142 (9.34%) had a university education while 951 (62.53%) were living with a partner. Most of them (61.34%) were over 18 years of age at first, and 43.19% never used a condom during sex. It is noteworthy that 40.89% of them had a history of STIs and 50.43% declared to be using contraception. Screening for precancerous lesions using VIA/VILI revealed 70 positive women (**Table 2**).

3.3 HR-HPV prevalence

The beta-globin gene used as an internal control was an essential factor for results validation in multiplex real-time PCR procedures for HR-HPV genotypes detection. Out of 118 CIN 2/3 tissue blocks samples, 43 positives for the beta-globin gene were considered valid while 65 samples were valid out of the 112 ICC specimens. Only valid samples were considered for the present study. HPV data were therefore available for 2264 valid samples out of 2386 recruited participants.

The prevalence of HR-HPV ranged from 15.63% to 72.31% based on the target population and nature of the samples. The overall prevalence was estimated at

Characteristic		**Target groups**		
		Childbearing age women $N = 1321$	**Teenage girls $N = 200$**	**Women in the general population $N = 1521$**
Educational level	Illiterate	433 (32.78%)	2 (1%)	435 (28.6%)
	Primary	293 (22.18%)	58 (29%)	351 (23.08%)
	Secondary	495 (37.47%)	98 (49%)	593 (38.98%)
	University	100 (7.57%)	42 (21%)	142 (9.34%)
Marital status	Married/ cohabiting Single	940 (71.16%)	11 (5.5%)	951 (62.53%)
	Widow	325 (24.60%)	189 (94.5%)	514 (33.79%)
		56 (4.24%)	—	56 (3.68%)
Age at first sexual intercourse	< 18 years	452 (34.22%)	102 (51%)	554 (36.42%)
	≥ 18 years	835 (63.21%)	98 (49%)	933 (61.34%)
	No answer	34 (2.57%)	—	34 (2.24%)
Condom use	Never	633 (47.92%)	24 (12%)	657 (43.19%)
	Rarely	263 (19.91%)	102 (51%)	365 (24%)
	Always	124 (9.39%)	74 (37%)	198 (13.02%)
	No answer	301 (22.78%)	—	301 (19.79%)
STIs history	Yes	605 (45.80%)	17 (8.5%)	622 (40.89%)
	No	716 (54.20%)	183 (91.5%)	899 (59.11%)
Use of means of contraception	Yes	605 (45.80%)	162 (81%)	767 (50.43%)
	No	716 (54.20%)	38 (19%)	754 (49.57%)
VIA/VILI[+]	Positive	58 (4.39%)	12 (6%)	70 (4.6%)

n = total number of participants.

Table 2.
Sociodemographic data and sexual behavior of the women general population.

39.05% (824/2264). As shown in **Figure 1**, a prevalence of 72.31% (*n* = 47) was observed in ICC cases, 63.90% (*n* = 117) in HIV-positive women, 53% (*n* = 106) in sex workers women, 48.80% (*n* = 21) in CIN 2/3 cases, 41.50% (*n* = 83) in adolescent girls, 35.40% (*n* = 468) in childbearing age women, 17.74% (n = 22) in men and 15.63% (*n* = 20) in otolaryngology cancers.

3.4 Prevalence and genotypic distribution of HR-HPV in target groups

The amplification kits used enabled us to essentially characterize the HR-HPV genotypes 16, 18, 31, 33, 35, 39, 45, 51, 52, 56, 58, 59, 66, and 68. **Table 3** shows the distribution of HR-HPV in descending order in the study population. Overall, varied distribution of HR-HPV genotypes was observed with predominance of non-HPV 16 and 18 genotypes (**Table 3**).

On the one hand, HPV 16 was particularly absent in childbearing age women from the Haut-Bassins region, in southwestern Burkina Faso, and in women with high-grade precancerous lesions (**Table 3**). On the other hand, HPV 18 was most common in ICC cases and HIV-positive women. In addition, HPV 56 was predominant in childbearing age women, otolaryngology cancers, and men. However, a predominance of HPV 68 was registered in sex workers and absent in ICC and otolaryngology cancers. It is noteworthy that HPV 56 was predominant in the general population as well as in the target groups (**Table 3**).

Table 4 shows the HR-HPV genotypes detected in the present study population and their prevalence in each target population. Considering the five most common HR-HPV genotypes found in the different target groups, HPV 16 presented a low proportion, especially in childbearing age women (1.82%), adolescent girls (5.2%), sex workers (2.7%), HIV + (4.9%), CIN 2/3 (0.0%). However, in decreasing order of frequency, it was the third genotype identified in otolaryngology cancers, the fourth in ICC, and the fifth in men. In HIV-positive women, a frequency of 2% of HPV6 infection was observed.

3.5 Prevalence of single and multiple infections in target groups

PCR screening in each target group revealed that among the 884 cases of HR-HPV infections, the number of genotypes per infected person ranged from 1 to 9 out of 14 genotypes tested. Single infection (isolated infection) ranged from 37.61 to 90.50% while multiple infection varied from 9.50 to 62.39% (**Table 5**).

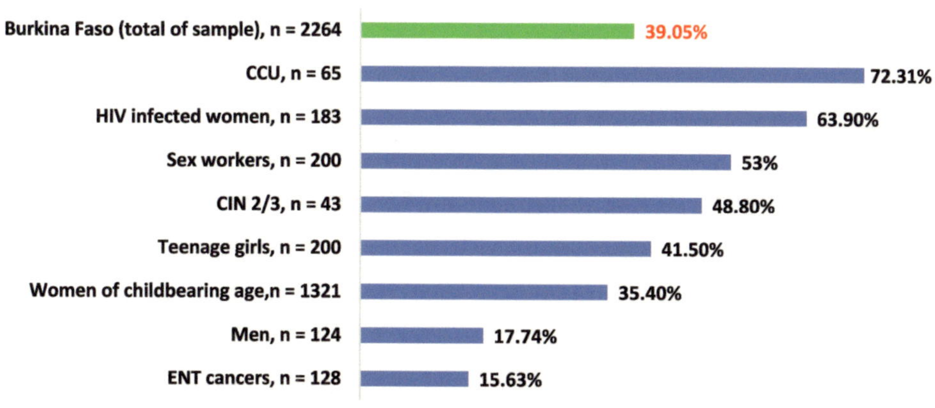

Figure 1.
Prevalence of HR-HPV according to the target groups and nature of the samples in the study population.

Target groups	Sample size	Prevalence of HR-HPV (CI 95%)	Most common HR-HPV	Absent genotypes
Childbearing age women in the general population	**1321**	**35.4%** (32.88–38.03)	**HPV 56; 52; 66; 59; 39;** 51; **18**; 35; 68; 58; 45; 31; 33; **16.**	HPV 16 absent in hauts-bassins
Teenage girls	**200**	**41.5%** (34.65–48.67)	**HPV 52; 59; 39; 51; 35**; 56; **16**; **18**; 58; 31; 45; 33	—
Sex workers	**200**	**53%** (45.84–60.04)	**HPV 68; 31; 52; 51; 56**; 66; 58; 35; 39; **18**; 45; 59; **16**; 33	—
HIV+ women	**183**	**63.9%** (56.48–70.80)	**HPV 18; 35; 31; 52; 58**; 56; 45; 59; 33; 51; **16**; 39	—
CIN 2/3	**43**	**48.8%** (33.56–64.32)	**HPV 39; 35; 45; 33; 51**; 52; 56; **18**; 31; 59; 68	HPV 16. 58. 66
ICC	**65**	**72.31%** (59.61–82.35)	**HPV 18; 31; 39**; 16; 45; 35; 58; 52; 51; 56; 59	HPV33; 66; 68
Otolaryngology cancers	**128**	**15.63%** (10.03–23.34)	**HPV 56; 33; 16; 18; 39.**; 45; 52	HPV31;35;51;58;59; 66 and 68
Men	**124**	**17.74%** (11.68–25.85)	**HPV 56; 31; 39; 68; 16**; 18; 33; 35; 51; 52; 45; 59; 66; 58	—
General population (women + men)	**1645**	**34.83%** (32.54–37.20)	**HPV 56; 52; 39; 59; 51**; 35; 31; 18; 68; 16; 66; 58; 45; 33	—
Target groups	**619**	**50.24%** (46.23–54.25)	**HPV 56; 18; 39; 45; 31; 35; 33; 52; 16; 51; 58; 68; 59; 66**	—
Burkina Faso (Bilan)	**2264**	**39.05%** (37.03–41.09)	—	—

NB: The general population consists of childbearing age women, adolescent girls, and men. The target population consists of sex workers, HIV+ women, CIN 2/3 cases, ICC cases, and otolaryngology cancers.

Table 3.
Genotypic distribution of HR-HPV in target groups.

3.6 Prevalence of HR-HPV genotypes targeted by bivalent, quadrivalent, and nonavalent HPV vaccines

The HR-HPV genotypes targeted by bivalent/quadrivalent HPV vaccines (HPV6/11/16/18) were identified in 7.83% of childbearing age women, 10.40% of adolescent girls, 8.90% of sex workers, 25.70% of HIV+ women, 4.30% of CIN 2/3, 38.57% of ICC cases, 14% of men, and 50% of otolaryngology cancer cases. The genotypes covered by the nonavalent vaccine (HPV6/11/16/18/31/33/45/52/58) were 36.22, 43.40, 44.90, 65.30, 39, 75.71, and 40%, respectively in childbearing

Prevalence of HR-HPV in each target group

Target groups	Sex workers	HIV+	CIN 2/3+	ICC	Otolaryngology cancers	Total
HR-HPV genotypes identified	HPV56 (7.60%)	HPV56 (7.80%)	HPV56 (8.70%)	HPV56 (1.43%)	HPV56 (45%)	70.53%
	HPV18 (6.20%)	HPV18 (18.80%)	HPV18 (4.30%)	HPV18 (25.71%)	HPV18 (10%)	65.01%
	HPV39 (6.20%)	HPV39 (2.60%)	HPV39 (21.70%)	HPV39 (12.86%)	HPV39 (5%)	48.36%
	HPV45 (5.80%)	HPV45 (6.20%)	HPV45 (13%)	HPV45 (12.86%)	HPV45 (5%)	42.86%
	HPV31 (12%)	HPV31 (10.70%)	HPV31 (4.30%)	HPV31 (15.71%)	HPV31 (0%)	42.71%
	HPV35 (7.10%)	HPV35 (13.30%)	HPV35 (13%)	HPV35 (7.14%)	HPV35 (0%)	40.54%
	HPV33 (1.80%)	HPV33 (5.80%)	HPV33 (8.70%)	HPV33 (0%)	HPV33 (20%)	36.30%
	HPV52 (9.30%)	HPV52 (8.80%)	HPV52 (8.70%)	HPV52 (2.86%)	HPV52 (5%)	34.66%
	HPV16 (2.70%)	HPV16 (4.90%)	HPV16 (0%)	HPV16 (12.86%)	HPV16 (10%)	30.46%
	HPV51 (8.90%)	HPV51 (5.20%)	HPV51 (8.70%)	HPV51 (1.43%)	HPV51 (0%)	24.23%
	HPV58 (7.10%)	HPV58 (8.10%)	HPV58 (0%)	HPV58 (5.71%)	HPV58 (0%)	20.91%
	HPV68 (14.60%)	HPV68 (0%)	HPV68 (4.30%)	HPV68 (0%)	HPV68 (0%)	18.90%
	HPV59 (3.10%)	HPV59 (5.80%)	HPV59 (4.30%)	HPV59 (1.43%)	HPV59 (0%)	14.63%
	HPV66 (7.60%)	HPV66 (0%)	HPV66 (0%)	HPV66 (0%)	HPV66 (0%)	7.60%

Prevalence of HR-HPV in each target group				
Target groups	**Childbearing age women in the study population**	**Teenage girls**	**Men**	**Total**
HR-HPV genotypes identified	HPV56 (15.94%)	HPV56 (8.80%)	HPV56 (20%)	44.74%
	HPV52 (12.73%)	HPV52 (22.80%)	HPV52 (6%)	41.53%
	HPV39 (8.25%)	HPV39 (13.20%)	HPV39 (11%)	32.45%
	HPV59 (10.91%)	HPV59 (14%)	HPV59 (3%)	27.91%
	HPV51 (7%)	HPV51 (10.30%)	HPV51 (6%)	23.30%
	HPV35 (5.45%)	HPV35 (10.30%)	HPV35 (6%)	21.75%
	HPV31 (3.36%)	HPV31 (3.60%)	HPV31 (11%)	17.96%
	HPV18 (6.01%)	HPV18 (5.20%)	HPV18 (6%)	17.21%
	HPV68 (5.17%)	HPV68 (0%)	HPV68 (11%)	16.17%
	HPV16 (1.82%)	HPV16 (5.20%)	HPV16 (8%)	15.02%
	HPV66 (11.05%)	HPV66 (0%)	HPV66 (3%)	14.05%
	HPV58 (5.17%)	HPV58 (4.40%)	HPV58 (0%)	9.57%
	HPV45 (5.03%)	HPV45 (1.50%)	HPV45 (3%)	9.53%
	HPV33 (2.10%)	HPV33 (0.70%)	HPV33 (6%)	8.80%

Table 4.
Prevalence of HR-HPV in risk population, precancerous lesions, and cancer cases.

Target groups	Presence of HR-HPV			Type of HR-HPV according to target groups		
	HR-HPV⁻	HR-HPV⁺	P-value	Single infections	Multiple infections	Number of HR-HPV genotypes per infected person
Childbearing age women n = 1321	64.57% (853/1321)	35.40% (468/1321)	< 0.001	63.68% (298/468)	36.32% (170/468)	1–6
Teenage girls, *n* = 200	58.5% (117/200)	41.50% (83/200)	0.001	57.80% (48/83)	42.20% (35/83)	1– 5
Sex workers, *n* = 200	47% (94/200)	53% (106/200)	0.230	46.20% (49/106)	53.80% (57/106)	1–9
HIV+, *n* = 183	36.06% (66/183)	63.90% (117/183)	< 0.001	37.61% (44/117)	62.39% (73/117)	1–7
CIN 2/3, *n* = 43	51.16% (22/43)	48.80% (21/43)	0.829	90.50% (19/21)	9.50% (2/21)	1–2
ICC, *n* = 65	27.69% (18/65)	72.31% (47/65)	< 0.001	65.96% (31/47)	34.04% (16/47)	1–4
Otolaryngology cancers, *n* = 128	84.37% (108/128)	15.63% (20/128)	0.722	90% (18/20)	10% (2/20)	1–2
Men, *n* = 124	82.26% (102/124)	17.74% (22/124)	< 0.001	—	—	—
Total, *n* = 2264	60.95% (1380/2264)	39.05% (884/2264)	<0.001			

n = total number of participants.

Table 5.
Prevalence of single and multiple infections in target groups.

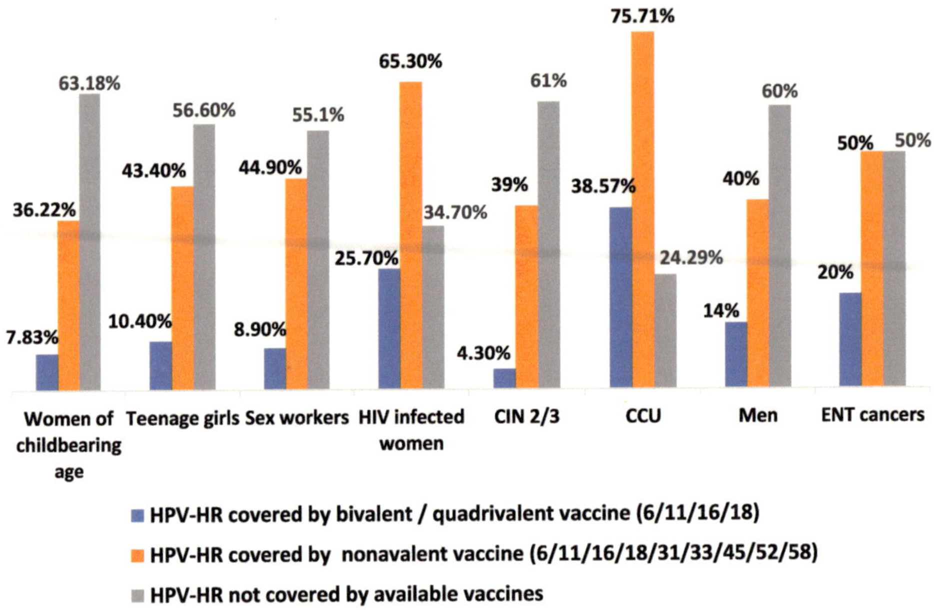

Figure 2.
Prevalence of HR-HPV identified in the target groups of our study according to their coverage by available vaccines.

age women, adolescent girls, sex workers, HIV-positive women, CIN 2/3, ICC, men, and otolaryngology cancer. HR-HPV not covered by bivalent, quadrivalent, or nonavalent HPV vaccines were observed with a higher prevalence in childbearing age women (63.18%), CIN 2/3 cases (61%), and men (60%) (**Figure 2**).

4. Discussion

HPV is one of the carcinogenic viruses, sexually transmitted, widespread in the world with a high prevalence in developing countries especially in Sub-Saharan Africa where socio-cultural and behavioral factors which promote transmission prevail in several regions. In the present epidemiological study, including 2386 samples out of which 2264 were valid using the PCR technique, the overall prevalence of HR-HPV was 39.05% (824/2264). This prevalence is in line with those reported in previous studies supporting a global prevalence of 10.4% of HR-HPV infection [20] which can reach 36.5% in some developing countries [21, 22].

Epidemiological studies suggested a difference in the prevalence and distribution of HR-HPV genotypes in infected women according to regions and risk groups throughout the world [23, 24]. Our results support this variable prevalence and distribution of HR-HPV according to target populations and sample types.

Indeed, the prevalence of 35.40% of infection observed in the population of childbearing age women was lower than that reported in some studies from Tanzania (74%) [25] and Ethiopia (83.2%) [26] almost similar to that of a study conducted in England (35%) [27].

HR-HPV is the main etiologic agent responsible for ano-genital cancers including ICC and a prevalence of 100% could be expected in ICC cases. The high prevalence of 72.31% of HR-HPV infection in ICC cases found in this study was lower than the 100% reported in Gabon [28], 90,7% in Nigeria [29], and 83,2% in Malaysia [30]. The difference in the methodologies used could support the existence of false-negative samples as reported in a previous study by Tan et al. [30] in Malaysia.

Furthermore, sex workers and men, an important active group for the maintenance of HPV in the population, showed a high prevalence of HR-HPV in our study. For instance, some studies reported a significant association between HPV infection, high number of sexual partners, and history of STIs [31]. The prevalence of 53% found among sex workers in our study was higher than those of 51.5% and 26% reported respectively in Côte d'Ivoire [32] and Ghana [7]. In contrast, the infection rate of 17.74% in the men of our study population was lower than the 32.4% observed by Zhu et al. [33] in men with genital warts. These results support the fact that sex workers and men constitute a reservoir for the transmission of HR-HPV, hence the importance of awareness-raising among these risk populations about the screening for HPV infection.

Data analysis also showed that 48.80% (21/43) of women with high-grade precancerous lesions (CIN2/3) were infected with HR-HPV; a lower prevalence than the 91.9% reported in another study in a similar population [34]. These results could be explained by the higher rate of infection in women under 30 years old, especially in those of 25–29 and 60 years and over [35–37]. For instance, the mean age of women with CIN 2/3 in our study was 41.5 ± 9.8 years (22–74 years) against was 45.7 years in the study of Wang et al. (21–83 years old).

Several studies reported a high prevalence of HPV infection in HIV+ women [7, 38] as HIV is a well-known factor associated with an increased risk of HR-HPV persistence and multiple infections, and therefore, promote the occurrence of anogenital cancers. The prevalence of 63.90% of HR-HPV observed in this target group of the present study was similar to 65.5% in Ghana [39] but higher than the 36% reported in Nigeria [40] and 33.3% in Brazil [41]. Compared to non-HIV infected women in the general population, this high prevalence could be explained by the immunosuppression and confirm the role of HIV infection as an additional risk factor for the persistence of HR-HPV.

The infection rate of 41.5% found in adolescent girls was lower than the 66.7% observed in South Africa [32]. The difference in age range (15 to 19 years in our study versus 16 to 22 in the South African study) could explain the prevalence variation between the two studies especially when previous studies support that HR-HPV infection is higher in those less than 30 years of age [37].

In our study, HPV 56 was the most common genotype in childbearing age women, men, and otolaryngology cancers with predominance in the general population as well as target groups. This genotype is not covered by any available HPV vaccine, although it has been found in ICC and CIN 2/3 cases [29]. The same is true for HPV 68 which was the most common genotype in sex workers and the fourth common in men.

Since sexual transmission is possible between men and women, the presence of these genotypes in ICC and CIN 2/3 cases suggests a low clearance of the latter HR-HPV genotype in Burkina Faso.

HPV 18 was more common in HIV-positive women and ICC cases with a high frequency of 18.8 and 25.71% respectively. It was also present in CIN 2/3 up to 4.3 and 10% in otolaryngology cancers. Our results are in line with those of studies reporting that this persistent genotype is one of the most commonly found in cervical cancers [29].

Immunodeficiency of HIV-infected women coinfected with HPV 18 promotes high-grade precancerous lesions and the occurrence of invasive cancer of the cervix. It would therefore be necessary to strengthen surveillance through screening, treatment, and vaccination of HIV-infected women.

In addition, unlike studies reporting HPV 16 as the most common genotype throughout the world, especially in cervical cancers [13, 28, 30, 42, 43], this genotype was classified among the less frequent HPVs in our study. However, in ICC

(12.86%), otolaryngology cancers (10%), and in men (8%), HPV 16 was not one of the most common genotypes but reached a frequency that required attention. The low prevalence of HPV-16/18 in our 2386 samples remains an enigma to be elucidated. It remains true that not only the distribution of the HPV genotypes would vary according to the continents, the zones, the countries, and the target populations but also the clearance and the borrowing of the pathway of the carcinogenesis induced by these viruses is modulated by genetic polymorphisms of their human hosts [44, 45]. Evidence from the literature support that the HPV16/18/31/33/35/45/52/58 genotypes are the most common genotypes found in 20% of cervical cancer cases worldwide [24].

The results of the present study also revealed a high prevalence of HR-HPV genotypes covered by the nonavalent vaccine (36.22–75.71%) as well as genotypes of HPV not covered by the vaccine (24.29–63,18%). It is noteworthy that some of the genotypes not covered by vaccine were found in high-grade precancerous lesions and cervical cancer cases [29, 46].

For effective prophylactic actions to control HPV infection, the present epidemiological study in Burkina Faso shows variable distribution of HR-HPV genotypes in the different target populations. Our results suggest that implementation of the nonavalent vaccine is important for HR-HPV infection control in Burkina Faso. Promotion of screening of men, especially for penile cancer and genital warts, and young boys vaccination programs are required since men are well-known reservoirs for HR-HPV dissemination.

5. Conclusion

The studies carried out in Burkina Faso show the circulation of fourteen high-risk HPV genotypes among different layers of the population. The prevalence of HPV infection and genotypes distribution varied among target groups with an overall predominance of non-HPV 16 and 18 genotypes. Moreover, the high-risk HPV genotypes found in Burkina Faso are not all covered by the available vaccines. It is however crucial and important to focus on vaccination using available and accessible vaccines for developing countries to reduce the disease incidence. Cervical cancer and other HPV-induced cancers remain a global public health concern. Strengthening the implementation of primary, secondary, and tertiary prevention strategies incorporating information-education-communication and awareness-raising, will allow effective control of HPV infection and its consequences in men and women.

Author details

Théodora Mahoukèdè Zohoncon[1,2,3], Rogomenoma Alice Ouedraogo[1,2], Florencia Wendkuuni Djigma[1,2], Lassina Traore[1,2], Teega-Wendé Clarisse Ouedraogo[1,2], Maimouna Ilboudo[1,2], Regine Ilboudo[1,2], Catherine Salambanga[1,2], Sindimalgdé Patricia Guigma[2], Sessi Frida Tovo[1,2], Mah Alima Esther Traore[1,2], Prosper Bado[1,2], Ali Kande[1,2], Cyrille Bisseye[2], Abdoul Karim Ouattara[1,2], Ina Marie Angèle Traore[1,2], Djeneba Ouermi[1,2], Tani Sagna[1,2], Albert Théophane Yonli[1,2], Wendyam Marie Christelle Nadembega[1,2], Dorcas Obiri-Yeboah[4], Yvette Marie Chantal Gyebre[5], Olga Mélanie Lompo[5], Charlemagne Marie Ragnag-Newende Ouedraogo[6] and Jacques Simpore[1,2]*

1 Laboratory of Molecular Biology and Genetics (LABIOGENE), Joseph KI-ZERBO University, Burkina, Faso

2 Pietro Annigoni Biomolecular Research Centre (CERBA), Burkina Faso

3 Faculty of Medicine, University Saint Thomas d'Aquin, Burkina Faso

4 Department of Microbiology and Immunology, University of Cape Coast, School of Medical Sciences, University Post Office, Accra, Ghana

5 Yalgado Ouedraogo University Hospital (CHU/YO), Burkina Faso

6 Obstetrician-Gynecologist, UFR/SDS, Joseph KI-ZERBO University, Burkina Faso

*Address all correspondence to: simpore93@gmail.com

References

[1] Saracci R, Wild CP. International Agency for Research on Cancer: The first 50 years, 1965-2015. France: International Agency for Research on Cancer; 2015. ISBN: 978-92-832-0441-1. Available from: https://www.iarc.who.int/wp-content/uploads/2018/07/IARC_50-years.pdf [Accessed 12-10-2021]

[2] Alain S, Hantz S, Denis F. Papillomavirus: les virus et la physiopathologie de l'infection. Médecine thérapeutique/Pédiatrie. 2010;**13**(1):5-19

[3] Bado P, Djigma Wendkuuni F, Zohoncon Théodora M, Obiri-Yeboah D,. Traoré Esther Mah A, Ouattara Abdoul K, et al. Polymorphism of MMP1 and MMP3 promoter regions and HR-HPV infection in women from Burkina Faso and Côte d'Ivoire. Biomol Concepts. 2020; **11**(1):116-124

[4] Doorbar J. The papillomavirus life cycle. Journal of Clinical Virology. 2005;**32**:7-15

[5] Zohoncon TM, Bisseye C, Djigma FW, Yonli AT, Compaore TR, Sagna T, et al. Prevalence of HPV high-risk genotypes in three cohorts of women in Ouagadougou (Burkina Faso). Mediterranean Journal of Hematology and Infectious Diseases. 2013;**5**(1):e2013059

[6] Bray F, Ferlay J, Soerjomataram I, Siegel RL, Torre LA, Jemal A. Global cancer statistics 2018: GLOBOCAN estimates of incidence and mortality worldwide for 36 cancers in 185 countries. CA: a Cancer Journal for Clinicians. 2018;**68**(6):394-424

[7] Adams AR, Nortey PA, Dortey BA, Asmah RH, Wiredu EK. Cervical human papillomavirus prevalence, genotypes, and associated risk factors among female sex workers in Greater Accra, Ghana. Journal of Oncology. 2019;**2019**:7. Article ID: 8062176. DOI: 10.1155/2019/8062176

[8] Zohoncon TM, Ouedraogo TC, Brun LVC, Obiri-Yeboah D, Djigma WF, Kabibou S, et al. Molecular epidemiology of high-risk human papillomavirus in high-grade cervical intraepithelial neoplasia and in cervical cancer in Parakou, Republic of Benin. Pakistan Journal of Biological Sciences: PJBS. 2016;**19**(2):49-56

[9] Bruni L, Albero G, Serrano B, Mena M, Gómez D, Muñoz J, et al. Human papillomavirus and related diseases in Mali. In: Summary Report. Barcelona: ICO/IARC Information Centre on HPV and Cancer (HPV Information Centre); 2019

[10] Damke E, Kurscheidt FA, Balani VA, Takeda KI, Irie MM, Gimenes F, et al. Male partners of infertile couples with seminal infections of human papillomavirus have impaired fertility parameters. BioMed Research International. 2017;**2017**:8. Article ID: 4684629. DOI: 10.1155/2017/4684629

[11] Foresta C, Pizzol D, Moretti A, Barzon L, Palù G, Garolla A. Clinical and prognostic significance of human papillomavirus DNA in the sperm or exfoliated cells of infertile patients and subjects with risk factors. Fertility and Sterility. 2010;**94**(5):1723-1727

[12] WH Organization. Human papillomavirus vaccines: WHO position paper, October 2014. Weekly Epidemiological Record = Relevé épidémiologique hebdomadaire. 2014;**89**(43):465-491

[13] ICO/IARC. Human Papillomavirus and Related Diseases in Burkina Faso. Barcelona: ICO/IARC Information Centre on HPV and Cancer (HPV Information Centre); 2018. p. 70

[14] Ilboudo M, Zohoncon TM, Traore EMA, Traore IMA, Kande A, Djigma FW, et al. Characterization of high-risk oncogenic human papillomavirus genotypes in histologically confirmed ear, nose and throat (Ent) cancers in Burkina Faso. Asian Pacific Journal of Cancer Prevention. 2019;**20**(11):3429-3435

[15] Traore IMA, Zohoncon TM, Djigma FW, Compaore TR, Traore Y, Simpore J. Association of TNF-α-308G/a and IL-18 polymorphisms with risk of HPV infection among sexually active women in Burkina Faso. Biomolecular Concepts. 2020;**11**(1):97-101

[16] Sagna T, Djigma F, Zeba M, Bisseye C, Karou SD, Ouermi D, et al. Human papillomaviruses prevalence and genital co-infections in HIV-seropositive women in Ouagadougou (Burkina Faso). Pakistan Journal of Biological Sciences. 2010;**13**(19): 951-955

[17] Yamada R, Sasagawa T, Kirumbi LW, Kingoro A, Karanja DK, Kiptoo M, et al. Human papillomavirus infection and cervical abnormalities in Nairobi, Kenya, an area with a high prevalence of human immunodeficiency virus infection. Journal of Medical Virology. 2008;**80**(5):847-855

[18] Soohoo M, Blas M, Byraiah G, Carcamo C, Brown B. Cervical HPV infection in female sex workers: A global perspective. The Open AIDS Journal. 2013;**7**:58

[19] Stratton KL, Culkin DJ. A contemporary review of HPV and penile cancer, Oncology (Williston Park, NY). 2016; **30**(3):245-249

[20] De Sanjosé S, Diaz M, Castellsagué X, Clifford G, Bruni L, Muñoz N, et al. Worldwide prevalence and genotype distribution of cervical human papillomavirus DNA in women with normal cytology: A meta-analysis. The Lancet Infectious Diseases. 2007;**7**(7):453-459

[21] Ouedraogo RA, Zohoncon TM, Guigma SP, Angèle Traore IM, Ouattara AK, Ouedraogo M, et al. Oncogenic human papillomavirus infection and genotypes characterization among sexually active women in Tenkodogo at Burkina Faso, West Africa. Papillomavirus Research. 2018;**6**:22-26

[22] Bao Y-P, Li N, Smith J, Qiao Y-L. Human papillomavirus type distribution in women from Asia: A meta-analysis. International Journal of Gynecologic Cancer. 2008;**18**(1):71-79. DOI: 10.1111/j.1525-1438.2007.00959.x

[23] Zohoncon TM, Djigma WF, Ouattara AK, Traore IM, Ouedraogo RA, Traore EM, et al. Mapping of fourteen high-risk human papillomavirus genotypes by molecular detection in sexually active women in the West African sub-region. International Journal of Genetics and Molecular Biology. 2020; **12**(1):11-21

[24] Clifford GM, Smith JS, Plummer M, Munoz N, Franceschi S. Human papillomavirus types in invasive cervical cancer worldwide: A meta-analysis. British Journal of Cancer. 2003;**88**(1): 63-73

[25] Watson-Jones D, Baisley K, Brown J, Kavishe B, Andreasen A, Changalucha J, et al. High prevalence and incidence of human papillomavirus in a cohort of healthy young African female subjects. Sexually Transmitted Infections. 2013;**89**(5):358-365

[26] Wolday D, Derese M, Gebressellassie S, Tsegaye B, Ergete W, Gebrehiwot Y, et al. HPV genotype distribution among women with normal and abnormal cervical cytology presenting in a tertiary gynecology referral Clinic in Ethiopia. Infectious Agents and Cancer. 2018;**13**:28

[27] Howell-Jones R, Bailey A, Beddows S, Sargent A, de Silva N, Wilson G, et al. Multi-site study of HPV type-specific prevalence in women with cervical cancer, intraepithelial neoplasia and normal cytology, in England. British Journal of Cancer. 2010;**103**(2):209-216

[28] Zoa-Assoumou S, Ndjoyi-Mbiguino A, Mabika BM, Belembaogo E, Khattabi A, Ennaji MM. Human papillomavirus genotypes distribution in cervical cancer cases in Gabon. Infectious Agents and Cancer. 2016;**11**(1):1-5

[29] Okolo C, Franceschi S, Adewole I, Thomas JO, Follen M, Snijders PJ, et al. Human papillomavirus infection in women with and without cervical cancer in Ibadan, Nigeria. Infectious Agents and Cancer. 2010;**5**(1):1-4

[30] Tan SC, Ismail MP, Duski DR, Othman NH, Ankathil R. Prevalence and type distribution of human papillomavirus (HPV) in Malaysian women with and without cervical cancer: An updated estimate. Bioscience Reports. 2018;**38**(2):BSR20171268

[31] Mbulawa ZZ, Van Schalkwyk C, Hu N-C, Meiring TL, Barnabas S, Dabee S, et al. High human papillomavirus (HPV) prevalence in south African adolescents and young women encourages expanded HPV vaccination campaigns. PLoS One. 2018;**13**(1):e0190166

[32] Tovo SF, Zohoncon TM, Dabiré AM, Ilboudo R, Tiemtoré RY, Obiri-Yeboah D, et al. Molecular epidemiology of human papillomaviruses, Neisseria gonorrhoeae, chlamydia trachomatis and mycoplasma genitalium among female sex Workers in Burkina Faso: Prevalence, coinfections and drug resistance genes. Tropical Medicine and Infectious Disease. 2021;**6**(2):90

[33] Zhu C, Wang Y, Mao W, Zhang H, Ma J. Prevalence and distribution of HPV types in genital warts in Xi'an, China: A prospective study. BMJ Open. 2019;**9**(5):e023897

[34] Wang J, Tang D, Wang K, Wang J, Zhang Z, Chen Y, et al. HPV genotype prevalence and distribution during 2009-2018 in Xinjiang, China: baseline surveys prior to mass HPV vaccination. BMC Women's Health. 2019;**19**(1):1-14

[35] Aziz H, Iqbal H, Mahmood H, Fatima S, Faheem M, Sattar AA, et al. Human papillomavirus infection in females with normal cervical cytology: Genotyping and phylogenetic analysis among women in Punjab, Pakistan. International Journal of Infectious Diseases. 2018;**66**:83-89

[36] Hooi DJ, Lissenberg-Witte BI, Kenter G, de Koning MN, Gomes Bravio I, Ardts K, et al. Human papillomavirus (HPV) prevalence and associated risk factors in women from Curaçao. PLoS One. 2018;**13**(7): e0199624

[37] Mutombo AB, Benoy I, Tozin R, Bogers J, Van Geertruyden J-P, Jacquemyn Y. Prevalence and distribution of human papillomavirus genotypes among women in Kinshasa, the Democratic Republic of the Congo. Journal of Global Oncology. 2019;5:1-9

[38] Djigma FW, Ouédraogo C, Karou DS, Sagna T, Bisseye C, Zeba M, et al. Prevalence and genotype characterization of human papillomaviruses among HIV-seropositive in Ouagadougou, Burkina Faso. Acta Tropica. 2011;**117**(3):202-206

[39] Obiri-Yeboah D, Akakpo PK, Mutocheluh M, Adjei-Danso E, Allornuvor G, Amoako-Sakyi D, et al. Epidemiology of cervical human papillomavirus (HPV) infection and squamous intraepithelial lesions (SIL) among a cohort of HIV-infected and uninfected Ghanaian women. BMC Cancer. 2017;**17**(1):688

[40] Akarolo-Anthony SN, Al-Mujtaba M, Famooto AO, Dareng EO, Olaniyan OB, Offiong R, et al. HIV associated high-risk HPV infection among Nigerian women. BMC Infectious Diseases. 2013;**13**(1):1-6

[41] Travassos AG, Netto E, Xavier-Souza E, Nóbrega I, Adami K, Timbó M, et al. Predictors of HPV incidence and clearance in a cohort of Brazilian HIV-infected women. PLoS One. 2017;**12**(10):e0185423

[42] Yuan X-W, Li Y-J, Qiu Q, Luo Z-Y, Zhao X-F. Prevalence and genotype distribution of human papillomavirus among 9945 women from the Nanhai area of Foshan. BMC Infectious Diseases. 2019;**19**(1):71

[43] Rossi PG, Sideri M, Carozzi FM, Vocaturo A, Buonaguro FM, Tornesello ML, et al. HPV type distribution in invasive cervical cancers in Italy: Pooled analysis of three large studies. Infectious Agents and Cancer. 2012;**7**(1):1-10

[44] Stanczuk G, Sibanda E, Tswana S, Bergstrom S. Polymorphism at the–308-promoter position of the tumor necrosis factor-alpha (TNF-α) gene and cervical cancer. International Journal of Gynecologic Cancer. 2003;**13**(2):148-153

[45] Yang X, Qiu M-T, Hu J-W, Jiang F, Li M, Wang J, et al. Association of Interleukin-18 gene promoter– 607 C> a and– 137G> C polymorphisms with cancer risk: A meta-analysis of 26 studies. PLoS One. 2013;**8**(9):e73671

[46] Félix A, Alemany L, Tous S, de Sanjosé S, Bosch FX. HPV distribution in cervical cancer in Portugal. A retrospective study from 1928 to 2005. Papillomavirus Research. 2016; **2**:41-45

Chapter 9

Perspective Chapter: Cervical Cancer Elimination by 2030—The W.H.O Goal: Neo Challenges and Next Gen Solutions "TIT for TAT"—The Community Competency Model of Raj ©

Rajamanickam Rajkumar

Abstract

Cervical Cancer is the fourth most common cancer among women, worldwide. It accounts for 600,000 new cases per year, and 340,000 deaths globally (WHO 2020 data). It causes a lot of maladies and suffering for women, in the age group of 30–60 years, especially in the poor community of developing countries. Cervical cancer is a great public health problem and is a cause of grave concern for the health system in Low-Middle-Income Countries—LMIC. But cervical cancer is amenable for early detection and successful treatment of precancer stages. Human Papilloma Virus—HPV vaccines offer a high level of primordial prevention, against cervical cancer. Therefore, the World Health Organization, in 2018, has called for "Elimination of Cervical Cancer by 2030." The objective is to reduce the incidence rate of cervical cancer to below 4/100,000, by the year 2030. This leads to many "Neo Challenges" and also opens the door for "Next Gen Solutions". The author, with vast experiences in his Cervical Cancer Screening Projects of IARC/ WHO, at Tamil Nadu, India, during 2000–2007, advocates a strategy called "TIT for TAT—The Community Competency model of Raj©."

Keywords: cervical cancer screening, pre cancer treatment, HPV vaccination, elimination

1. Introduction

Cervical Cancer accounts for about 600,000 incident cases and 340,000 cause specific deaths, per year, worldwide, according to IARC/WHO, for the year 2020 [1]

Cervical Cancer ranks 7th among the most common cancers in general and among women, it is ranking as the 4th highest, worldwide, as per the data available with the WHO, for the year 2020 [2].

As far as Mortality is concerned, it is the 9th most common cancer-causing deaths among all cancers and the 4th leading among cancers in women, during 2020 [3].

2. Methodology

2.1 Efforts towards elimination of cervical cancer: the favorable features of the disease

The Human Papilloma Virus—HPV, is the known causal factor for the Cervical Cancer. HPV consists of more than 180 strains. But only a few are oncogenic. The HPV 16, 18 are the high-risk oncogenic strains. When a woman enters sexual life, she is exposed to the HPV infections. But these infections undergo self-clearance, due to the good immunity that may exist in the woman. In some cases, the HPV infection persists for a long time, even up to 10 years. If there are oncogenic strains like the HPV 16, 18, the cervical cells undergo a pathological process called dysplasia or Cervical Intra epithelial Neoplasia—CIN. These are the Pre cancer lesions. At this stage, the disease is detectable by the application of screening tests.

The screening tests which are available:

1. Visual Inspection with—Acetic acid VIA, Lugol's Iodine VILI

2. Pap smear test

3. HPV tests (DNA—Hybrid capture—Genotyping)

These tests have acceptable levels of Sensitivity and Specificity to detect CIN lesions.

2.2 Precancer lesions: diagnosis and management protocols

2.2.1 See & treat

The Health care provider, who does the screening, subjects the woman to VIA testing. If the VIA test is positive, then the woman is treated by Cryotherapy/Thermal ablation/Cold coagulation/Laser/Cold knife conization/LEEP or LLETZ.

2.2.2 See: test & treat

The woman is subjected to VIA testing. If the result is positive, another screening test is applied, by means of Pap smear or HPV testing. Even if one of these tests is positive, the woman undergoes Precancer treatment, by modalities listed above.

2.3 The 3 eligibility criteria for elimination, are fulfilled by cervical cancer

2.3.1 Criteria 1: effective vaccines

The HPV Vaccines which are available in the Health care system are the Bivalent, Quadravalent and Nonovalent vaccines. They are prophylactic vaccines given to Girls between the age group 9–15 years, in doses as recommended by their Health care providers. The protective value of these vaccines are claimed to be more than 70%.

2.3.2 Criteria 2: early diagnosis at precancer stages

Various screening methods are available for the early diagnosis of Cervical Cancer, especially in the Precancer stages. The methods are VIA, Pap smear and HPV tests. These tests have high accuracy with acceptable levels of Sensitivity and Specificity. Further confirmation is done by Colposcopy and Cervical Biopsies. Hence, sure methods for diagnosis of pre cancer stages are available and the effective treatment of these lesions, prevent the stages of invasive Cervical Cancer. This is an important criterion for fulfilling the eligibility of Cervical cancer, for Elimination.

2.3.3 Criteria 3: effective treatment for cervical precancer

The various treatment modalities available for the treatment of cervical precancer lesions:

1. Cryotherapy

2. Cold coagulation

3. Thermal ablation—electric cautery

4. Laser ablation

5. Cold knife conization

6. Loop Electrosurgical Excision Procedure—LEEP/Large Loop Electrosurgical Excision of Transformation Zone—LLETZ

All the above methods are very efficient for the treatment of Cervical precancers, resulting in Cure rates, up to 80–90%.

3. The WHO declares cervical cancer Elimination by 2030

3.1 Milestones

1. May, 2018—The Director General of WHO, gave a call at WHA for "Elimination of Cervical Cancer by 2030" [4].

2. November 2020, The WHO launched the Global strategy to "Accelerate the Elimination of Cervical Cancer".

3. Signatory countries should achieve an Incidence rate of < 4 per 100,000 women per year, by 2030.

4. The IARC/WHO provides all the support needed to achieve this goal by 2030.

3.2 The targets set by WHO, for cervical cancer elimination by 2030

3.2.1 HPV vaccination

90% of girls to be fully vaccinated with the HPV vaccine by the age of 15 years [4].

3.2.2 Cervical cancer screening

70% of women to be screened by VIA/Pap smear /HPV tests, by the age of 35 years, and again by the age of 45 years.

3.2.3 Precancer and cancer treatment

90% of women with precancer lesions, to be treated. 90% of women with invasive cancer to be treated and offered Palliative care.

3.2.4 Challenges for cervical cancer screening, in low- and middle-income countries

1. Low levels of Awareness.

2. Lack of Knowledge.

3. Indifferent and negative Attitude.

4. Poor Health seeking Behavior.

5. Very poor levels of Translation of Knowledge into Practice.

6. Screening—Acceptability, Availability, Affordability.

7. Pre cancer Treatment—the availability and problems in utilization.

8. Socio Economic barriers.

9. Cultural and Political barriers.

4. Discussion

Cervical Cancer Elimination by 2030
Neo Challenges and Next Gen Solutions
"TIT for TAT"
The Community Competency Model of Raj ©
"TIT"
Trained manpower—Indigenous resources—Translational research—**TIT**
"TAT"
Targets achievement—Action plan—Transformational research—**TAT**

The author recommends

"TIT" as the Next Gen solutions
"TAT" as the Neo challenges
The Community Competency Model of Raj ©, for achieving Cervical Cancer Elimination by 2030.

These recommendations are based on the "Proof of Concept ", Cervical Cancer Screening project of IARC/WHO, at Christian Fellowship Community Health Center, Ambilikai, Dindigul district, Tamil Nadu, India, during 2000–2007. The Author was the Principal Investigator of this project, which achieved a reduction in the

Cervical Cancer Incidence by 25% and mortality due to Cervical Cancer by 35%, in a period of 5 years [5].

Brief description of the model "TIT for TAT":
NEXT GEN SOLUTIONS—"TIT"
"TIT"
T = **T**rained manpower
I = **I**ndigenous resources
T = **T**ranslational research
NEO CHALLENGES—"TAT"
"TAT"
T = **T**arget achievement
A = **A**ction plan
T = **T**ransformational research

4.1 Next gen solutions = "TIT"

4.1.1 T = Trained manpower

It is very important and prudent, to have the entire team, trained in their role, from authorized persons/organizations, and get certified, which are approved and accepted by the implementing authorities. Assessment exams are to be conducted at the start, concurrent and terminal levels to assure Internal Quality Control and Quality Assurance.

4.1.1.1 Doctors

To be trained in Colposcopy, Cryotherapy and LEEP/LLETZ, procedures. The author had his trainings with the fellowship from IARC/WHO, at RCSI—Dublin, RCOG—London, SCCPS—Singapore and served as a Hon. Consultant to the Cervical Cancer Screening Program of The Ohio State University Medical Center.

4.1.1.2 Nurses/female health workers

To be trained in Visual Inspection methods with Acetic acid—VIA, Lugol's Iodine—VILI Pap smear techniques, Endocervical curettage, Colposcopy guided Biopsy techniques, Cervical cells collection for HPV testing, technical assistance during treatment procedures and Counseling methods. Maintenance of clinical instruments, equipment, sterilization, autoclaving and laundry, which are very important tasks for the nurses.

4.1.1.3 Lab technicians

To be trained in Cervical Pathology and HPV testing procedures. The Medical Records staff needs to be trained in appropriate computer applications, Data management, data analysis, interpretation and publishing techniques.

4.1.1.4 Health educators/counselor

The participation of women for the Cervical Cancer Programs and compliance with the treatment and follow-up procedures, largely depends upon the level of Knowledge, Attitude and Practice. Even though, they may have adequate knowledge regarding Cervical Cancer and its prevention, the proportion of women who will translate "Knowledge into Practice" is relatively small.

4.1.1.5 Knowledge—present/practice—absent

The main barriers to achieving the above ambitious goal, are the lacunae and deficiencies in the conversion of knowledge into practice, by the women, who are otherwise well informed about the prevention of Cervical Cancer, as a result of massive inputs in the field of Health Education. Thus, the screening participation and compliance to precancer treatment remain low. This barrier in *translational knowledge* should be overcome efficiently. The author, by the virtue of his vast experiences, in planning and implementing one of the largest cervical cancer screening programs in India, has conceptualized "**The STAR P6 Health Education Model of Raj**© (6), for successful conversion of "Knowledge into Practice".

The STAR P6 Health Education Model of Raj© (**Figure 1**) [6].

4.1.1.6 The "P 6" concepts

The STAR approach can be better explained under 6 aspects of the program:

1. Projection
2. Perception
3. Promotion
4. Performance
5. Perseverance
6. Pursuit

The sole motive of the STAR approach is to encourage young women and girls for the HPV Vaccination and Screening of Cervical Cancer, applying the above mentioned 6 criteria, which involves a series of programmed and tailored steps in Health Education.

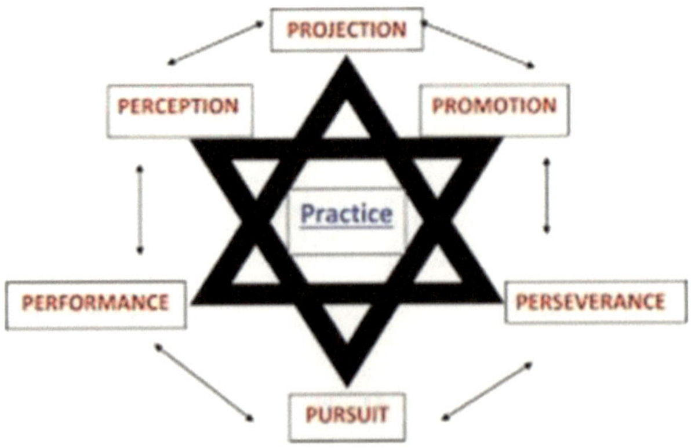

Figure 1.
The STAR P6 Health Education Model of Raj© [6].

4.1.2 I = Indigenous

4.1.2.1 Indigenous resources

The stability and sustainability of the Cervical Cancer Screening programs largely depend upon the **Availability and Affordability of Resources**. Instead of depending on distant and foreign resources which may be very costly and unaffordable, it is always prudent to develop locally available and affordable **Indigenous resources**, which would be functional and effective, even in limited and low resource settings. Some of the examples, that the Author has used in his WHO project are listed below:

1. Puppet shows and Role plays instead of Electronic media, especially in the hilly, mountainous, tribal areas, which are non-motorable and where electricity is not available. The programs are conducted with the help of Generators which are diesel fuelled.

2. Colposcopes are binocular and locally made, rather than sophisticated, hi-tech digital Colposcopes. Spectacles with a magnifying lens, were tried for examination of the Cervix, and it was satisfactory and successful (**Figure 2**).

3. Cryotherapy equipment which are locally made and uses Carbon di Oxide or Nitrous Oxide, under high pressure, targeted with a Gun, for freezing the cervical dysplasia lesions (**Figure 3**).

4. Silver nitrate crystals for hemostasis after Cervical biopsy, as a substitute to Monsel's paste, which is not available in many places and also is very costly for the limited budget programs.

5. Development of Pathology Laboratory, exclusively for the screening program, with a well-trained technician, in Cervical Pathology.

4.1.3 T = Translational research

The flow of knowledge, skills, technology, training, manpower, money and materials from a resource-rich organization, to resource poor and resource needed organization, is envisaged in Translational Research.

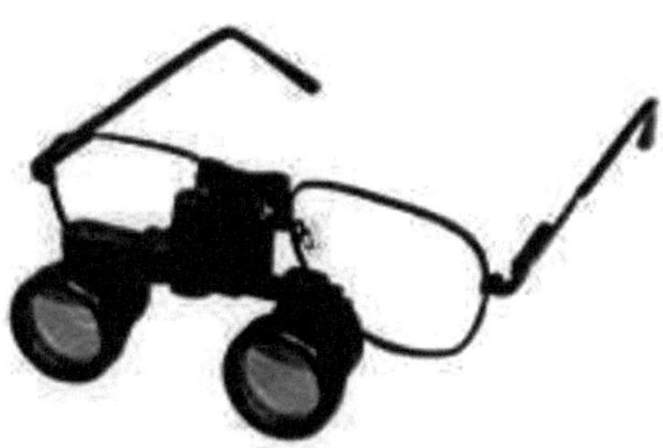

Figure 2.
Spectacles with lens attached—Indigenous Cervix scope.

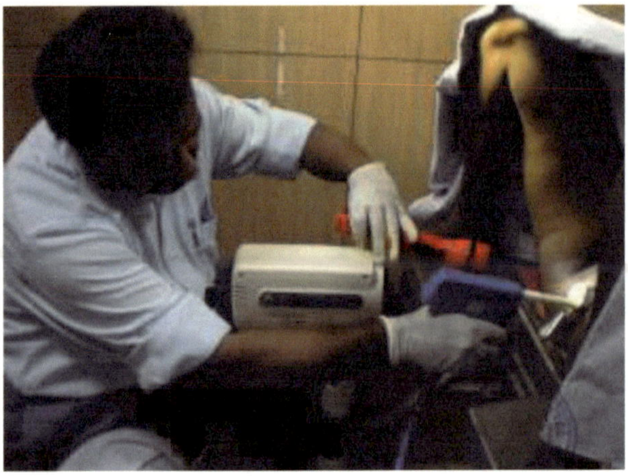

Figure 3.
Indigenous Colposcope and Cryotherapy Gun.

The author mobilized resources from Ireland, UK, France, Singapore and USA, to get trained in Cervical Cancer Screening and treatment procedures. Experts from these countries, came to the project sites of the Author, in Tamil Nadu, India, to conduct workshops and Community Based Screening programs in the villages.

Thus the 3 concepts of "TIT"—Trained manpower—Indigenous resources—Translational research, were the Neo Gen solutions.

4.2 Neo challenges = "TAT"

4.2.1 T = Targets achievement

The WHO has set the Goal of Cervical Cancer Elimination by 2030. More than 190 countries are signatories to this declaration and have committed to the achievement of the Targets, set as follows:

1. The first is for 90% of girls to be fully vaccinated against the human papillomavirus (HPV) by the age of 15 years.

2. The second is to ensure that 70% of women are screened using a high-performance test by the age of 35, and again by age 45.

3. The final target is that, 90% of women with pre-cancer receive treatment and for 90% of women with invasive cancer to have proper treatment and palliative care.

4.2.2 A = Action plan

4.2.2.1 For the successful implementation of "Cervical Health Evolution Cascade—CHEC"

1. Every 30,000 population, should have a "Community Health Center—CHC". This should be accessible to all, and equipped with basic equipment, instruments, essential drugs for Primary Health Care.

2. Each CHC should have 2 Female Community Health Nurses—CHN.

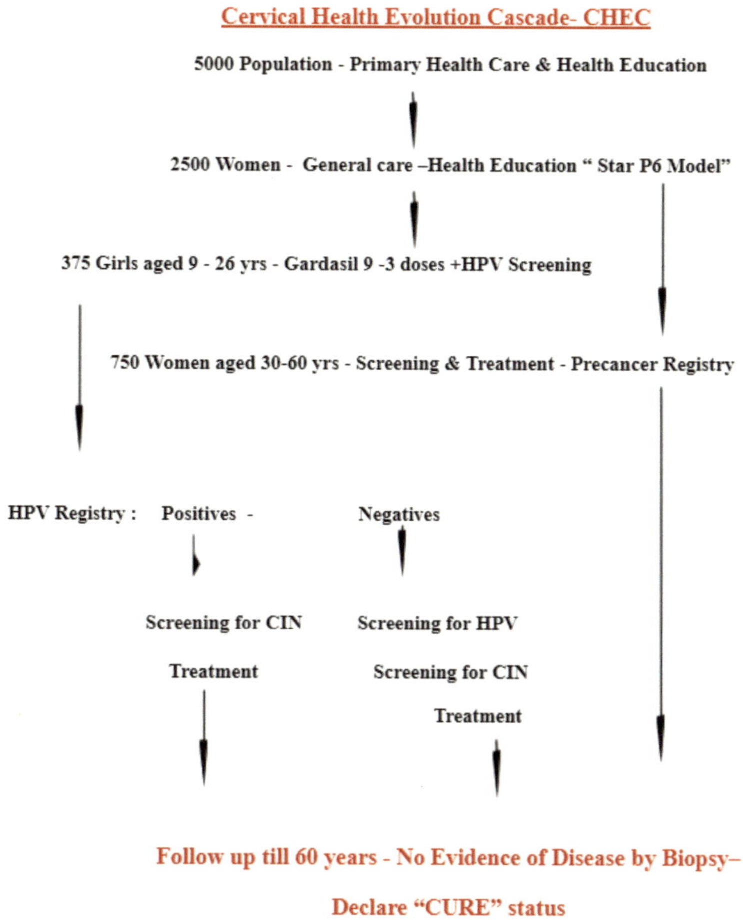

Figure 4.
Cervical Health Evolution Cascade—CHEC.

3. From every 5000 population, 2 Female Community Health Volunteers—CHV, should be identified and well trained in the practical aspects of Cervical Cancer screening and treatment (**Figure 4**).

4.2.3 T = Transformational research

> *"Start from what you know, Build on what you have and Achieve on what you should" ....Raj—the Author*

The Health Care System tilts towards the Prevention of Diseases and Promotion of Health from the Curative and Remedial care (**Figure 5**).

5. Conclusion

The main focus of this chapter is "Papilomaviridae Infections and Cervical Cancer—The Neo Challenges and Next Gen Solutions." The take home message is that HPV prevalence varies among region to region, communities to communities. The strains which infect the women are also multiple, varying in different countries and communities. The oncogenic strains of HPV are highly prevalent in Africa, Asia

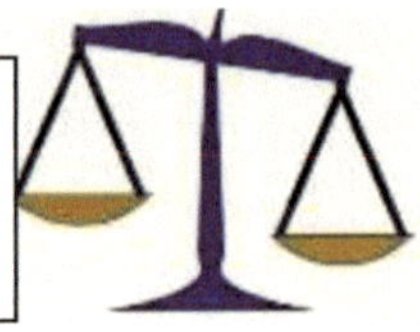

EXISTING HEALTH SYSTEM TREATMENT BASED	TRANSFORMED HEALTH SYSTEM PREVENTION BASED
Diseases Based	Health Based
Treatment centered	Prevention centered
Specialists dependent	Doctors - Nurses dependent
High tech Equipments	Low cost Simple Equipments
High Trained Technicians	Basics Trained Technicians – Digital & AI
Costly medicines / procedures	Essential medicines / Office procedures
Out of pocket expenditures	Insurance - Planned budgeting
Unstable personnel – Migratory job	Stable – Native personnel
Uncertain future	Certainty through Community Ownership
No sustainability	Sustainability by Community Contribution, Savings,Investments and Insurance
No consolidation of gains	Consolidation of gains by the Local infrastructure & Governance
Program ceases	Program expands by Collaborations based on Trustworthiness

Figure 5.
The tilted balance for "Transformational Research".

and American regions. Therefore, Cervical Cancer has a high incidence in these continents. The WHO has initiated a Goal—Elimination of Cervical Cancer by 2030.

The Neo challenges faced are listed under the phrase "TAT" (Target—Action plan—Transformation).

T—Targets are the 90-70-90 of WHO. 90% of the girls in age group 9–15 to be fully immunised against HPV. 70% of the eligible women to undergo Screening for Cervical Cancer. 90% of the Precancers to be treated and palliative care to be offered for Cervical Cancer patients.

A—Action plan to create Primary Health Care infrastructure, in the communities through their full participation, contribution and ownership

T-Transformational Research, which shifts the paradigm of Health Services from Treatment based to Prevention focused, by use of Appropriate Technology for Health.

The Next Gen solutions are listed under the phrase "TIT".

(Trained manpower—Indigenous resources—Translational research).

T—Trained manpower emphasizes on adequate training for the locally available and permanently employed Doctors, Nurses, Lab technicians, Health educators, Counselors and other paramedical staff of the programs, rather than relying on the specialists and temporary staff from external sources.

I—Indigenous resources, equipment, instruments and technology, are the accessible, affordable and available infrastructures for the efficient functioning of the programs, on a long-term basis.

T—Transformational research is based on shifting of the paradigm of Health care services from Treatment mode to Prevention mode.

Therefore, for the achievement of the WHO Goal of "Elimination of Cervical Cancer by 2030", the author, strongly recommends the TIT for TAT—The Community Competency Model of Raj© which effectively addresses the "Papilloma viridae infections and Cervical Cancer—The Neo Challenges and Next Gen solutions", both at regional and Global levels.

Acknowledgements

The author records his boundless love to Mary Ethalya Thiarathi, granddaughter, a baby angel of 2 years, for allowing him to write this chapter amidst so much pampering and playing. My sincere thanks to my family Ms. Celin Rani, Er. Rixon Raj, Dr. Rijula Raj, Er. Pavith Raj, for their excellent care and support, during my long hours of work, for editing this book and compiling this chapter.

The author is pleased to serve as Chief Editor, for his 7th book in this series, with the InTech Open Access Publishers. Their combination has the credentials of contributing to the "Advances in Academics and Revolution in Research", in the most pertinent, high priority fields of, "Cervical Cancer Prevention and HPV Vaccination", thus serving the Science and Society at Supreme levels.

We thank the Almighty, for keeping us safe and healthy, in these difficult times of war and pandemics, to serve for the community, in thoughts, words and deeds.

Conflict of interest

"The authors declare no conflict of interest."

Author details

Rajamanickam Rajkumar
Meenakshi Medical College Hospital and Research Institute MAHER, Kanchipuram, Tamil Nadu, India

*Address all correspondence to: rajcfchc@gmail.com

References

[1] Available from: https://www.iarc.who.int/wp-content/uploads/2021/01/CCAM_Tile_01_zoom.jpg

[2] Available from: iarc.who.int/wp-content/uploads/2021/01/CCAM_Tile_02_zoom.jpg

[3] Available from: https://www.iarc.who.int/wp-content/uploads/2021/01/CCAM_Tile_03_zoom.jpg

[4] Available from: https://iarc.who.int/featured-news/iarc-marks-cervical-cancer-awareness-month-2022/

[5] Rengaswamy S, Okkuru EP, Rajamanickam R, Richard M, Rajaraman S, Sivanandam S, et al. Effect of visual screening on cervical cancer incidence and mortality in Tamil Nadu, India: A cluster-randomized trial. Lancet. 2007;**370**(9585):398-406

[6] Rajkumar R. HPV and Cervical Cancer Control Programs: Effective Translation of Knowledge in to Practice; IntechOpen; 2020. DOI: 10.5772/intechopen.91313. Available from: https://www.intechopen.com/online-first/hpv-and-cervical-cancer-control-programs-effective-translation-of-knowledge-into-practice

Chapter 10

Association between Human Papillomavirus and Urological Cancers: An Update

Mehmet Sarier

Abstract

Human papillomavirus (HPV) is currently the most common sexually transmitted pathogen in the world, and as such imposes a substantial global burden due to its oncogenic properties. The significant association of HPV with anogenital and head and neck carcinomas is well established. In terms of urological malignancies, only the association between HPV and penile cancer has been well defined; despite close anatomical proximity, its relationship with bladder, prostate, kidney, and testicular cancers has remained unclear. With technological advances in the nucleic acid amplification tests used to detect HPV over the last two decades, the results of new studies have led to the need to reexamine these relationships. This brief review aims to evaluate the association between urological malignancies and HPV infection in light of recent data.

Keywords: HPV, penile cancer, prostate cancer, kidney cancer, bladder cancer, testicular cancer

1. Introduction

The human papillomavirus (HPV) is a double-stranded DNA virus whose only host is humans. It is the most common sexually transmitted pathogen in the world today. Epidemiological studies indicate the global prevalence of HPV is close to 12% [1]. The main reason for this high prevalence is that HPV infection is usually asymptomatic. The clinical course of HPV infection is divided into three periods—the latent, subclinical, and clinical phases [2]. Up to 90% of HPV infections are controlled by host adaptive immunity, thereby remaining in the latent phase and eventually becoming undetectable. However, 10% of cases progress to intraepithelial neoplasia or condylomatous lesions, and 1% transform into invasive cancer [3]. While over 200 HPV types have been identified to date, only 40 of them cause anogenital infections and HPV-associated malignancies [4]. Unlike many other viruses, HPVs are classified according to genetic sequence rather than antigenic structures. Therefore, instead of serotypes, they are numbered by genotype and in the order of discovery [5]. Despite its largely benign nature, HPV is a high-profile public health issue and poses a substantial socioeconomic burden due to its oncogenic properties. HPV and Epstein–Barr virus (EBV) are responsible for the most frequent virus-related cancers [6], with HPV linked to nearly 10% of cancers globally [7]. Based on their oncogenic potential, HPVs are divided into high-risk (HR-HPV) and low-risk (LR-HPV) types. HR-HPVs disrupt the cell cycle via their E6 and E7 oncoproteins, preventing progression from G1 to S phase [8]. The E6 oncoprotein inhibits the function of tumor suppressor protein p53. This increases the risk of cell transformation due to a lack of genetic stability and inhibition of apoptosis. The E7 oncoprotein inactivates another tumor suppressor protein, retinoblastoma (Rb). This results in the uncontrolled synthesis of the proteins necessary for cell cycle progression, and the cell enters a state of continuous proliferation [9]. Unlike HR-HPVs, the E6 and E7 oncoproteins of LR-HPVs do not inactivate p53 and Rb to the same degree [10].

Because HPV shows epithelial tropism, squamous cell carcinoma is the most common histologic type of HPV-related cancer. HPV association has been reported in 96% of cervical carcinomas, 75% of vulvar carcinomas, 41% of oropharyngeal carcinomas, and 36% of anal carcinomas [11–13]. The results of meta-analyses suggest that the presence of HPV is a favorable prognostic factor in anogenital and head and neck cancers [13–15]. Although it is not clear how the presence of HPV improves prognosis in these carcinomas, it was reported that HPV-negative primary cancers showed high metastatic potential and had more aggressive p53 mutations, resulting in more severe deregulation of normal growth control and poorer prognosis compared to HPV-positive cancers [16].

Considering the close anatomical proximity to anogenital carcinomas, researchers have investigated the relationship between HPV and urological malignancies for approximately three decades. Among these cancers, only penile cancer has been clearly associated with HPV. The relationship between HPV and other urological malignancies such as prostate, kidney, bladder, and testicular cancers remains controversial today. This lingering uncertainty is the result of limitations arising from methodological differences in past publications. These limitations can be summarized as small case series, lack of fresh tissue sampling, the use of serological tests for HPV detection, and the inadequacy of case–control studies [17–19]. In recent years, however, remarkable advances in polymerase chain reaction (PCR) assay technology have enabled the identification of more genotypes in a single sample, and DNA extraction from formalin-fixed, paraffin-embedded (FFPE) tissues, has become more efficient. Therefore, it is clear that results obtained two to three decades ago must be reevaluated.

2. Penile cancer and HPV

Penile cancer is rare, accounting for approximately 0.5% of all cancers in men, with a peak prevalence in the sixth decade of life [20]. The incidence of penile cancer varies by geographical region depending on the hygienic, cultural, and religious characteristics of the population. Its incidence is between 0.3 and 1 per 100,000 in developed countries, while it reaches 4 per 100,000 in developing countries [1]. At present, the main known risk factors are phimosis, chronic inflammation of the penis, poor personal hygiene, smoking, polygamy, and HPV infection. Histopathologically, 95% of penile cancers are different variations of squamous cell carcinoma [21]. The fact that HPV-associated cancers are of squamous histology led to the early discovery of the relationship between HPV and penile carcinomas. Although there are methodological differences in HPV detection among published studies, the prevalence of HPV in penile cancers is reported to be between 39.7% and 59.3% [22]. According to a recent meta-analysis evaluating 2531 patients in 270 studies, the prevalence of HPV-DNA in patients with penile cancer was 48% (confidence interval [CI]: 40.0%–57.0%) [7]. HPV type 16 is the dominant type identified in HPV-associated penile cancers, with more than half of cases attributed to this type alone [23]. The second most common strain detected in penile carcinomas is HPV type 18, and together these two types are responsible for more than 70% of HPV-associated penile carcinomas [24].

Penile intraepithelial neoplasia (PIN) is a penis cancer precursor lesion similar to cervical intraepithelial neoplasia (CIN). The extent to which the natural course of PIN mirrors that of CIN is unclear, and its clinical management is less standardized compared to CIN [25]. However, the link between PIN and HPV is noteworthy. Studies have indicated 70–100% association between HPV and PIN, much stronger than its relationship with penile carcinoma [26]. An important biomarker currently being studied in HPV-associated carcinomas is $p16^{INK4a}$, a protein whose expression is stimulated by the E7 oncoprotein [27]. Numerous recent studies suggest that $p16^{INK4a}$ expression can be used as an alternative marker of infection in cervical and other HPV-associated carcinomas due to its association with HR-HPV carcinogenesis [27]. Martins et al. reported that the expression of $p16^{INK4a}$ was significantly associated with the presence of HR-HPV in penile cancers, and could serve as a marker of HPV in penile cancer [28]. A recent meta-analysis by Olesen et al. investigating $p16^{INK4a}$ positivity in penile cancers and PIN yielded the interesting finding that the rate of $p16^{INK4a}$ positivity was 79.6% in HPV-positive patients with penile cancer but only 49.5% among those with PIN [29]. In this meta-analysis, of the histological subtypes of HPV-related penile squamous cell carcinomas, the highest prevalence of HPV was reported to be 84% in basaloid squamous cell carcinoma, followed by 75.7% in warty-basaloid squamous cell carcinoma.

There is little information in the literature regarding the relationship between HPV and tumor grade in penile squamous cell carcinoma. However, tumor grade and lymph node metastasis are the most important prognostic factors for disease-free survival [30]. Hölters et al. observed an association between HPV and histological grade in their study, reporting that the prevalence of HR-HPV types was higher in poorly differentiated grade 3 tumors [31]. Similarly, a recent study also demonstrated a positive correlation between HR-HPV and high-grade penile squamous cell carcinoma, especially in HPV-related basaloid and warty-basaloid carcinomas [32]. In light of these findings, it can be speculated that unlike cervical, anal, and oropharyngeal carcinomas, the presence of HPV may be a negative prognostic factor in penile carcinomas.

Circumcision is known to be an important protective factor against penile cancer, though it is not clear whether circumcision protects against HPV infection. Van Howe et al. determined that the prevalence of HPV did not differ between circumcised and uncircumcised men but reported a longer HPV clearance time in men who were uncircumcised [33]. In a study by Lu et al., viral clearance was higher for HR-HPV types in circumcised men than uncircumcised men, while there was no significant difference between the two groups in the clearance of LR-HPV types [34]. Gray et al. showed that circumcision reduced transmission of both HR-HPV and LR-HPV types [35]. In the latest report from Davis et al., male circumcision was found to reduce HR-HPV viral load in female partners, leading the authors to recommend circumcision for the reduction of HPV infection in both men and women [36].

3. Bladder cancer and HPV

Bladder cancer is the fourth most common malignancy in men and the eighth most common in women, causing an estimated 400,000 new cases and 186,000 deaths per year worldwide [37]. Important known risk factors include age, ethnicity, smoking tobacco, chemical exposure (aromatic amines and hydrocarbons), and in some regions, schistosomiasis. Histologically, more than 90% of bladder cancers are urothelial cell carcinoma. The incidence of bladder cancer has shown a marked increase over the last three decades, and despite extensive efforts, it is still difficult to predict tumor progression, optimal treatment, and final clinical outcomes [38]. Over the same period, the relationship between HPV and bladder cancer has also been investigated and two hypotheses have been proposed to explain their association. The first hypothesis is that the urethra is the first point of contact during sexual transmission of the virus and serves both as a viral reservoir and direct connection between the urinary bladder and genital area, possibly providing a natural route of viral migration. The second hypothesis is based on the natural epithelial tropism of HPV [39]. In a pooled meta-analysis of 2855 cases in 52 studies, the prevalence of HPV in bladder cancer samples ranged between 0% and 100% [40]. However, this extremely wide range of HPV prevalence is open to interpretation. In the past, extracting DNA from FFPE tissue was a challenge, and most publications stating that there is no relationship between HPV and bladder cancer were conducted in FFPE tissues using older technologies in HPV research [41–43]. Li et al. emphasized this in their meta-analysis, noting that the prevalence of HPV was higher in studies using fresh tissue than in studies using FFPE and suggesting that FFPE tissues may yield false-negative results. In the same meta-analysis, it was also determined that the HPV prevalence in patients with bladder cancer was 16.88% and HPV types 16 and 18 were the major types detected [40]. Another meta-analysis by Jimenez-Pacheco et al. including 20 controlled studies of HPV-DNA revealed a significant association between HPV presence and bladder cancer, with a pooled odds ratio (OR) of 2.19 (95% CI: 1.40–3.43) [44]. Most recently, Sarier et al. conducted a case–control study using fresh tissue and demonstrated a strong correlation between urothelial carcinoma of the bladder and HPV infection (OR: 4.24, 95% CI: 1.63–12.34) [45].

Although squamous cell carcinoma of the bladder accounts for 2% of all bladder cancers, scientific interest in its relationship with HPV has persisted due to its histological structure [46]. However, because it is rare cancer, published series are small and studies have yielded conflicting results [47–49]. In a recent study by Collins et al. investigating the presence of p16 and HR-HPV in 33 patients with squamous cell carcinoma of the bladder using in situ hybridization (ISH), P16 expression was detected in 28% of the patients, while HR-HPV was not detected in any patient [50].

Tumor grade is an important factor in terms of bladder cancer progression. However, the literature also includes conflicting reports regarding the relationship between tumor grade and HPV. An association between HPV and low-grade tumors was reported by Tenti et al. [51], while an association with high-grade tumors was observed by Cai et al. [52]. In contrast, Sarier et al. observed no significant correlation between tumor grade and HPV in their study [45].

Tumor recurrence is an important and common event in bladder cancer. Exposure to infectious agents is recognized as one of the risk factors for urological malignancies, especially those with a high tumor recurrence rate [53]. Although the literature data on the relationship between HPV and bladder tumor recurrence are limited, the results are impressive and largely consistent among studies. Badawi et al. reported a significant association between HPV type 16 and tumor recurrence rate [54]. Moghadam et al. found that HPV was significantly associated not only with tumor recurrence but also with tumor stage [55]. In their 2-year follow-up study, Sarier et al. observed higher tumor recurrence rates in patients with bladder tumors associated with HPV-DNA [56].

4. Prostate cancer and HPV

Prostate cancer is the second most common cancer and a fourth most common cause of cancer deaths in men and therefore poses a serious burden worldwide [57]. The most important risk factors are age over 50 years, ethnicity, family history of prostate cancer, diet, and infection, although the available data are limited. There is evidence to suggest that chronic inflammation of the prostate is quite common in adults and may directly contribute to the development and progression of prostate malignancy [58]. This inflammation forms the basis of the main hypothesis for the relationship between HPV and prostate cancer. Epithelial damage caused by chronic inflammation may result in loss of tolerance to normal prostate-associated antigens, thereby triggering a sustained autoimmune reaction [59]. The immune evasion strategies of viruses contribute to persistent viral infection and induce chronic inflammation through cytokines. This presents a mechanism by which HPV may trigger chronic inflammation of the prostate glandular epithelium [59].

In fact, numerous studies have investigated the relationship between infection and prostate cancer. Taylor et al. demonstrated a significant association between prostate cancer risk and infection with any sexually transmitted disease-related agents in their meta-analysis of 29 studies including 6022 prostate cancer patients and 7320 control cases [60].

As with bladder cancer, a wide range has been reported for the prevalence of HPV in prostate cancer (0–100%). Again, methodological approaches are the major limitation. The use of serology-based tests for HPV detection is controversial. These tests identify general exposure to HPV infection but are not able to identify HPV infection in specific organs, such as the prostate. Although ISH is an effective method for detecting HPV, PCR is considered the gold standard [61]. By using multiple degenerate primary pairs in the amplification reaction, the PCR assay can easily be adapted to detect most HPV types associated with anogenital tract disease. A recent meta-analysis by Lawson et al. is valuable in this regard. In the part of their study evaluating 14 serology-based studies including 5149 prostate cancer patients and 7794 benign prostate controls, HPV antibodies were detected in 20% of both groups. Based on this finding, they stated that when evaluated serologically, there is no difference in the prevalence of HPV antibodies between men with and without prostate cancer. However, in another part including only PCR-based studies conducted after the year 2000 (including 1071 prostate cancer patients and 1103 benign prostate controls), the HPV prevalence was found to be 21.6% in prostate cancer patients and 6.7% in controls ($p = 0.001$) [17]. The authors concluded from this meta-analysis that HR-HPV has a causal role in prostate cancer. Other meta-analyses conducted in the last decade using different parameters also showed similar results. In a meta-analysis by Sasidharanpillai et al. evaluating the relationship between HPV and oropharyngeal and anogenital cancers based on recent molecular studies (nine studies, 876 men), significant HPV association was reported in prostate cancer tissue specimens (19%, CI: 10–29%) [7]. Yin et al. also determined that HPV was associated with an increased risk of prostate cancer (OR: 2.27) in their meta-analysis of 24 case–controlled studies including 971 prostate cancer and 1085 benign prostate patients [62]. In a meta-analysis of 26 tissue-based case–control studies conducted by Yang et al., the prevalence of HPV infection was found to be 18.93% and overall HPV positivity in prostate tissues was associated with a significantly higher risk of prostate cancer (OR: 1.79, 95% CI: 1.29–2.49) [57]. Moghoofei et al. reported that the two major genotypes associated with prostate cancer were HPV types 16 and 18, respectively [63].

Gleason score is an important pathological parameter for the prognosis of prostate cancer. However, the data on the relationship between HPV and Gleason score are controversial. Singh et al. reported that Gleason score was high (≥ 8) in 74% of patients with HPV-related prostate cancer ($p = 0.003$), whereas Moghadam et al. found no significant difference in Gleason score in his patient group [64].

Glenn et al. published an interesting study regarding HPV and prostate cancer. The researchers identified HR-HPVs in the benign prostate tissue specimens of patients who developed prostate cancer 1–10 years later. A remarkable finding from their study was that E7 oncoprotein expression was detected in 82% of samples at the time of benign prostatic hyperplasia diagnosis but only 29% of prostate cancer specimens were from the same patients. The authors suggested that HPV has an oncogenic role in the early stage of prostate tumorigenesis [65].

5. Kidney cancer and HPV

Kidney cancer is responsible for an estimated 2% of global cancer diagnoses and deaths, and its global burden is expected to increase [66]. The two most common subtypes are renal cell carcinoma and urothelial cell carcinoma. However, there are few studies on its possible association with HPV in the literature, and based on the evidence to date, the relationship between kidney cancers and HPV remains unclear. In a PCR-based study of 28 patients with kidney cancer, Grce et al. did not detect HPV in any patient [67]. Similarly, Hodges et al. did not detect HPV in any of their 62 patients with renal tumors by using ISH, leading the authors to conclude that HPV appears to have no oncogenic role in benign or malignant renal tumors [68]. In contrast, in their small case–control study (49 renal cell carcinoma cases, 16 controls), Salehipor et al. determined using PCR that the prevalence of HPV was 14.3% in the patient group and 0% in the control group [69]. Kamel et al. evaluated 56 patients with renal cell carcinoma using ISH and determined the prevalence of HPV to be 52% [70]. Although this is a remarkable finding, the fact that the study was not case-controlled can be seen as an important limitation. More recently, Farhadi et al. investigated the presence of HPV in 122 patients with renal cell carcinoma and demonstrated HPV association in 30.3%, with HPV type 18 being the most common type identified [71]. In terms of the case series, an important study by Koury et al. based on the Cancer Genome Atlas Database, which includes 3775 malignant neoplasms, indicated that there was no relationship between HPV infection and kidney cancer [72].

6. Testicular cancer and HPV

Although testicular cancers represent only 1% of all malignancies in men, they are the most common organ malignancy in men between 20 and 40 years of age [73]. The main known risk factors for testicular cancer are undescended testes, a family history of testicular cancer, and the presence of germ cell cancer in the opposite testicle [74]. While testicular tumors are still relatively uncommon, there has been an unexplained increase in their incidence over the last two decades [75]. Researchers have recently focused on the potentially important role of inflammation in the formation and progression of testicular cancer, as seen in the pathogenesis of other cancers [76]. In fact, the relationship between viral infections and testicular cancer was first investigated approximately 40 years ago [77]. Unfortunately, few studies have been published on the relationship between HPV and testicular cancer in the intervening period. In their study of 39 testicular cancer and 48 control cases, Strickler et al. determined the prevalence of HPV to be 5% in testicular cancer specimens and 4% in the control group [78]. A PCR-based study evaluating the presence of HPV in 19 testicular cancer patients and one control case was not able to demonstrate a relationship between HPV infection and testicular cancer [79]. Similarly, Bertazzoni et al. reported that HPV was not detected by PCR in any specimens from 61 seminomas and 23 control cases [80]. Finally, in a meta-analysis of 20 studies and 265,057 patients to evaluate the relationship between testicular cancer and viral infections, Garolla et al. determined that testicular cancer was not associated with HPV, cytomegalovirus, or parvovirus b-19 infections, whereas EBV and HIV infections were significantly associated with a higher risk of developing testicular germ cell tumors (OR: 7.38, 95% CI: 1.89–28.75, OR: 1.71, 95% CI: 1.51–1.93, respectively) [81]. An important point to keep in mind when evaluating the relationship between testicular germ cell neoplasms and HPV is that HPV shows epithelial tropism, and germ cell neoplasms of the testicle do not arise from the epithelium.

7. Conclusion

The link between penile cancers and HPV is now well known. In this regard, the significant relationship between HPV and tumor grade should be taken into consideration and further studies should be conducted to elucidate the prognostic significance of HPV presence in penile cancers. The association between HPV and urothelial carcinoma of the bladder has become clearer in recent years with the use of molecular tests in HPV diagnosis and the findings of studies conducted with fresh tissue. In bladder cancer, the significant relationship between HPV and tumor recurrence should be kept in mind. The development of PCR technology has had a major impact on our understanding of the link between HPV and prostate cancer. Compared to previous serology-based studies, the results obtained using nucleic acid amplification tests such as PCR are noteworthy and show that a reevaluation of this relationship is needed. A key point here may be studied on the relationship between HPV and inflammation in the pathophysiology of prostate cancer. In contrast, it is premature to talk about an association between kidney cancer and HPV based on the limited evidence available today. Case-controlled studies with larger patient series will be elucidating. The existing evidence regarding testicular cancer indicates no association with HPV infection.

Abbreviations

CI	Confidence interval
EBV	Epstein–Barr virus
FFPE	Formalin-fixed, paraffin-embedded
HR	High-risk
HPV	Human papillomavirus
ISH	in situ hybridization
LR	Low-risk
OR	Odds ratio
PCR	Polymerase Chain Reaction
PIN	Penile intraepithelial neoplasia
Rb	Retinoblastoma

Author details

Mehmet Sarier[1,2]

1 Department of Urology, Istinye University, Istanbul, Turkey

2 Department of Urology, Medical Park Hospital, Antalya, Turkey

*Address all correspondence to: drsarier@gmail.com

References

[1] Tolstov Y, Hadaschik B, Pahernik S, Hohenfellner M, Duensing S. Human papillomaviruses in urological malignancies: A critical assessment. Urologic Oncology. 2014;**32**(1):46.e19-46.e27. DOI: 10.1016/j.urolonc.2013.06.012

[2] Schneider A. Pathogenesis of genital HPV infection. Genitourinary Medicine. 1993;**69**(3):165-173. Available from: http://www.ncbi.nlm.nih.gov/pubmed/8392965 [Accessed date: 15 April 2019]

[3] Andersen ES, Thorup K, Larsen G. The results of cryosurgery for cervical intraepithelial neoplasia. Gynecologic Oncology. 1988;**30**(1):21-25. Available from: http://www.ncbi.nlm.nih.gov/pubmed/3366393 [Accessed date: 15 April 2019]

[4] Sarier M, Ozel E, Duman I, Yuksel Y, Demirbas A. HPV type 45-positive condyloma acuminata of the bladder in a renal transplant recipient. Transplant Infectious Disease. 2017;**19**(2):e12667. DOI: 10.1111/tid.12667

[5] Sarier M, Ceyhan AM, Sepin N, et al. HPV infection in urology practice. International Urology and Nephrology. 2020;**52**(1):1-8. DOI: 10.1007/s11255-019-02302-2

[6] Cobos C, Figueroa JA, Mirandola L, et al. The role of Human Papilloma Virus (HPV) infection in non-anogenital cancer and the promise of immunotherapy: A review. International Reviews of Immunology. 2014;**33**(5):383-401. DOI: 10.3109/08830185.2014.911857

[7] Sasidharanpillai S, Ravishankar N, Kamath V, Bhat PV, Bhatt P, Arunkumar G. Prevalence of human papillomavirus (HPV) DNA among men with oropharyngeal and anogenital cancers: A systematic review and meta-analysis. Asian Pacific Journal of Cancer Prevention. 2021;**22**(5):1351-1364. DOI: 10.31557/APJCP.2021.22.5.1351

[8] Heidegger I, Borena W, Pichler R. The role of human papilloma virus in urological malignancies. Anticancer Research. 2015;**35**(5):2513-2519. Available from: http://www.ncbi.nlm.nih.gov/pubmed/25964524 [Accessed date: 30 November 2018]

[9] Kraus I, Molden T, Holm R, et al. Presence of E6 and E7 mRNA from human papillomavirus types 16, 18, 31, 33, and 45 in the majority of cervical carcinomas. Journal of Clinical Microbiology. 2006;**44**(4):1310-1317. DOI: 10.1128/JCM.44.4.1310-1317.2006

[10] Longworth MS, Laimins LA. Pathogenesis of human papillomaviruses in differentiating epithelia. Microbiology and Molecular Biology Reviews. 2004;**68**(2):362-372. DOI: 10.1128/MMBR.68.2.362-372.2004

[11] Rakislova N, Saco A, Sierra A, Del Pino M, Ordi J. Role of human papillomavirus in vulvar cancer. Advances in Anatomic Pathology. 2017;**24**(4):201-214. DOI: 10.1097/PAP.0000000000000155

[12] Assmann G, Sotlar K. HPV-associated squamous cell carcinogenesis. Pathologe. 2011;**32**(5):391-398. DOI: 10.1007/s00292-011-1442-2

[13] Urbute A, Rasmussen CL, Belmonte F, et al. Prognostic significance of HPV DNA and p16 INK4a in anal cancer: A systematic review and meta-analysis. Cancer Epidemiology, Biomarkers & Prevention. 2020;**29**(4):703-710. DOI: 10.1158/1055-9965.epi-19-1259

[14] Li P, Tan Y, Zhu LX, et al. Prognostic value of HPV DNA status

in cervical cancer before treatment: A systematic review and meta-analysis. Oncotarget. 2017;**8**(39):66352-66359. DOI: 10.18632/oncotarget.18558

[15] Liu H, Li J, Zhou Y, Hu Q, Zeng Y, Mohammadreza MM. Human papillomavirus as a favorable prognostic factor in a subset of head and neck squamous cell carcinomas: A meta-analysis. Journal of Medical Virology. 2017;**89**(4):710-725. DOI: 10.1002/jmv.24670

[16] Goyal S, Singh UR, Sharma S, Kaur N. Correlation of mitotic indices, AgNor count, Ki-67 and Bcl-2 with grade and stage in papillary urothelial bladder cancer. Urology Journal. 2014;**11**(1):1238-1247. DOI: 10.22037/uj.v11i1.1500

[17] Lawson JS, Glenn WK. Evidence for a causal role by human papillomaviruses in prostate cancer - A systematic review. Infectious Agents and Cancer. 2020;**15**(1):1-11. DOI: 10.1186/s13027-020-00305-8

[18] Gutiérrez J, Jiménez A, de Dios LJ, Soto MJ, Sorlózano A. Meta-analysis of studies analyzing the relationship between bladder cancer and infection by human papillomavirus. The Journal of Urology. 2006;**176**(6 Pt 1):2474-2481. discussion 2481. DOI: 10.1016/j.juro.2006.07.157

[19] Gould VE, Schmitt M, Vinokurova S, et al. Human papillomavirus and p16 expression in inverted papillomas of the urinary bladder. Cancer Letters. 2010;**292**(2):171-175. DOI: 10.1016/j.canlet.2009.11.022

[20] Bleeker MCG, Heideman DAM, Snijders PJF, Horenblas S, Dillner J, Meijer CJLM. Penile cancer: Epidemiology, pathogenesis and prevention. World Journal of Urology. 2009;**27**:141-150. DOI: 10.1007/s00345-008-0302-z

[21] Cai T, Di Vico T, Durante J, Tognarelli A, Bartoletti R. Human papilloma virus and genitourinary cancers: A narrative review. Minerva Urologica e Nefrologica. 2018;**70**(6):579-587. DOI: 10.23736/S0393-2249.18.03141-7

[22] Backes DM, Kurman RJ, Pimenta JM, Smith JS. Systematic review of human papillomavirus prevalence in invasive penile cancer. Cancer Causes & Control. 2009;**20**(4):449-457. DOI: 10.1007/S10552-008-9276-9

[23] Heideman DAM, Waterboer T, Pawlita M, et al. Human papillomavirus-16 is the predominant type etiologically involved in penile squamous cell carcinoma. Journal of Clinical Oncology. 2007;**25**(29):4550-4556. DOI: 10.1200/JCO.2007.12.3182

[24] Kidd LC, Chaing S, Chipollini J, Giuliano AR, Spiess PE, Sharma P. Relationship between human papillomavirus and penile cancer-implications for prevention and treatment. Translational Andrology and Urology. 2017;**6**(5):791-802. DOI: 10.21037/TAU.2017.06.27

[25] Ferrándiz-Pulido C, Masferrer E, De Torres I, et al. Identification and genotyping of human papillomavirus in a Spanish cohort of penile squamous cell carcinomas: Correlation with pathologic subtypes, p16INK4a expression, and prognosis. Journal of the American Academy of Dermatology. 2013;**68**(1):73-82. DOI: 10.1016/J.JAAD.2012.05.029

[26] Marchionne E, Perez C, Hui A, Khachemoune A. Penile squamous cell carcinoma: A review of the literature and case report treated with Mohs micrographic surgery. Anais Brasileiros de Dermatologia. 2017;**92**(1):95-99. DOI: 10.1590/abd1806-4841.20175009

[27] Steinestel J, Al Ghazal A, Arndt A, et al. The role of histologic subtype,

p16INK4a expression, and presence of human papillomavirus DNA in penile squamous cell carcinoma. BMC Cancer. 2015;**15**(1):1-9. DOI: 10.1186/S12885-015-1268-Z

[28] De Andrade MV, Pinho JD, Júnior AALT, et al. P16INK4a expression in patients with penile cancer. PLoS One. 2018;**13**(10):e0205350. DOI: 10.1371/JOURNAL.PONE.0205350 [Published: 2018 Oct 12]

[29] Olesen TB, Sand FL, Rasmussen CL, et al. Prevalence of human papillomavirus DNA and p16 INK4a in penile cancer and penile intraepithelial neoplasia: A systematic review and meta-analysis. The Lancet Oncology. 2019;**20**(1):145-158. DOI: 10.1016/S1470-2045(18)30682-X

[30] Aita GA, Zequi S de C, Costa WH da, Guimarães GC, Soares FA, Giuliangelis TS. Tumor histologic grade is the most important prognostic factor in patients with penile cancer and clinically negative lymph nodes not submitted to regional lymphadenectomy. International Brazilian Journal of Urology 2016;42(6):1136-1143. doi:10.1590/S1677-5538.IBJU.2015.0416

[31] Hölters S, Khalmurzaev O, Pryalukhin A, et al. Challenging the prognostic impact of the new WHO and TNM classifications with special emphasis on HPV status in penile carcinoma. Virchows Archiv. 2019;**475**(2):211-221. DOI: 10.1007/S00428-019-02566-0

[32] de Araújo LA, AAP DP, da SC de PH, et al. Human papillomavirus (HPV) genotype distribution in penile carcinoma: Association with clinic pathological factors. PLoS One. 2018;**13**(6):e0199557. DOI: 10.1371/JOURNAL.PONE.0199557

[33] Van Howe RS. Human papillomavirus and circumcision: A meta-analysis. The Journal of Infection. 2007;**54**(5):490-496. DOI: 10.1016/J.JINF.2006.08.005

[34] Lu B, Wu Y, Nielson CM, et al. Factors associated with acquisition and clearance of human papillomavirus infection in a cohort of US men: A prospective study. The Journal of Infectious Diseases. 2009;**199**(3):362-371. DOI: 10.1086/596050

[35] Gray RH, Serwadda D, Kong X, et al. Male circumcision decreases acquisition and increases clearance of high-risk human papillomavirus in HIV-negative men: A randomized trial in Rakai, Uganda. The Journal of Infectious Diseases. 2010;**201**(10): 1455-1462. DOI: 10.1086/652184

[36] Davis MA, Gray RH, Grabowski MK, et al. Male circumcision decreases high-risk human papillomavirus viral load in female partners: A randomized trial in Rakai, Uganda. International Journal of Cancer. 2013;**133**(5):1247-1252. DOI: 10.1002/IJC.28100

[37] Siegel RL, Miller KD, Jemal A. Cancer statistics, 2018. CA: A Cancer Journal for Clinicians. 2018;**68**(1):7-30. DOI: 10.3322/CAAC.21442

[38] Stein JP, Grossfeld GD, Ginsberg DA, et al. Prognostic markers in bladder cancer: a contemporary review of the literature. The Journal of Urology. 1998;**160**(3 Pt 1):645-659. Available from: http://www.ncbi.nlm.nih.gov/pubmed/9720515 [Accessed date: November 24, 2018]

[39] Visalli G, Facciolà A, Aleo FD, et al. Hpv and urinary bladder carcinoma: A review of the literature. WCRJ. 2018;**5**(1):1-12

[40] Li N, Yang L, Zhang Y, Zhao P, Zheng T, Dai M. Human papillomavirus infection and bladder cancer risk: A meta-analysis. The Journal of Infectious Diseases. 2011;**204**(2):217-223. DOI: 10.1093/infdis/jir248

[41] Knowles MA. Human papillomavirus sequences are not detectable by Southern blotting or general primer-mediated polymerase chain reaction in transitional cell tumours of the bladder. Urological Research. 1992;**20**(4):297-301. Available from: http://www.ncbi.nlm.nih.gov/pubmed/1324541 [Accessed date: November 26, 2018]

[42] Chang F, Lipponen P, Tervahauta A, Syrjänen S, Syrjänen K. Transitional cell carcinoma of the bladder: Failure to demonstrate human papillomavirus deoxyribonucleic acid by in situ hybridization and polymerase chain reaction. The Journal of Urology. 1994;**152**(5 Pt 1):1429-1433. Available from: http://www.ncbi.nlm.nih.gov/pubmed/7933176 [Accessed date: 26 November 2018]

[43] Ben Selma W, Ziadi S, Ben Gacem R, et al. Investigation of human papillomavirus in bladder cancer in a series of Tunisian patients. Pathology, Research and Practice. 2010;**206**(11): 740-743. DOI: 10.1016/j.prp.2010.06.005

[44] Jimenez-Pacheco A, Exposito-Ruiz M, Arrabal-Polo M, Lopez-Luque A. Meta-analysis of studies analyzing the role of human papillomavirus in the development of bladder carcinoma. Korean Journal of Urology. 2012;**53**(4):240-247. DOI: 10.4111/KJU.2012.53.4.240

[45] Sarier M, Sepin N, Keles Y, et al. Is there any association between urothelial carcinoma of the bladder and human papillomavirus? A Case-Control Study. Urologia Internationalis. 2020;**104**(1-2):81-86. DOI: 10.1159/000500467

[46] Jørgensen KR, Jensen JB. Human papillomavirus and urinary bladder cancer revisited. APMIS. 2020;**35**(8): 1-8. DOI: 10.1111/apm.13016

[47] Westenend PJ, Stoop JA, Hendriks JGM. Human papillomaviruses 6/11, 16/18 and 31/33/51 are not associated with squamous cell carcinoma of the urinary bladder. BJU International. 2001;**88**(3):198-201. DOI: 10.1046/J.1464-410X.2001.02230.X

[48] Alexander RE, Hu Y, Kum JB, et al. P16 expression is not associated with human papillomavirus in urinary bladder squamous cell carcinoma. Modern Pathology. 2012;**25**(11):1526-1533. DOI: 10.1038/MODPATHOL. 2012.103

[49] Chapman-Fredricks JR, Cioffi-Lavina M, Accola MA, et al. High-risk human papillomavirus DNA detected in primary squamous cell carcinoma of urinary bladder. Archives of Pathology & Laboratory Medicine. 2013;**137**(8):1088-1093. DOI: 10.5858/ARPA.2012-0122-OA

[50] Collins K, Hwang M, Hamza A, Rao P. Prevalence of high-risk human papillomavirus in primary squamous cell carcinoma of urinary bladder. Pathology, Research and Practice. 2020;**216**(9):153084 epub. DOI: 10.1016/J.PRP.2020.153084

[51] Tenti P, Zappatore R, Romagnoli S, et al. p53 overexpression and human papillomavirus infection in transitional cell carcinoma of the urinary bladder: correlation with histological parameters. The Journal of Pathology. 1996;**178**(1): 65-70. DOI: 10.1002/(SICI)1096-9896(199601)178:1<65::AID-PATH451>3.0.CO;2-W

[52] Cai. Human papillomavirus and non-muscle invasive urothelial bladder cancer: Potential relationship from a pilot study. Oncology Reports. 2011;**25**(2):485-489. DOI: 10.3892/or.2010.1083

[53] Alibek K, Karatayeva N, Bekniyazov I. The role of infectious agents in urogenital cancers. Infectious Agents and Cancer. 2012;**7**(1):35. DOI: 10.1186/1750-9378-7-35

[54] Badawi H, Ahmed H, Ismail A, et al. Role of human papillomavirus types 16, 18, and 52 in recurrent cystitis and urinary bladder cancer among egyptian patients. Medscape Journal of Medicine. 2008;**10**(10):232. Available from: /pmc/articles/PMC2605136/ [Accessed: 07 October 2021]

[55] Ohadian Moghadam S, Mansori K, Nowroozi MR, Afshar D, Abbasi B, Nowroozi A. Association of human papilloma virus (HPV) infection with oncological outcomes in urothelial bladder cancer. Infectious Agents and Cancer. 2020;**15**(1):4-11. DOI: 10.1186/s13027-020-00318-3

[56] Sarier M, Usta SS, Turgut H, et al. Prognostic value of HPV DNA in urothelial carcinoma of the bladder: A preliminary report of 2-year follow-up results. Urology Journal. 28 Apr 2021. DOI: 10.22037/uj.v18i.6429

[57] Yang L, Xie S, Feng X, et al. Worldwide prevalence of human papillomavirus and relative risk of prostate cancer: A meta-analysis. Scientific Reports. 2015;**5**:14667 epub. DOI: 10.1038/SREP14667

[58] Sfanos KS, De MAM. Prostate cancer and inflammation: The evidence. Histopathology. 2012;**60**(1):199-215. DOI: 10.1111/J.1365-2559.2011.04033.X

[59] Nahand JS, Khanaliha K, Mirzaei H, et al. Possible role of HPV/EBV coinfection in anoikis resistance and development in prostate cancer. BMC Cancer. 2021;**21**(1):1-19. DOI: 10.1186/s12885-021-08658-y

[60] Taylor ML, Mainous A, Wells B. Prostate cancer and sexually transmitted diseases: A meta-analysis. Undefined. Family Medicine. 2005;**37**(7):506-512

[61] Kösel S, Burggraf S, Mommsen J, Engelhardt W, Olgemöller B. Type-specific detection of human papillomaviruses in a routine laboratory setting--improved sensitivity and specificity of PCR and sequence analysis compared to direct hybridisation. Clinical Chemistry and Laboratory Medicine. 2003;**41**(6):787-791. DOI: 10.1515/CCLM.2003.119

[62] Yin B, Liu W, Yu P, et al. Association between human papillomavirus and prostate cancer: A meta-analysis. Oncology Letters. 2017;**14**(2):1855-1865. DOI: 10.3892/OL.2017.6367

[63] Moghoofei M, Keshavarz M, Ghorbani S, et al. Association between human papillomavirus infection and prostate cancer: A global systematic review and meta-analysis. Asia-Pacific Journal of Clinical Oncology. 2019;**15**(5):e59-e67. DOI: 10.1111/AJCO.13124

[64] Moghadam SO, Nowroozi MR, Nowroozi A, Rezaei P. Infection with human papillomavirus as a potential risk factor for prostate cancer: A case-control study. Archives of Clinical Infectious Diseases. 2021;**16**(1):16-20. DOI: 10.5812/archcid.107137

[65] Glenn WK, Ngan CC, Amos TG, et al. High risk human papilloma viruses (HPVs) are present in benign prostate tissues before development of HPV associated prostate cancer. Infectious Agents and Cancer. 2017;**12**(1):1-10. DOI: 10.1186/s13027-017-0157-2

[66] Padala SA, Barsouk A, Thandra KC, et al. Epidemiology of renal cell carcinoma. World Journal of Oncology. 2020;**11**(3):79-87. DOI: 10.14740/WJON1279

[67] Grce M, Furcić I, Hrascan R, et al. Human papillomaviruses are not associated with renal carcinoma. Anticancer Research. 1997;**17**(3C):2193-2196

[68] Hodges A, Talley L, Gokden N. Human Papillomavirus DNA and P16INK4A are not detected in renal

tumors with immunohistochemistry and signal-amplified in situ hybridization in paraffin-embedded tissue. Applied Immunohistochemistry & Molecular Morphology. 2006;**14**(4):432-435. DOI: 10.1097/01.PAI.0000205059.42421.CB

[69] Salehipoor M, Khezri A, Behzad-Behbahani A, et al. Role of viruses in renal cell carcinoma. Saudi Journal of Kidney Diseases and Transplantation. 2012;**23**(1):53-57. Available from: http://www.sjkdt.org [Accessed date: 08 October 2021]

[70] Kamel D, Turpeenniemi-Hujanen TV, K, Pääkkö P, Soini Y. Proliferating cell nuclear antigen but not p53 or human papillomavirus DNA correlates with advanced clinical stage in renal cell carcinoma. Histopathology. 1994;**25**(4):339-347. DOI: 10.1111/J.1365-2559.1994.TB01352.X

[71] Farhadi A, Behzad-Behbahani A, Geramizadeh B, Sekawi Z, Rahsaz M, Sharifzadeh S. High-risk human papillomavirus infection in different histological subtypes of renal cell carcinoma. Journal of Medical Virology. 2014;**86**(7):1134-1144. DOI: 10.1002/JMV.23945

[72] Khoury JD, Tannir NM, Williams MD, et al. Landscape of DNA virus associations across human malignant cancers: Analysis of 3,775 cases using RNA-Seq. Journal of Virology. 2013;**87**(16):8916-8926. DOI: 10.1128/JVI.00340-13

[73] Ferlay J, Soerjomataram I, Dikshit R, et al. Cancer incidence and mortality worldwide: Sources, methods and major patterns in GLOBOCAN 2012. International Journal of Cancer. 2015;**136**(5):E359-E386. DOI: 10.1002/ijc.29210

[74] Sarier M, Tunç M, Özel E, et al. Evaluation of histopathologic results of testicular tumors in antalya: Multi center study. Bulletin of Urooncology. 2020;**19**(2):64-67. DOI: 10.4274/uob.galenos.2019.1412

[75] Cheng L, Albers P, Berney DM, et al. Testicular cancer. Nature Reviews. Disease Primers. 2018;**4**(1):29. DOI: 10.1038/s41572-018-0029-0

[76] Elinav E, Nowarski R, Thaiss CA, Hu B, Jin C, Flavell RA. Inflammation-induced cancer: Crosstalk between tumours, immune cells and microorganisms. Nature Reviews. Cancer. 2013;**13**(11):759-771. DOI: 10.1038/nrc3611

[77] Algood CB, Newell GR, Johnson DE. Viral etiology of testicular tumors. The Journal of Urology. 1988;**139**(2):308-310. DOI: 10.1016/S0022-5347(17)42394-9

[78] Strickler HD, Schiffman MH, Shah KV, et al. A survey of human papillomavirus 16 antibodies in patients with epithelial cancers. European Journal of Cancer Prevention. 1998;**7**(4):305-313. DOI: 10.1097/00008469-199808000-00006

[79] Rajpert-De Meyts E, Hørding U, Nielsen H, Skakkebaek N. Human papillomavirus and Epstein-Barr virus in the etiology of testicular germ cell tumours. APMIS. 1994;**102**(1):38-42. DOI: 10.1111/J.1699-0463.1994.TB04842.X

[80] Bertazzoni G, Sgambato A, Migaldi M, et al. Lack of evidence for an association between seminoma and human papillomavirus infection using GP5+/GP6+ consensus primers. Journal of Medical Virology. 2013;**85**(1):105-109. DOI: 10.1002/JMV.23431

[81] Garolla A, Vitagliano A, Muscianisi F, et al. Role of viral infections in testicular cancer etiology: Evidence from a systematic review and meta-analysis. Frontiers in Endocrinology (Lausanne). 2019;**10**(JUN):355. DOI: 10.3389/FENDO.2019.00355

Chapter 11

Cervical Cancer Induced by Human Papillomaviruses in the Context of Africa: Contribution of Genomics

Florencia Wendkuuni Djigma,
Fidèle Tiendrebeogo, Lassina Traore,
Théodora Mahoukèdè Zohoncon, Augustin Tozoula Bambara,
Pegdwendé Abel Sorgho, Hierrhum Aboubacar Bambara,
Abdou Azaque Zoure, Dorcas Obiri-Yeboah,
Bagora Bayala, Teega-Wendé Clarisse Ouedraogo,
Prosper Bado, Rogomenoma Alice Ouedraogo,
Ina Marie Angèle Traore, Mah Alima Esther Traore,
Isabelle Touwendpoulimdé Kiendrebeogo,
Albert Théophane Yonli,
Charlemagne Marie Ragnag-Néwendé Ouedraogo
and Jacques Simpore

Abstract

In recent years, Africa has been increasingly involved in biotechnology and genomics. However, this interest is much more accentuated in the field of agriculture. From published studies, we know that biotechnology and genomics can be of great interest in the health field. Africa would, therefore, benefit from investing in these disciplines, especially since the continent is facing several pandemics and epidemics. The objective of this chapter is to make a review of the applications in genomics already existing in Africa, particularly in Burkina Faso, to show the interest of genomics in the field of health by taking into account the context of developing countries and to specify the possible applications of genomics in the fight against papillomaviridae and their associated cancer.

Keywords: genomics, papillomaviridae infection, cancer, Africa

1. Introduction

Advances in molecular biology and genomics, combined with computer and technological development, artificial intelligence, and significant improvement in the production and processing of NGS data, will increasingly have an impact on strategic sectors such as agriculture, breeding, energy, and health. Since the advent of modern biotechnology, it is increasingly evident that the solutions to the major challenges of our world will undoubtedly come from bio-innovation. As the world understands the importance of new technologies, more and more startups are investing in specific areas of health such as oncology, infectious diseases, immunology, metabolism, etc.

While the rest of the world has understood the challenges of current innovations and tries to use them for its population, it remains a great challenge for Sub-Saharan Africa. The intellectual, scientific, and political elite understood the challenges of the biological sciences and new technologies, but this elite often faces external constraints that affect the priorities to be defined for the countries concerned. The consequence is a very low representation of African researchers in the global dynamics of biotechnological innovations. Very often, research funding is provided by external mechanisms and this is still not sufficient to take into account all research concerns. African scientists, including those from Burkina Faso, are then forced to fight for the minimum amount of capital in order to finance their own research.

Located in the heart of West Africa, Burkina Faso covers an area of 274,000 km^2 with a population of 20,244,080 inhabitants in 2018 [1]. Burkina Faso is a landlocked country, with neighboring countries Mali to the north and west, Niger to the east, Benin to the south-east, Togo and Ghana to the south, and Côte d'Ivoire at the south west. Burkina Faso's economic outlook remains strong; the economy has remained resilient despite difficult security and health environment. However, like many African countries, the part of the budget allocated to research remains low, at 0.9% in 2019 [2]. However, since the advent of SARS-COV2, the interest in research has increased for the population and also for political leaders. Initiatives to enhance the research activities carried out in the country and also to enhance the multidisciplinary nature of research have been started. funding from the President of Burkina Faso has been granted to researchers to conduct research on the topics of COVID-19 and infectious diseases. This constitutes a very good opportunity to promote a new dynamic and perspective for research in the country. In addition, there is today an improvement at the national level in the fight against cancer through the intensification of prevention activities and improvement of the technical platform through the construction of cancer and radiotherapy centers. Despite COVID-19 and insecurity staying the major problems, this dynamic remains. And the boost given to research in this context of the coronavirus pandemic will undoubtedly benefit cancer research.

The objective of our reflection in this chapter is to make concrete proposals on the contribution of genomics in the fight against cancers, especially cervical cancer caused by the human papillomavirus (HPV) in the context of African countries such as Burkina Faso.

The part attributable to infections in the occurrence of cancer in resource-limited countries such as Burkina Faso is around 26%, compared to 7% in developed countries. Among these infections are the human papillomavirus (HPV) and hepatitis B virus (HBV). The fight against infectious diseases would therefore constitute an important element in the cancer control strategy in African countries.

This chapter will focus on three points: a brief overview of the contribution of genomics in infectious diseases in general and HPV in particular, a review of human papillomavirus and associated cancers in Africa, and finally, a study of the contribution of genomics in the fight against papillomavirus and cervical cancer in Africa, and in Burkina Faso in particular.

2. Contribution of genomics in the fight against papillomaviridae and related cancers

2.1 Contribution of genomics in the fight against infectious diseases

Since the rediscovery of Mendel's work in 1900, the progress of science has been considerable. The discovery of DNA as a carrier of genetic information, the discovery of RNA, as well as the elucidation of the molecular mechanisms of replication, transcription, and the cell cycle, all of this combined with the rapid development of techniques of molecular biology have deeply opened the fields of application of the biological sciences. All these potentials have led researchers to move very quickly from "classical" genetics to genomics. Genomics, which appeared in the 1990s, was born out of a change in the scale of molecular genetics, from studying a single gene or a small fraction of the genome to studying the genome as a whole. Its objective is to understand the functioning of living organisms in all their complexity. An anonymous source said: "If creating human beings is only about aligning sequences of nucleotides, we geneticists would be able to create humans. Fortunately, there is the notion of epigenetics that must be taken into account. And it forces us to recognize how perfect a human is. "New scientific discipline at the crossroads of biology, new analytical techniques, robotics, computer science, and genomics requires us to take epigenetics into account in understanding the mechanisms of infectious and noninfectious diseases. Genomics has opened up new therapeutic possibilities for the treatment of certain diseases: knowledge of genes predisposing to major pathologies makes it possible to provide very specific treatments in addition to increasingly sensitive screening tests at a lower cost. Likewise, the identification of the genes responsible for various diseases offers researchers the possibility of determining the exact targets on which the drugs should act. In recent years, advances in genomics have transformed the therapeutic research and strategy of most of the major pharmaceutical groups. 'recombinant' drugs can be more effective and their development faster, and therefore it could be less expensive.

People are often exposed to viruses, bacteria, and parasites. Some of these microorganisms are sources of infection, epidemics, and even pandemics. During the previous centuries, these infectious diseases have negatively impacted the life expectancy of the population in the long term. With the discovery of microorganisms by Louis Pasteur, humans seemed to have learned to "control" infectious diseases through the enhancement of personal and public hygiene, and access to vaccines and antibiotics. Unfortunately, over the past few decades, we have seen more and more so-called "emerging or reemerging" infectious diseases. In developing countries, infectious diseases were responsible for 6 of 10 deaths between 2000 and 2019. This is in contrast to the rest of the world where it is noncommunicable diseases that cause the most health challenges. The World Health Organization estimates that nearly a quarter of deaths worldwide or nearly thirteen million persons die per year, and this is still directly linked to infectious diseases. This shows how infectious diseases remain a major public health problem in Africa. The fight against infectious diseases requires the establishment of an effective awareness and prevention strategy, reliable diagnostic tools, and a rapid response. Already, after the publication of the results of the sequencing of the whole human genome, the WHO report entitled "Genomics and World Health" indicated that a better knowledge of the genomics of pathogens and their vectors would greatly contribute to the fight against these infections [3].

Prevention of infectious diseases: Since it was understood that infectious diseases were caused by microorganisms, it became evident that to guard against these pathologies, it was necessary to combine a healthy lifestyle and vaccination. Hygiene also involves the implementation of barrier measures and to develop these measures, it is necessary to have a good knowledge of the germ, its mode of transmission, its target in the body, and also its mode of multiplication. Providing an effective vaccine also requires a very good knowledge of the germ and its genetic material. Since the advent of sequencing and bioinformatics, much information on the genetics of microorganisms is now available in international databases and accessible to all. Likewise, nowadays, the development of sequencing tools gives researchers the ability to sequence any genome in few hours, analyze the sequencing data, and even make comparisons and classify organisms. More and more studies show that human genetic factors play a major role in susceptibility to infections. We notice, for example, that different populations, confronted with the same germ, react differently to infection. Genomic studies take into account factors related to the germ, the host, and the environment in understanding the dynamics of disease occurrence following microbial infection.

Diagnosis of infectious diseases: A good diagnosis, made early, can reduce the transmission of a disease. For a long time, the diagnosis of a disease depended on knowing the clinical signs and symptoms presented by the patient. It was quickly realized that different diseases could have almost the same symptoms; moreover, between contact with the germ and the onset of the first symptoms, a person can infect many other people. It, therefore, became evident that diagnostic tests were needed to confirm the presence of the germ as early as possible. Hence, the emergence of indirect diagnostic tests and later direct diagnostic tests, which target the pathogenic organism. But setting up these tests required very advanced knowledge of the microorganism. It, therefore, required more time for the provision of these tests. With the appearance of new molecular biology technologies and the genomic knowledge of germs, it is becoming easier and faster to make a diagnostic test accessible to populations.

The response to infectious diseases: A rapid response to a disease requires a synergy of action involving several skills at the same time. The response is different depending on whether you are dealing with a new disease or an "old disease." The example of the COVID-19 pandemic shows us how genomics can revolutionize the management of infectious diseases. The accumulated knowledge, as well as the pooling of skills and the availability of ultra-modern technologies, have enabled the world to have diagnostic tests only a few weeks after the appearance of the virus and a vaccine less than a year later. At the same time, this made it possible to develop response mechanisms on a global and continental level against the virus. Knowledge of the molecular mechanisms of resistance of pathogens to drugs would certainly help save lives by making it possible to precisely prescribe the most effective drug to treat a specific disease. This is called pharmacogenomics. According to the European Agency for the Evaluation of Medicinal Products, pharmacogenomics can be defined as the study of the variability in the expression of different genes in relation to the response to drugs, whether this expression is assessed at the cell, tissue, individual, or population level [4]. It is a science that allows the identification of genomic expression profiles involved in the therapeutic response, whether in the expression of drug efficacy or toxicity. Genomics also allows the monitoring of different pathogen variants. Currently, the technological capacity in terms of genomics facilitates the traceability of the variants of SARS-COV2 and anticipates the availability of vaccines and also the transmission of the virus throughout the world.

In addition to infectious diseases being a major concern in terms of mortality in developing countries, some of them are also a source of cancer, such as HPV, the subject of our study.

2.2 Human papillomavirus and associated cancers in Africa

HPVs are DNA viruses, belonging to the papillomaviridae family. HPV transmission occurs primarily through direct skin-to-skin or mucous-to-mucous membrane contact, indirectly through contaminated objects or from mother to child. Sexual transmission is the most common mode. This virus is responsible for cancer of the cervix and also for other types of cancers, such as of the penis, anus, ear, nose, throat, etc.

2.2.1 HPV and cervical cancer

HPVs are further subdivided into high-risk and low-risk oncogenic types. High-risk HPVs cause high-grade lesions and invasive cervical cancers. In the mucous membranes, the onset of a high-grade lesion or cancer is usually preceded by the appearance of a low-grade lesion. If the persistence of infection by an HPV is an essential factor in the progression to cancer, infection with a high-risk HPV and the existence of cofactors linked to the field is a fundamental phenomenon in the genesis of related cancers to these viruses. The determinants of persistence are both viral and linked to environmental factors such as immune response, genetics, and carcinogens. In the cervix, the vast majority of HPV is eliminated spontaneously in 18 months on average. Cohort studies show that only 10% of genital mucosal HPV infections progress to a high-grade lesion and cancer, between 10 and 20 years. However, in some cases, the period of progression from mild dysplasia to high-grade lesion may be short, one to two years, and some lesions may turn out to be high-grade straight away, progressing very quickly to cancer [5]. The contribution of HPVs in cervical cancer depends on the genotypes of the virus. HPV16 and 18 contribute to more than 70% of all cases of cervical cancer, between 41% and 67% for high-grade cervical lesions and 16 to 32% for low-grade cervical lesions [6]. This is due to their higher carcinogenic capacity than other HPV genotypes [7]. The other six most commonly detected HPV genotypes in the world after HPV16 and 18 were HPV31, 33, 35, 45, 52, and 58 [8]. They are thought to be responsible for an additional 20% of cervical cancers worldwide [6]. However, this global distribution could vary from region to region or from study to study (study type and population). In Burkina Faso, the prevalence of HPV was estimated at 58.33% and 59.6% in two populations of HIV-positive women, with HPV50'S, HPV18, and HPV30'S as the most prevalent [9, 10]. In women with normal cytology in general populations who attended gynecological services, the prevalence of HPV infection in studies carried out in Burkina Faso was 40.4%, 25.3%, and 34.1% [11–13]. These prevalences were also variable according to the locality. In high-grade lesions and cancer cases, the prevalence was 48.8% and 72.31%, respectively [14, 15].

Cervical cancer is the most common cancer in women worldwide in 45 countries and kills more women than all other forms of cancer in 55 countries. These countries include many countries of Sub-Saharan Africa, Asia (especially India), and some countries of Central and South America. Cervical cancer accounts for over 80% of cancers attributable to HPV infection [16]. The number of cervical cancer cases worldwide is 569,847 with 311,365 deaths. It is the 3rd leading cause of death in the world, and the 2nd most common cause of cancer and death in women aged 15 to 44 [17]. In Africa, where cervical cancer is the second leading cause of cancer in women after breast cancer, 119,284 cases are diagnosed each year. It is also the leading cause of cancer death (81,687 deaths) in Africa according to 2018 estimates [6]. Among women aged 15 to 44, cervical cancer is the most common cause of cancer death (2nd rank) [6], West and East Africa are the most affected. Each year in West Africa, there are approximately 31,955 cases of cervical cancer with 23,529 deaths. And specifically, depending on the country, the estimates are 783 cases and 652 deaths in Benin; 2517 cases and 2081 deaths in Burkina Faso (a leading cause of cancer); 1789 cases and 1448 in Côte d'Ivoire; 2206 cases and 1704 deaths in Mali (a leading cause of cancer); 543 cases and 476 deaths in Niger; 568 cases and 414 deaths in Togo [6, 18, 19].

2.2.2 Anal cancer and HPV in Africa

Similar to cervical cancer, anal cancer is associated with HPV infection in approximately 88% of cases worldwide [17, 20]. It is frequently detected in both sexes and there are differences based on sexual orientation. The prevalence of HPV in anal infections is thought to be higher in male homosexuals and HIV-positive men. In women, a decrease in the prevalence of HPV with age has been observed, unlike that of heterosexual men [21–23]. According to a meta-analysis, the prevalence of anal HPV in homosexuals (men who have sex with men) is double that of women (58.8% against 30.7%); and the prevalence of the latter is thought to be double that of men who have sex with women (14.2%) [24]. According to HPV genotypes, HPV16 is the most common genotype (73% of all HPV positive tumors) followed by HPV18 (approximately 5% of cases). In precancerous anal lesions (AIN), HPV DNA is detected in 91.5% of AIN1 cases and 93.9% of AIN2/3 cases [17, 25]. Worldwide, the different prevalence of HPV in anal infections is 80.8% in Asia, 87.6% in Europe, 95.8% in the USA, 61.9% in West Africa [26], 97.1% in Australia [27], 100% in Germany [28], and 95.4% in Ukraine [29]. We lack data in Burkina Faso on anal cancer. However, a retrospective and cross-sectional study which involved patients seen during lower gastrointestinal endoscopy from the period between 09/29/1999 and 10/04/2008 in a hospital setting in Ouagadougou showed that anorectal malignancies (6, 9%) were in fourth place after hemorrhoidal disease (45.6%), anitis (21.1%), and fissures (13.9%) [30].

2.2.3 Vulvar cancer and HPV

HPV is responsible for 43% of vulvar cancer worldwide [20]. Vulvar cancer has two distinct histologic profiles: basaloid wart types more common in young women with an infection of about 86% HPV and keratinizing types, the frequency of which in older women is about 6%. HPV infection is frequently detected among high-grade VIN (VIN2/3) cases (85.3%). HPV16 was the most common type detected, followed by HPV33 [25]. HPV infections were detected in 70.8% of vulvar cancer cases in Africa, 28.7% in Asia [31], 90.0% in Australia [32], 50.0%, in the USA, and 19.3% in Europe [31].

2.2.4 Vaginal cancer and HPV

Cancer of the vagina in women may present with a history of other anogenital cancers, such as cervical cancer, which are frequently and simultaneously diagnosed. Invasive vaginal carcinomas where DNA of HPV was detected in 70% of cases and high-grade vaginal neoplasia (VaIN2/3) in 91% of cases. HPV16 was the most common type in high-grade vaginal neoplasia and is detected in at least 70% of HPV-positive carcinomas [17, 20, 25]. Several studies and meta-analyses allow some estimation of the prevalence in some regions of the world: 68.4% of HPV infection was observed in vaginal carcinomas in Africa, 71.1% in Europe, 78.0% in America, 97.6% in VaIN2 / 3 in Europe, and 92.5% in VaIN2/3 in America, still with a predominance of HPV16 [33].

2.2.5 Penile cancer and HPV

A prevalence of 50% of HPV DNA has been detected in penile cancers [12]. HPV16 was the most common type, followed by HPV18 and HPV types 6/11 [34]. A large majority of invasive penile cancers (over 95%) is squamous cell carcinomas (SCC). Keratinization (49%), mixed wart-basaloids (17%), verrucas (8%), and basaloids (4%) are the most common histological subtypes of penile SCC. HPV is commonly detected in basaloid and verrucous tumors, but it is less common in keratinizing and verrucous tumors. Still, with a higher prevalence of the HPV16 type, the prevalence of HPV was detected in 36.8% and 87.5% of penile cancer cases in Africa [35, 36], 13.4% in Asia, 32.2% in Europe, 36.5% in Latin America and the Caribbean, 18.8% in the USA [35], and 63.2% in Brazil [37]. In the cases of PeIN2/3, the prevalence of HPV was 18.8% in the USA and 89.1% in Europe [35].

2.2.6 Oropharyngeal and HPV cancers

The origin of head and neck cancer associated with HPV is an oral HPV infection, which, in the absence of clearance, persists and progresses to a neoplastic lesion. About 25.6% of all oropharyngeal cancers is attributable to HPV infection, with HPV16 the most common type [20]. In Africa, specifically in Burkina Faso, a prevalence of 54.84% of HPV6/11 infection has been attributed to laryngeal papillomatosis, 15.4% and 25% of high-risk HPV infections (HR-HPV) to cancers of mucous cells of the throat and nose, respectively [38, 39]. Worldwide, HPV infection ranges from 22.4% (19.9–25.0) for the oropharynx, 4.4% (3.3–4.8) for the oral cavity, to 3.5% (2.4–4.8) for the larynx, with a dominance of HPV16 [40]. Two meta-analyses of healthy individuals reported an oral HPV prevalence of 4.5% (3.9–5.1) and 7.5% (6.7–8.4) [41, 42]. In the United States, an oral HPV prevalence of 6.9% (5.7–8.3) was observed, with a significant difference between 10.1% males and 3.6% females [43].

In the rest of our study, we will mainly address the case of cervical cancer, which is the cancer with the highest incidence in Africa. Over the past 30 years, the incidence and death rate of cervical cancer has declined in countries where socioeconomic levels have improved. These decreases are largely the result of the implementation of secondary prevention measures, which include effective screening, early diagnosis, and treatment of precancerous lesions. Because of this situation, the contribution of genomics in the fight against HPV infections and cervical cancer could be an alternative for developing countries such as Burkina Faso. This strategy will undoubtedly save a lot of time and use less economic resources in this struggle.

2.3 Contribution of genomics in the fight against papillomavirus and cervical cancer in Africa

The fight against cervical cancer includes three main components: primary prevention, which consists of the elimination of HPV through sensitization, socio-behavioral change, communication, and importantly vaccination; secondary prevention consists mainly of screening to detect and treat precancerous lesions; and tertiary prevention, which consists of management of cervical cancer and palliative care. Tertiary prevention requires intensive therapeutic approaches, which still produces poor outcomes, especially in our countries with limited resources. WHO, therefore, recommends focusing control strategies on primary and secondary preventions. Most of the time, a high-risk oncogenic HPV infection progresses 10 to 20 years before cancer develops. This implies that if the tools for diagnostic strategies are put in place effectively, there would be a great chance of preventing the development of cancerous lesions. WHO recommends the use of molecular tests in combination with other techniques such as visual inspection with acetic acid or Lugol solution, cervico-vaginal smear, etc. Several screening strategies are recommended by the WHO for developing countries: the "screen-and-treat" strategy that consists of applying visual tests (IVA /IVL) and treating women who test positive without going through a viral detection diagnostic test; the "see-and-treat" strategy that consists of offering women who are screen positive by visual methods, a colposcopy examination before treatment. The diagnosis of the virus requires the use of molecular biology techniques such as the polymerase chain reaction (PCR), DNA/RNA hybridization, etc. Until fairly recent times, many people would have been said that the developing countries of the African continent are unable to utilize these molecular biology techniques nationwide. However, since the advent of COVID-19, developing countries have reorganized their testing laboratories to include PCR testing. Availability of equipment and skills should no longer be an obstacle for molecular HPV testing, but the issue of the cost of consumables and reagents remains. We will address this case in our specific analysis in Burkina Faso.

Another strategy for the use of genomics in the fight against HPV is the provision of effective vaccines at lower costs for the majority of the population. In the context of HPV, two vaccines are already available. They are: Cervarix®, which protects against HPV16 and 18, and Gardasil 9®, which protects against HPV 6, 11, 16, 18, 31, 33, 45, 52, and 58. However, these vaccines are not yet subsidized in all African countries and they do not cover all the high-risk genotypes encountered in these countries such as HPV56, 66, 59, 39, 51, 35, 68, and 45. However, some studies show that these genotypes are part of the "Top 5" of the most common HPVs. In addition to testing for the virus, African countries would benefit from testing for HPV genotypes circulating in cancer cases. This will allow them to make a wise choice in terms of the vaccine available and also to invest strategically in the design of a specific and more effective vaccine for their population. It should also be noted that genomics will accelerate the implementation of this vaccine development. It is increasingly becoming clear that HPV, like other viruses, does not always cause disease to develop in an infected person. The influence of genetic factors of the host on the susceptibility or resistance to this infection is suspected. It would, therefore, be very interesting to understand these mechanisms of susceptibility/resistance. This will help to protect vulnerable people and elucidate possible treatment pathways against HPV and associated cancers. Likewise, some low-grade lesions spontaneously progress to clearing while others progress to cancer. In addition to viral and environmental factors, genetic and epigenetic factors of the human host are also suspected. An investigation of these mechanisms could lead to the establishment of markers for monitoring or early diagnosis of cancer. HPV sequencing would also be an asset for identifying new viral variants, for molecular epidemiological surveillance of the virus, and for understanding the biology of the pathogen. A better knowledge of the biology of the virus will also allow a good understanding of the mechanisms of carcinogenesis.

Cancer is known to be a genetic disease, for it induces mutations in the genome or epigenome level. It is also known that people with the same type of cancer can have different mutations. And these mutations can influence a person's treatment. It is, therefore, evident that without the contribution of genomics, the analysis which enables these mutations to be identified, at some point clinicians are forced to treat patients "blind." If it is later found that the treatment is not working, it will need to be changed. And during this time, the disease physically, psychologically, and economically has a negative impact on the person. Therefore, for low-income countries, it would be more strategic to encourage pharmacogenomics, as this will reduce costs and also improve patient survival rate, especially, since there is undoubtedly a delay in diagnosis of cancers. These delays are most often due to a lack of money, inaccessibility to medical specialists, and the refusal to accept the disease. Thus, a genomic study of cancer cells will make it possible to offer adapted and personalized therapeutic protocols to people already suffering from cancer due to HPV.

2.4 Specific case of Burkina Faso

Burkina Faso is a landlocked country and, therefore, constitutes a crossroads for the populations of certain West African countries. This position is advantageous from an economic point of view, but from a health point of view, it can be a way for rapid transmission of infectious diseases. According to estimates from the West African Economic and Monetary Union (WAEMU), 2 out of 5 people (41.4%) lived in poverty in 2018. The country was victim of several terrorist attacks, which claimed the lives of several thousands of people and caused the internal displacement of more than one million people. In addition to this insecure situation, we have the COVID-19 pandemic and its health and economic consequences. This situation of insecurity prompted the government to initiate capacity building for the defense forces in order to provide an effective response to the security issue. This puts pressure on public finances with a budget deficit of nearly 5% of GDP in 2018 against 7.5% in 2017.

In terms of health, the Burkinabè live longer now than in previous decades. Life expectancy at birth has increased from 53.8 years in 1996 to 60.4 years in 2016. This is mainly attributed to the improvement of living conditions, better access to health services, reduction of diseases preventable by vaccination, and better management and treatment of malaria and infectious diseases such as pneumonia, tuberculosis, and HIV/AIDS.

Burkina Faso has a Ministry of Health, Public Hygiene and Well-being and a Ministry of Higher Education, Research and Innovation for the implementation of its policies in health and research. We will develop below, the organization of these two ministries.

2.4.1 Organization of the health system

Burkina Faso's national health system includes the public subsector, the private subsector, and the traditional medicine/pharmacopeia. The leadership of the Ministry of Health (MoH) is reflected in the adoption of policies and standards, the adoption of laws and other conventions relating to health, the increase in resources for health through the development of the partnership, implementation of the common basket, and better structural and functional organization. The organization of the health system takes into account the organization of administrative services and the organization of care services. Administratively, Burkina's health system comprises three levels, namely the central, intermediate, and peripheral levels: the central level is made up of central structures organized around the cabinet of the Minister and the General Secretariat; the intermediate level includes 13 regional health directorates; the peripheral level is made up of 70 health districts. The health district is the operational unit of the national health system. The provision of care is provided by public and private structures. Public health care structures are organized into three levels which provide primary, secondary, and tertiary care. The first level has medical centers (CM): 71, health and social promotion centers (CSPS): 2041, isolated dispensaries and maternities: 120, infirmary: 187. The second level of care is the medical center with a surgical unit (CMA): 46. It is the reference center for health facilities at the first level of the district. The second level of care is represented by the regional hospital center (CHR) which serves as a reference for the CMAs. There are a total of nine (09) CHR in the country. The third level consists of the university hospital center, numbering six (06) in 2020. These structures constitute the highest reference level. In addition to these structures, there are pharmacopeia, traditional medicine, and community-based health which also contribute to the provision of health services to the population. The population/health center ratio makes it possible to assess the country's health coverage. It is estimated at 9662 inhabitants for 01 CSPS in 2019 and efforts still need to be made to bring the country closer to the standard defined by WHO which recommends 01 CSPS for 5000 inhabitants. The number of nurses in public health facilities in 2019 was 8613, i.e., a ratio of 41 nurses per 100,000 inhabitants, which is higher than the WHO standard which recommends 2 nurses per 10,000 inhabitants. Malaria remains the main reason for consultation and hospitalization, and the leading cause of death in health facilities. In 2018, deaths attributed to malaria were 16.4%. Overall, the Burkinabé health system still faces enduring bottlenecks including geographic and financial accessibility, low availability of drugs and trained personnel, quality of care, and socio-cultural acceptability.

The National Institute of Health is a public health establishment created by decree No. 2018–0618/ PRES/PM/MINEFID/MS/MESRI of 06/18/2018, which depends on the Ministry of Health. It is made up of 6 technical departments namely: the Direction of the MURAZ Center (CM), the Direction of the National Center for Research and Training on Malaria (CNRFP), the Direction of the Nouna Health Research Center (CRSN), the Direction of the Health Emergency Response Operations Center (CORUS), the Directorate of the National Population Health Observatory (ONSP), and the Directorate of the Central Reference Laboratory (LCR). Both public and private medical biology laboratories are organized into a network and coordinated by the laboratory management. The network architecture is as follows: the national reference laboratories (NRLs) which report directly to the LCR; national-level laboratories (located in the CHU and research centers); intermediate or regional level laboratories (located in CHR), and peripheral level laboratories (located in CM/CMA). Each laboratory level has clear texts that specify its organization and missions, so that all laboratory activities are well coordinated.

The part of the national budget allocated to health was relatively stable between 2015 and 2016, standing at 12.15% and 12.4%, respectively. Nevertheless, we note a downward trend in 2017 and 2018, i.e., 11.89% and 10.70%, respectively, probably attributable to the security situation. The country adopted Law N ° 060–2015/CNT establishing a single and compulsory universal health insurance scheme (RAMU) as part of the strengthening of inclusiveness, solidarity, and social protection. The establishment of this insurance scheme will improve the well-being of the population and help to considerably reduce the direct health costs in the household budget. Funding for health research is an area that will need to be strengthened because it is practically nonexistent.

2.4.2 Research organization

As a member country of the West African Economic and Monetary Union (WAEMU), Burkina Faso had 20.5 million inhabitants, of which 51.7% were women in 2019 according to the preliminary results of the RGPH 2019. The average annual rate of population growth remained at 2.9%. Those under 20 years represented 55.8% of the total population. The urbanization rate was 26.3%. This urbanization is concentrated between the cities of Ouagadougou (administrative capital) and Bobo-Dioulasso (economic capital), which alone absorbs 62.1% of the urban population. In 2019, Burkina Faso was ranked 182nd out of 189 countries with an HDI of

0.452 according to the 2020 UNDP Sustainable Human Development Report. This index improved from the previous year when it was 0.434. The value of the HDI in 2019 places Burkina Faso in sixth place in the WAEMU area.

From a structural point of view, research activities are mainly carried out in public and private research centers, public universities, and public hospitals. In 2019, the total number of research facilities was 45, including 15 research centers, 9 research institutes, 8 research stations, and 13 universities. All the structures have 2272 researchers and teacher-researchers, 17.1% of whom are women. The private and international sectors only account for 2.9% and 2.5% of researchers. In a population of 1,000,000 inhabitants, the number of researchers is 111. In terms of funding, 151 research projects/agreements were registered in 2019 for a total funding of 13,636,364 US dollars. The part of the national budget allocated to research represents 0.9% of all the budget and 24.3% of that of the Ministry of Higher Education, Scientific Research and Innovation (MESRSI). The contributory share of external research aid was 85.4% and that of the state 7.8%. In 2019, expenditure other than projects/programs of research structures amounted to 16,138,182 US dollars. Salary costs represented 36.8%, functionary costs 50.9%, spending on investments represented 7.7%. The budget devoted to expenditure other than projects and programs of research structures represented 33.6% and the contribution of external partners 24.7%. The expenditure on own resources is the highest and represented 41.7%. The research sector is one of the 14 planning sectors of the National Economic and Social Development Plan (PNDES). Thus, to boost this sector and improve scientific output, the government has instituted, among other things, the prize for excellence in scientific research, the International Symposium on Science and Technology (SIST). Also, to provide a secure framework for funding research and innovation activities, the government has in recent years increased the budget of the National Fund for Research and Innovation for Development (FONRID). Most of the specific research infrastructures, listed in 2019, belonged to public structures. Indeed, the public owns 78.3% of the infrastructures against 12.0% for the private sector. In 2019, all the researchers and teacher-researchers produced 1787 publications. Publications by public research structures represent 85.5%. Private and international structures respectively account for 5.4% and 9.1% of published research results. The average number of publications per researcher ratio in 2019 is less than one publication per researcher (0.8). The highest ratio is recorded in international organizations where it is nearly three publications per researcher. Scientific articles (34.4%), technical reports (29.5%), and scientific communications (13.3%) are the most common scientific publications.

Overall, it appears that research is very poorly funded in Burkina Faso. Most of the research activities done are carried out with external capital. This calls into question the country's sovereignty in the field of research. However, an effort is being made in the area of valorization of research results. This effort remains very insufficient, especially in universities where there are very few documents of vulgarization and technical reports compared to research centers and institutes.

We were unable to obtain sufficient data on the part of health research funding in the national budget or external funding. But nevertheless, given the meager part of research funding in general, we can assume that health research funding remains very low.

2.5 Possible strategy

At this point, we will make concrete proposals for Burkina Faso, and therefore, for the other countries of Sub-Saharan Africa which have similar problematic management mechanisms in terms of health and research. For efficiency in the implementation of contribution strategies of genomics in the fight against cervical cancer induced by papillomaviruses, we will address aspects of governance, capitalization of existing structures, human resources, and equipment.

2.5.1 The governance

The fight against HPV and associated cancers will not happen without a political commitment as strong as that seen for the fight against COVID-19. One of the great strengths of the Burkina Faso Ministry of Health is that it is very well organized. And this is due to the gains made over the decades. However, in this fight against HPV and associated cancers, it will absolutely be necessary for this ministry to work in close collaboration with the Ministry of Higher Education, Research and Innovation because most of the human skills and equipment of genomics are located in research centers which work under this ministry. There is, therefore, a need for a synergy of inter-ministerial action. Let us not forget either the Ministry of Finance which is the "portfolio" of the government and therefore responsible for financing all the activities that will be initiated by the other two ministries. We propose that the government create a "cell" under the first ministry. This cell could be called "medicine and genomics" for example. It should be constituted from clinicians, researchers, and academic-researchers working in the field of genomics or teaching-hospital-university teachers, bio-ethicists (to take ethical aspects into account in decisions), and sociologists (for taking sociological aspects into account in decisions). The first ministry will then have to work to make available organizational and functional texts of this "cell" and to allocate the necessary resources to achieve its objectives. This unit should also be able to mobilize external resources to finance its activities.

2.5.2 Capitalization of healthcare and research structures and equipment

Several research structures are currently working in the field of health. These structures work under the Ministry of Health or the Ministry of Research. In addition, the structuring of the Ministry of Health has made it possible to set up national reference laboratories. Among these NRLs is the National Reference Laboratory for HPV (LNR-HPV) hosted by the Pietro Annigoni Biomolecular Research Center (CERBA). This structure could be the technical arm of the "medicine and genomics cell" in the implementation of its activities, particularly dedicated to HPV and associated cancers. CERBA also has an efficient technical platform for genotyping, sequencing, and anticancer tests in vitro. Likewise, certain structures such as the Muraz Center, the plant virology and biotechnology laboratory of the Institute for the Environment and Agricultural Research, etc., also have state-of-the-art equipment which can contribute to the fight against these diseases. Knowing that these structures have more or less developed cooperative relations, but in a sometimes informal way, it will just be necessary to strengthen and formalize the partnerships in order to make them more fruitful. Certain structures such as the IRSS and the Laboratory of Animal Physiology at Joseph KI-ZERBO University will be able to make an excellent contribution to clinical trials. The laboratories of the department of pharmacy of Joseph KI-ZERBO University and the IRSS would contribute to the pharmacology, toxicology part. Results of a study carried out by CERBA's team have shown that essential oils of Cymbopogon nardus, a medicinal plant from Burkina Faso, have quite interesting properties on cervical cancer cells in culture [44].

The cell will therefore have to create diversified partnership agreements with several national structures for carrying out genomic analysis and also for the research activities necessary to understand the mechanisms of infection and carcinogenesis. It should also be noted that this kind of partnership network could be used for any pathology other than HPV and cervical cancer.

Referral hospitals will be encouraged to set up patient cohorts for better organization of clinical and research activities. And also for better patient follow-up like has been done with HIV.

2.5.3 Capitalization of human resources

Burkina Faso has skilled human resource in the field of molecular biology, genetics, and biotechnology. Unfortunately, these human resources are not sufficient to effectively implement a large national program in genomics and medicine. However, the country could approach Burkinabès living outside even part-time. Some countries such as China and India have experimented with this approach and it has enabled them to boost research and also to draw on the skills of their compatriots living and working in developed countries.

3. Conclusions

HPVs and their associated cancers constitute a public health problem in our African countries. This is a shame since it is a preventable cancer if screening is done systematically and also on time. Burkina Faso, like many other countries in Sub-Saharan Africa, has many health and security challenges to overcome. These countries have very few financial resources and they would benefit from focusing on new sciences such as molecular biology, biotechnology, bioinformatics, and genomics. This will allow them to make a considerable leap in the fight against infectious diseases and also against cancer. Very often, there are competent human resources in these countries, advanced equipment too, but due to a lack of optimal coordination, this is not valorized. We suggest in this analysis, a pooling of skills and equipment already available and above all a common organization of research and health with a unique vision driven by political leaders. It would be a shame if African countries failed to enter the field of genomics as they did in other fields.

Author details

Florencia Wendkuuni Djigma[1*], Fidèle Tiendrebeogo[2], Lassina Traore[1], Théodora Mahoukèdè Zohoncon[3], Augustin Tozoula Bambara[1], Pegdwendé Abel Sorgho[4], Hierrhum Aboubacar Bambara[1], Abdou Azaque Zoure[2], Dorcas Obiri-Yeboah[5], Bagora Bayala[6], Teega-Wendé Clarisse Ouedraogo[4], Prosper Bado[4], Rogomenoma Alice Ouedraogo[4], Ina Marie Angèle Traore[2], Mah Alima Esther Traore[2], Isabelle Touwendpoulimdé Kiendrebeogo[4], Albert Théophane Yonli[4], Charlemagne Marie Ragnag-Néwendé Ouedraogo[1] and Jacques Simpore[1]

1 University Joseph KI-ZERBO, Ouagadougou, Burkina Faso

2 Scientific and Technological Research Center, Ouagadougou, Burkina Faso

3 University Saint Thomas d'Aquin, Ouagadougou, Burkina Faso

4 Biomolecular Research Center Pietro Annigoni, Ouagadougou, Burkina Faso

5 University of Cape Coast, Ghana

6 École Normale Supérieure (ENS), Koudougou, Burkina Faso

*Address all correspondence to: florencia.djigma@gmail.com

References

[1] INSD. Tableau de bord de la gouvernance. 2020. Available from: http://www.insd.bf/

[2] DGESS/MESRSI. Enquête statistique annuelle: tableau de bord 2019 de la recherche scientifique. 2021. Available from: www.mesrsi.gov.bf

[3] World Health Organization. Advisory Committee on Health Research. Genomics and world health: Report of the Advisory Committee on Health Research. World Health Organization. 2002. Available from: https://apps.who.int/iris/handle/10665/42453

[4] CPMP. Terminology in Pharmacogenetics. The European Agency for the Evaluation of Medicinal Products Evaluation of Medicines for Human Use. 2002

[5] Alain S, Hantz S, Denis F. Papillomavirus : Les virus et la physiopathologie de l'infection. Med. Ther. Pediatr. 2010;**13**:5-19. DOI: 10.1684/mtp.2010.0275

[6] Bruni L, Albero G, Serrano B, Mena M, Gómez D, Muñoz J, et al. ICO/IARC information Centre on HPV and Cancer (HPV information Centre). Human papillomavirus and related diseases in the World. In: Summary Report 2 February 2022. 2019a. Available from: www.hpvcentre.net [Accessed: November 04, 2019]

[7] Khan MJ, Castle PE, Lorincz AT, Wacholder S, Sherman M, Scott DR, et al. The elevated 10-year risk of cervical precancer and cancer in women with human papillomavirus (HPV) type 16 or 18 and the possible utility of type-specific HPV testing in clinical practice. Journal of the National Cancer Institute. 2005;**97**:1072-1079

[8] Clarisse OT, Djigma FW, Idani B, Zohoncon TM, Sorgho PA, Bado P, et al. Impact of glutathione S-transferase genes polymorphisms on human papillomavirus infection and precancerous lesions in west African women. Intern. J. of Genetic and molecular Biol. 2020;**12**(2):59-70

[9] Sagna T, Djigma WF, Zeba M, Bisseye C, Karou S, Ouermi D, et al. Human papillomaviruses prevalence and genital co-infections in HIV-seropositive women in Ouagadougou (Burkina Faso). Pakistan Journal of Biological Sciences. 2010;**13**:951

[10] Djigma F, Ouedraogo C, Karou D, Sagna T, Bisseye C, Zeba M, et al. Prevalence and genotype characterization of human papillomaviruses among HIV-seropositive in Ouagadougou, Burkina Faso. Acta Tropica. 2011;**117**:202-206

[11] Ouédraogo C, Rahimy R, Zohoncon T, Djigma F, Yonli A, Ouermi D, et al. Épidémiologie et caractérisation des génotypes à haut risque de Papillomavirus humain dans une population d'adolescentes sexuellement actives à Ouagadougou. Journal de Gynécologie Obstétrique et Biologie de la Reproduction. 2015;**44**:715-722

[12] Traore IMA, Zohoncon TM, Dembele A, Djigma FW, Obiri-Yeboah D, Traore G, et al. Molecular Characterization of High-Risk Human Papillomavirus in Women in Bobo-Dioulasso. Burkina Faso: BioMed Research International; 2016. p. 2016

[13] Ouedraogo RA, Zohoncon TM, Guigma SP, Traore IMA, Ouattara AK, Ouedraogo M, et al. Oncogenic human papillomavirus infection and genotypes characterization among sexually active women in Tenkodogo at Burkina Faso, West Africa. Papillomavirus Research. 2018;**6**:22-26

[14] Ouédraogo C, Zohoncon TM, Traoré EM, Ouattara S, Bado P, Ouedraogo CT, et al. Distribution of high-risk human papillomavirus genotypes in precancerous cervical lesions in Ouagadougou, Burkina Faso. Open Journal of Obstetrics and Gynecology. 2016;**6**:196

[15] Zohoncon T, Bado P, Ouermi D, Traoré EM, Ouattara S, Djigma F, et al. Molecular characterization of high-risk human papillomavirus genotypes involved in invasive cervical cancer from formalin-fixed, paraffin-embedded tissues in Ouagadougou, Burkina Faso. International Journal of Current Research. 2016;**8**:39314-39318

[16] De Martel C, Plummer M, Vignat J, Franceschi S. Worldwide burden of cancer attributable to HPV by site, country and HPV type. International Journal of Cancer. 2017;**141**:664-670

[17] Bruni L, Albero G, Serrano B, Mena M, Gómez D, Muñoz J, et al. ICO/IARC information Centre on HPV and Cancer (HPV information Centre). In: Human Papillomavirus and Related Diseases in the World. Summary Report 17 June 2019. 2019b

[18] Bruni L, Albero G, Serrano B, Mena M, Gómez D, Muñoz J, et al. ICO/IARC information Centre on HPV and Cancer (HPV information Centre). In: Human Papillomavirus and Related Diseases in Burkina Faso. Summary Report 10 December 2018. 2018. Version posted at www.hpvcentre.net [Accessed November 04, 2019]

[19] Bruni L, Albero G, Serrano B, Mena M, Gómez d, Muñoz J, et al. ICO/IARC information Centre on HPV and Cancer (HPV information Centre). In: Human Papillomavirus and Related Diseases in Africa Summary Report 17 June 2019. 2019c

[20] De Martel C, Ferlay J, Franceschi S, Vignat J, Bray F, Forman D, et al. Global burden of cancers attributable to infections in 2008: A review and synthetic analysis. The Lancet Oncology. 2012;**13**:607-615

[21] Schim Van Der Loeff MF, Mooij SH, Richel O, De Vries HJ, Prins JM. HPV and anal cancer in HIV-infected individuals: A review. Current HIV/AIDS Reports. 2014;**11**:250-262

[22] Giuliano AR, Nyitray AG, Kreimer AR, Pierce Campbell CM, Goodman MT, Sudenga SL, et al. EUROGIN 2014 roadmap: Differences in human papillomavirus infection natural history, transmission and human papillomavirus-related cancer incidence by gender and anatomic site of infection. International Journal of Cancer. 2015;**136**:2752-2760

[23] Bruni L, Barrionuevo-Rosas L, Albero G, Serrano B, Mena M, Gómez D, et al. ICO/IARC information Centre on HPV and Cancer (HPV information Centre). In: Human Papillomavirus and Related Diseases in Montenegro. Summary Report 27 July 2017. 2017. Available from: http://www.hpvcentre.net/index.php

[24] Serrano B, Brotons M, Bosch FX, Bruni L. Epidemiology and burden of HPV-related disease. Best Practice & Research Clinical Obstetrics & Gynaecology. 2018;**47**:14-26

[25] De Vuyst H, Clifford GM, Nascimento MC, Madeleine MM, Franceschi S. Prevalence and type distribution of human papillomavirus in carcinoma and intraepithelial neoplasia of the vulva, vagina and anus: A meta-analysis. International Journal of Cancer. 2009;**124**:1626-1636

[26] Alemany L, Saunier M, Alvarado-Cabrero I, Quiros B, Salmeron J, Shin HR, et al. Human papillomavirus DNA prevalence and type distribution in anal carcinomas

worldwide. International Journal of Cancer. 2015;**136**:98-107

[27] Hillman RJ, Garland SM, Gunathilake MP, Stevens M, Kumaradevan N, Lemech C, et al. Human papillomavirus (HPV) genotypes in an Australian sample of anal cancers. International Journal of Cancer. 2014;**135**:996-1001

[28] Rödel F, Wieland U, Fraunholz I, Kitz J, Rave-Fränk M, Wolff HA, et al. Human papillomavirus DNA load and p16INK4a expression predict for local control in patients with anal squamous cell carcinoma treated with chemoradiotherapy. International Journal of Cancer. 2015;**136**:278-288

[29] Baricevic I, He X, Chakrabarty B, Oliver AW, Bailey C, Summers J, et al. High-sensitivity human papilloma virus genotyping reveals near universal positivity in anal squamous cell carcinoma: Different implications for vaccine prevention and prognosis. European Journal of Cancer. 2015;**51**:776-785

[30] Nanelin GA, Sombié RA, Bougouma A. Les tumeurs malignes anorectales en milieu hospitalier à Ouagadougou: aspects épidémiologiques et diagnostiques. Pan African Medical Journal. 2014;**18**(1):26. Available from: https://www.ncbi.nlm.nih.gov/pmc/articles/PMC4214564/#

[31] De Sanjose S, Alemany L, Ordi J, Tous S, Alejo M, Bigby SM, et al. Worldwide human papillomavirus genotype attribution in over 2000 cases of intraepithelial and invasive lesions of the vulva. European Journal of Cancer. 2013;**49**:3450-3461

[32] Tan SE, Garland SM, Rumbold AR, Zardawi I, Taylor-Thomson D, Condon JR, et al. Investigating a cluster of vulvar cancers in young women: Distribution of human papillomavirus and HPV-16 variants in vulvar dysplastic or neoplastic biopsies. Sexual Health. 2013;**10**:18-25

[33] Alemany L, Saunier M, Tinoco L, Quiros B, Alvarado-Cabrero I, Alejo M, et al. Large contribution of human papillomavirus in vaginal neoplastic lesions: A worldwide study in 597 samples. European Journal of Cancer. 2014;**50**:2846-2854

[34] Miralles-Guri C, Bruni L, Cubilla AL, Castellsague X, Bosch FX, De Sanjose S. Human papillomavirus prevalence and type distribution in penile carcinoma. Journal of Clinical Pathology. 2009;**62**:870-878

[35] Alemany L, Cubilla A, Halec G, Kasamatsu E, Quiros B, Masferrer E, et al. Role of human papillomavirus in penile carcinomas worldwide. European Urology. 2016;**69**:953-961

[36] Lebelo RL, Boulet G, Nkosi CM, Bida MN, Bogers JP, Mphahlele MJ. Diversity of HPV types in cancerous and pre-cancerous penile lesions of south African men: Implications for future HPV vaccination strategies. Journal of Medical Virology. 2014;**86**:257-265

[37] IDB DS, FCB V, JPC BV, GCF DM, Do DSBNM, LMO B. Prevalence of human papillomavirus in penile malignant tumors: Viral genotyping and clinical aspects. BMC Urology. 2015;**15**:13-13

[38] Ilboudo M, Zohoncon TM, Traore EMA, Traore IMA, Kande A, Djigma FW, et al. Characterization of high-risk oncogenic human papillomavirus genotypes in histologically confirmed ear, nose and throat (Ent) cancers in Burkina Faso. Asian Pacific Journal of Cancer Prevention. 2019a;**20**:3429-3435

[39] Ilboudo M, Zohoncon TM, Traore IMA, Traore EMA, Kande A, Obiri-Yeboah D, et al. Implication of low risk human papillomaviruses, HPV6 and

HPV11 in laryngeal papillomatosis in Burkina Faso. American Journal of Otolaryngology. 2019b;**40**:368-371

[40] Castellsagué X, Alemany L, Quer M, Halec G, Quirós B, Tous S, et al. HPV involvement in Head and Neck cancers: Comprehensive assessment of biomarkers in 3680 patients. Journal of the National Cancer Institute. 2016;**108**:djv403

[41] Kreimer AR, Bhatia RK, Messeguer AL, González P, Herrero R, Giuliano AR. Oral human papillomavirus in healthy individuals: A systematic review of the literature. Sexually Transmitted Diseases. 2010;**37**:386-391

[42] Wood ZC, Bain CJ, Smith DD, Whiteman DC, Antonsson A. Oral human papillomavirus infection incidence and clearance: A systematic review of the literature. Journal of General Virology. 2017;**98**:519-526

[43] Gillison ML, Broutian T, Pickard RK, Tong Z-Y, Xiao W, Kahle L, et al. Prevalence of oral HPV infection in the United States, 2009-2010. JAMA. 2012;**307**:693-703

[44] BAYALA B, NADEMBEGA C, GUENNÉ S, BUÑAY J, Mahoukèdè Zohoncon T, Wendkuuni Djigma F, et al. Chemical composition, antioxidant and cytotoxic activities of Hyptis suaveolens (L.)Poit. Essential oil on prostate and cervical cancers cells. Pakistan Journal of Biological Sciences. 2020;**23**(9):1184-1192. DOI: 10.3923/pjbs.2020.1184.1192

Chapter 12

Vaccination against Human Papillomavirus (HPV) in Vulnerable Populations – Sexual Minorities

Elsa Díaz López

Abstract

The human papillomavirus (HPV) is one of the most frequent sexually transmitted infections worldwide, causing cancers including cervical cancer and diseases such as genital warts and oral papillomatosis, these diseases affect both men and women. HPV vaccination has been one of the main tools to decrease the burden of HPV disease. In many countries, national vaccination programs do not provide for their application to boys, men, as well as adults, although their efficacy and immunogenicity has been demonstrated. There are vulnerable populations such as the LGBTTTIQA population (Lesbian, Gay, Bisexual, Transgender, Transvestite, Intersex, Queer and Asexual) in which HPV immunization should be emphasized since they present greater risks of infection and, they face not only social stigmatization but also often that coming from medical services resulting in cases with more advanced cancers and little primary prevention. When talking about sexual and reproductive health, points of inequity that require their resolution must be analyzed, initiating this, from a bioethical analysis.

Keywords: HPV, HPV vaccination, sexual diversity, sexual minories

1. Introduction

The social content of sexual and reproductive rights is directed more towards the procreation aspect and society frequently ignores the rights towards a sexual, healthy, and pleasant life. Sexuality and reproduction are linked to the dignity of the person, so it is necessary to guarantee in all aspects (social, economic, legal, political strategy and universal health) the physical and mental integrity of the person, of equality gender and universal access to health services, this was raised 20 years ago when the commitment was created at the meeting in Cairo and Beijing [1].

The World Health Organization (WHO) defines the right to sexual health as a: "State of physical, mental, emotional and social well-being in relation to sexuality; it is not just the absence of disease, dysfunction, or weakness. Sexual health requires a respectful and positive approach towards sexuality and sexual relations, as well as towards the possibility of having pleasant and safe sexual relations, free from coercion, discrimination, and violence. Sexual rights must be respected, protected and satisfied in order to achieve and maintain sexual health for all people" [2].

The exercise of sexuality carries risks and one of them is the acquisition of pathogens that are transmitted sexually. There are more than 25 different organisms that can be acquired this way. The consequences of these infections are infertility, ectopic pregnancies, abortions, surgical medical emergencies, such as ruptured pelvic abscesses, cancer and often social discrimination, this aspect is often due to the historical forms in which sexually transmitted infections have been symbolized. In the West, sexually transmitted infections were "feminized" since they considered women as the source of venereal diseases and men as the acquiring, but not infectious, part, in addition, another characteristic was added, the perception that they are not women generally those who transmit them, but only the "promiscuous" and women were penalized for the risk they presented to health, excluding men [3]. At another time, in the 1970s, AIDS (Acquired Immune Deficiency Syndrome) was in the center of the developed world (United States) [3]. In the health measures taken for the prevention of AIDS, genders were underestimated, it was considered a "disease of men ... homosexuals", with results such as the loss of opportunities for protection and prevention of vulnerable populations such as infected women and children with a great impact of public health.

2. Vulnerability

Scientific development has caused several changes and transformations in social relations, giving rise to various ethical dilemmas showing socioeconomic disparities, which leads to a great challenge, the vulnerability of the human being, it is applied to the existential condition of the individual and population groups in certain circumstances of helplessness [4] which forces governments, medical services, and society to protect their individual and social integrity. In the Helsinki declaration, integrity appears as a part of the inviolability of the person [5].

Vulnerability refers to the possibility of being harmed, all human beings are vulnerable, fragile, and not only individually, but there will also be human groups that are more exposed and less capable of defending themselves against abuse and mistreatment such as orphans, women, children, migrants, pregnant women, immunosuppressed patients. Prisoners, disabled, people with gender diversity, LGBTTTIQA (Lesbian, Gay, Bisexual, Transgender, Transgender, Transvestite, Intersex, Queer and Asexual) [6] among the most susceptible to being harmed, therefore, it is necessary to speak of social vulnerability, where we cannot lose the context; cultural, customs, historical situation, social and economic condition, affected gender, ethnic population, where factors such as public policies, availability of services, accessibility of both physical and human resources, existing beliefs and prejudices intervene.

Despite non-discrimination policies and programs, LGBTTTIQA people suffer from discrimination and health disparities as well as lack of communication between patients and health providers with consequences that affect health care with health inequities.

The health risks of lesbian (women who have sex with women, WSW) and bisexual (women who have sex with women and WSWM men) differ from heterosexual women in terms of risks, health behaviors and how they experience health contact [7]. This group frequently faces sexually transmitted infections (STIs), including Human Papillomavirus (HPV) infections. Studies have shown that half of lesbian and bisexual women suffer from a genital HPV infection and one third of them have a high-risk HPV infection [8]. In addition, WSWs face a screening that has not been able to reach optimal levels and where the uptake of patients with genital neoplastic disease often reaches more advanced stages compared to the heterosexual population [9, 10].

Barker [11] mentions some risk factors that can increase the rate of cervical cancer in bisexual women and men such as; increased exposure to smoking, unprotected sex generally during adolescence and inconsistent condom use, and, as previously mentioned, poor attendance at cervical cancer screening and testing for other sexually transmitted infections. Another situation that Baker points out is the low influx of patients with sexual diversity to health services as they perceive discrimination from health personnel coupled with a history of marginalization they have faced due to their sexual preference [11].

When speaking of vulnerability, global bioethics intervenes in the analysis of the circumstances of risk of harm for an individual or population group and the search for new approaches that include different points of solution or avoid current and future bioethical problems, but it will always take care to promote the interests of patients by reinforcing their fundamental rights based on human dignity and human rights.

3. Health services in LGBTTTIQA

All people need medical service, for some groups such as those with sexual diversity, health care can be difficult to access due to inequities in health resources, discrimination, bullying, rejection, violence and stigma, as well as health personnel not trained in the management of people with sexual diversity [12].

One of the studies that show evidence on the perception of health personnel in the health care of lesbian patients in Israel noted; stigmatization is pointed out in the caregivers' relationships and communication with lesbian women since they consider this group as one with which the nursing personnel do not identify themselves psychologically as members of the same gender. This negative bias has been related to rejection, disrespect, isolation, prejudice, and negatively affected relationships and communication with lesbian, gay, bisexual, and transgender women [13].

LGBTTTIQA people face rejection and stigma from health personnel, which can make it difficult to apply health measures for their comprehensive protection [10]. In this group, high rates of drug, tobacco and alcohol consumption are observed, which favor risky sexual behaviors, on the other hand, there is discrimination in job opportunities with a decrease in the possibility of access to insurance or institutional medical coverage, employment, housing, and economic stability.

4. Human papilloma virus infection

Human papillomavirus (HPV) infection is one of the most common sexually transmitted infections in the world, causing cancers in both men and women [14]. This infection affects at least five areas of the human body; in women; cervix, vulva, vagina, anus and head and neck, while in men anus, penis and head and neck [14, 15] and although genital warts [16] and respiratory papillomatosis are not a malignant pathologies, they are responsible for a great emotional, dysfunctional, sexual and economic impact.

4.1 HPV in lesbian women

In the study of the situational diagnosis of LGBTIQ people in Mexico, they obtained these results; 80% of lesbian women and 81% of bisexual women stated that they had not used any protection during sexual intercourse. 71% of them report having had sexual activity with men [15]. 53% of lesbian women and 35% of bisexual women surveyed in Mexico City reported having children.

In this other study [16] 830 women were identified like gay lesbian sexual activity between 20 and 59 years were analyzed, they found that 53% of women were infected with any type of human papillomavirus, 37% of them with a high-risk human papillomavirus, who by having five or more sexual partners in their lifetime were more likely to become infected with a high-risk type of human papillomavirus. When the group of lesbian women was compared with the heterosexual group, it was observed that in the former there was a lower rate of human papillomavirus infections. HPV infection was more frequent among younger women. The infection remained common among women of all ages.

It is necessary to guarantee sexual minority women, regardless of their age, receive prevention services against HPV and cervical cancer, as well as to inform about the risks of acquisition and pathology associated with HPV in this group. And constantly work with health personnel on the risks present in this group.

4.2 HPV in men

The incidence of anal cancers and others related to the human papilloma virus have increased in the general population, even more in those people who suffer from a human immunodeficiency, such as those affected by HIV.

Anal infection, and anal intraepithelial neoplasia are very common in HIV-negative men who have sex with men (MSM) and to a greater extent are HIV carriers, as well as genital warts.

The disease burden associated with human papillomavirus infection in men is not only the diseases that they can develop; (anal genital, oral cancer, respiratory papillomatosis, and genital warts), another situation is the possibility of infecting women through the sexual route. Lesions of the penis can often be observed in sexual partners of women suffering from cervical epithelial neoplasia. Other aspect that we must not forget is the role of men in cervical cancer, several studies have shown that the husbands of women with cervical cancer do not have a higher prevalence of human papillomavirus than the husbands of control women [17].

There are several studies that demonstrate the impact of the protection and prevention of diseases associated with the human papilloma virus in men with the quadrivalent vaccine [17]. In 86% reduction in persistent infections due to the viral types included in the vaccine in the external genital area has also been observed in boys and heterosexual men and men who have sex with men, in response to this and in response to the Food Drug Administration (FDA) and the Advisory Committee on Immunization Practices (ACIP) approved and recommended routine vaccination of the quadrivalent and nonvalent vaccine in children 9 to 26 years of age for the prevention of human papillomavirus infection [14].

An 86% reduction in persistent infections by the viral types that are included in the vaccine in the external genital area has been observed in boys and heterosexual men as well as those men who have sex with men, in response to the Food Drug Administration (FDA) and the Advisory Committee on Immunization Practices (ACIP) respectively approved and recommended routine vaccination of the quadrivalent and nonvalent vaccine in children 9 to 26 years of age for the prevention of human papillomavirus infection [14].

This scheme shows risk factors that favor the acquisition of HPV in men [13, 18–20] so it is necessary to reassess the impact on their health, and on those of their partners. (This scheme was carried out by Elsa Díaz MD)

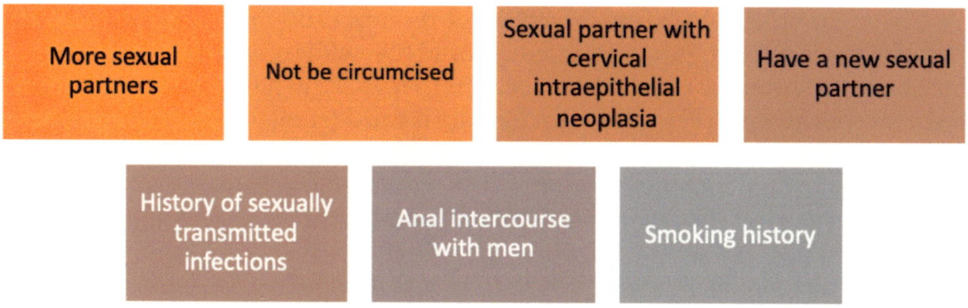

MSM have a high risk of HPV infection. An example is anal cancer, with which an association of 44 times more was found in MSM compared to the general population [21, 22].

4.3 HPV vaccination

Currently there are safe and effective vaccines for the prevention of serious diseases such as cervical cancer, however these have proven their impact in the prevention of other malignant neoplasms such as vaginal, vulvar, anus, penis, head, and neck cancer [20, 21] the quadrivalent and nonvalent vaccines have also proven their effectiveness in preventing benign lesions such as genital warts.

In the multicenter study conducted by Dr. Silvia de San José, which evaluates the potential impact of vaccines against human papillomavirus in reducing diseases associated with the human papillomavirus, an estimate of a reduction of close to 90% in cervical cancer was concluded and a global reduction of 50% of all the cases HPV-related cancer sites [23].

Regarding vaccination in men, studies have been carried out that have proven the safety and efficacy of the quadrivalent vaccine in boys and men, its efficacy has been demonstrated in reducing the 86% in persistent infection in the external genital area in children and straight men and men who have sex with men. Likewise, the 90% efficacy of reducing the incidence of external genital lesions has also been proven [17].

We often have vulnerable patients exposed to HPV infection that can lead to serious complications or fatal outcomes when we have a primary prevention tool such as vaccination.

We have three prophylactic vaccines [19, 20] that prevent human papillomavirus infection; the bivalent vaccine containing virus-like particles of serotypes 16 and 18, quadrivalent; (6, 11, 16, 21) and the nonvalent (16, 18, 31, 33, 45, 52, 58, 6 y 11). Currently, serotypes 16 and 18 are identified as responsible for 70% of cancers attributable to HPV.

Vaccination against HPV has been carried out for 14 years with bivalent and quadrivalent vaccines. In 2009 the FDA approved the quadrivalent vaccine for boys and men ages 9-26 [14]. Later in 2014 the nonavalent vaccine was added, all have proven to be effective in the long term and show persistence of their immunogenicity [24].

The results observed have been short and long term; reduction of the disease burden associated with human papillomavirus, reduction of cervical disease and anogenital dysplasia in different clinical studies and with high effectiveness not only in the population of the initial protocols such as those carried out with the quadrivalent vaccine in the cities of Denmark, Iceland, Norway and Sweden in addition to the open population, where the great impact of the frank decrease in genital warts in addition to dysplasia and cervical cancer has been observed, as has been the case in Australia [25], United States, Canada to mention just a few countries.

One of the objectives in the elimination of cervical cancer proposed by the WHO [26] is to reach 90% of girls vaccinated against HPV, while only 7 countries have included gender-neutral vaccination, on the other hand, in national immunization programs not an age group older than 15 years is considered, which is the age where sexual life generally begins and their behavior is defined.

The efficacy and immunogenicity of HPV vaccination in men during adolescence and even after starting their sexual life has been demonstrated in several studies [21].

One of the fundamental goals of vaccination is to stop the transmission of an infectious agent such as HPV. Maintaining coverage only to women is an insufficient process if you want to eradicate the diseases associated with this virus, especially in those men who have a greater chance of acquiring it and with a greater risk of transforming it into cancer, especially if they have immunosuppression or sexual behavior higher risk such as MSM or bisexual activity [14, 21, 27].

When bioethical analyzes is carried out regarding vaccination and a utilitarian current is applied; the decisions are often made based on the search for the greatest good for the greatest number of people and only the social good is considered. Are individuals being forgotten as people as unique and individual beings? [24].

Vaccination against HPV in men protects them against the pathology associated with the human papillomavirus but at the same time has the potential to protect women through herd or herd immunity for the same reason that female vaccination can protect women. The men [14].

On the other hand, the economic budget that HPV vaccination coverage represents is another important factor in vaccination strategies in a population, especially in those with a low human development index. Let us give an example about vaccination and herd effect, in men who have only sex with men, could they have any immune benefit? if men are not included in vaccination programs. In the study carried out by Hammad Ali et al. In Australia [25], in which they refer to a significant decrease in the proportion of genital warts in young women five years after the application of the vaccine and an impact on the decline of lesions o genital warts in heterosexual men because of herd immunity, but not in bisexual men. Clinical practice is strongly linked to medical ethics, it is required to guide decisions based on principles such as non-maleficence, beneficence, autonomy, and justice. These principles are complementary, not opposed.

Public health starts from a social reality and faces bioethical challenges, which must be analyzed; focus on the problems that society presents and place health at the center of social justice [28], for this, an approach is required that analyzes differences, gender, ethnic and population group, life cycles and social determinants. Bioethics must play a fundamental role in guiding decisions in public health [29] through the articulation of social reality; Identify their needs and those vulnerable groups that may not benefit from making public health policies and stop actions aimed at deepening inequities and the search for social and individual protection.

5. Conclusions

When talking about sexual and reproductive health, it is necessary to point out the existence of inequities, the lack of prevention programs and specific timely detection towards the heterosexual male population and the LGTTTIQA population. There are clinics for patients with sexual diversity, but these are insufficient. The application of vaccination against human papillomavirus should not only be aimed at women, it must be extended to men since they play a fundamental role not only in the transmission of human papillomavirus infection but also in the development of diseases associated with this virus, especially in MSM, this vulnerable and high-risk population group.

Women with gay lesbian activity are a group susceptible to contracting human papillomavirus infection, which requires strategies such as information campaigns on HPV prevention in them and in health professionals, promoting non-stigmatizing communication in health services. Health about sexually transmitted diseases. Improve the screening according to the established guidelines, if these improvements are made, we can prevent them from reaching the heterosexual population with more advanced cervical cancer compared to the heterosexual population.

Bioethics is a field of reflection on ethical problems and dilemmas in medicine and life sciences as well as their relationship with the technologies applied to the human being and what surrounds him; which leads us to rationality, coherence, justice and the recognition of the dignity of each person and therefore to ensure the protection of the most vulnerable such as the poor, the sick, patients with immunosuppression, the disabled, children, women, the elderly, pregnant women and people with sexual diversity who, due to their risks, will require our attention and personalization and individualization in the attention to their sexual and reproductive health.

In the text of Boaventura de Souza [6] "The counter-hegemonic use of law" he mentioned that we are in a historical moment of great technological advances but with societies that show greater inequality and exclusion than ever, which leads to an intense task of reinvention from the scientific, social, politics where values revolve around people and society, and values such as; freedom, equality, autonomy, justice and solidarity do not have a different meaning for each individual.

Author details

Elsa Díaz López[1,2]

1 Faculty of Bioethics, Anahuac University, Mexico

2 GESFEM SC (Specialized Group in Women's Health SC), Mexico

*Address all correspondence to: elsa.diazlo@anahuac.mx

References

[1] Cairo y Beijing El rostro Humano de los derechos. 2004

[2] lucía MCM. Derechos Sexuales y Reproductivos de las mujeres. In: Diputados LLC, editor. 1a ed. MéxicoJulio; 2015

[3] Gayet C. Infecciones de transmisión sexual en México. Una mirada desde la historia y el género. Censida; 2015. pp. 20-372

[4] Pedro CADMTSM. Los conceptos de vulnerabilidad humana y la integridad individual para la bioética. Revista de Bioética. 2017;**25**:311-319

[5] Emanuel E. Siete requisitos éticos. In: Pautas Éticas de Investigación en Sujetos Humanos: Nuevas Perspectivas. pp. 2-14

[6] Santos BS. El uso contra - hegemónico del Derecho en la lucha por una globalización desde abajo. In: Suárez AF, editor. 2005. pp. 363-420

[7] Meads C, Hunt R, Martin A, Varney J. A systematic review of sexual minority women's experiences of health care in UK. International Journal of Environmental Research and Public Health. 2019;**16**:1-24

[8] Manuel GO. Riesgos de vulneración de los derechos fundamentales de las personas con discapacidad en relación con las crisis sanitarias. Revista de bioética y derecho. 2020;**50**:369-383

[9] Robinson KGK, Bewley S, Meads C. Lesbian and bisexual women's gynaecological conditions: A systematic review and exploratory meta-analysis. BJOG: An International Journal of Obstetrics and Gynaecology. 2017;**124**(3):381-392

[10] Ángel P. La idea de solidaridad en la ética de la salud pública. Rev de Bioética y Derecho. 2017;**40**:33-47

[11] Barker MRC, Jones R, Bowes C. The Bisexuality Report. Bisexual Inclusion in LGTBT. Equality and Diversity. The Open University; 2012. pp. 1-42

[12] programs N. How Discrimination Impacts LGBTQ Healthcare. St. Catherine University; 2021

[13] Morris BJ. Male Circumcision Protects against HPV Infection and Cervical Cancer. HPV Today; 2020

[14] Giuliano AR, Palefsky JM, Goldstone S, Moreira ED Jr, Penny ME, Aranda C, et al. Efficacy of quadrivalent HPV vaccine against HPV infection and disease in males. The New England Journal of Medicine. 2011;**364**: 401-411

[15] Mendoza Juan Carlos OHL, Román R. Principales resultados del diagnóstico situacional de personas lesbianas gays bisexuales transgénero tras travestis transexuales intersexuales y queers (LGBTIQ) de México 1a parte [Internet]. 2015. Unidad Xochimilco. México. Available from: http://www2.xoc.uam.mx/oferta-educativa/divisiones/cbs/ciencias/materiales/11.pdf

[16] Branstetter AJ, McRee AL, Reiter PL. Correlates of human papillomavirus infection among a national sample of sexual minority women. Journal of Women's Health. 2017;**26**:1004-1011

[17] Palefsky JM. Human papillomavirus-related disease in men: Not just a women's issue. Journal of Adolescent Health. 2010;**46**:S12-S19

[18] Laurent JS, Luckett R, Feldman S. HPV vaccination and the effects on rates of HPV-related cancers. Current Problems in Cancer. 2018;**42**:493-506

[19] Manual de vacunas en línea, (Actualización 2021)

[20] Jacquline H. Disparities in HPV vaccination rates and HPV prevalence in the United States: A review of the literature. Human vaccines and Immunotherapeutics. 2019;**15**: 146-155

[21] Giuliano AR, Isaacs-Soriano K, Torres BN, Abrahamsen M, Ingles DJ, Sirak BA, et al. Immunogenicity and safety of Gardasil among mild adult aged men (27-45 years)—The MAM study. Vaccine. 2015;**33**:5640-5646

[22] Machalek DA, Poynten M, Jin F, et al. Anal human papillomavirus infection and associated neoplastic lesions in men who have sex with men: A systematic review and meta-analysis. The Lancet Oncology. 2012;**13**:487-500

[23] de SanJosé S, Serrano B, Tous S, et al. Burden of human papillomavirus (HPV)-related cancers attributable to HPVs 6/11/16/18/31/33/45/52 and 58. JNCI Cancer Spectrum. 2019;**2**:1-11

[24] Kjaer SK, Nygard M, Sundström K, Dillner J, et al. Final analysis of a 14 year long term follow up study of the effectiveness and immunogenicity of the quadrivalent human papillomavirus vaccine in women from four nordic countries. EClinical Medicine. 2020;**23**:1-11

[25] Canfell KHM, Simms K, Smith M, Saville M. Australia on-Track to be the First Country to Achieve Cervical Cancer Elimination. HPVWorld; 2018

[26] Simms Kate TSJ, Michael C, et al. Impact of scaled up human papillomavirus vaccination and cervical screening and the potential for global elimination of cervical cancer in 181 countries, 2020-99: A modelling study. Lancet Oncology. 2019:394-407

[27] CastellsaguÉ Xavier BFX, Muñoz Nubia MD. The role in cervical cancer. Salud Pública de México. 2001;**45**: 345-352

[28] R MLG. Bioética y Salud pública. In: Academia Mexicana de Cirugía M, editor. IV Encuentro Nacional de Bioética6-7 Mayo. 2019. pp. 1-9

[29] declaración universal sobre bioética y derechos humanos. 2005